Occupational Pulmonology

Editors

CARRIE A. REDLICH
PAUL D. BLANC
MRIDU GULATI
WARE G. KUSCHNER

CLINICS IN
CHEST MEDICINE

www.chestmed.theclinics.com

December 2012 • Volume 33 • Number 4

ELSEVIER

1600 John F. Kennedy Boulevard • Suite 1800 • Philadelphia, Pennsylvania 19103

http://www.theclinics.com

CLINICS IN CHEST MEDICINE Volume 33, Number 4
December 2012 ISSN 0272-5231, ISBN-13: 978-1-4557-4905-8

Editor: Katie Saunders
Developmental Editor: Donald E. Mumford

Clinics in Chest Medicine (ISSN 0272-5231) is published quarterly by Elsevier Inc., 360 Park Avenue South, New York, NY 10010-1710. Months of issue are March, June, September, and December. Periodicals postage paid at New York, NY and additional mailing offices. Subscription prices are $316.00 per year (domestic individuals), $506.00 per year (domestic institutions), $151.00 per year (domestic students/residents), $347.00 per year (Canadian individuals), $621.00 per year (Canadian institutions), $431.00 per year (international individuals), $621.00 per year (international institutions), and $211.00 per year (international and Canadian students/residents). International air speed delivery is included in all Clinics subscription prices. All prices are subject to change without notice. **POSTMASTER:** Send address changes to Clinics in Chest Medicine, Elsevier Health Sciences Division, Subscription Customer Service, 3251 Riverport Lane, Maryland Heights, MO 63043. **Customer Service: Telephone: 1-800-654-2452** (U.S. and Canada); **1-314-447-8871** (outside U.S. and Canada). **Fax: 1-314-447-8029. E-mail: journalscustomerservice-usa@elsevier.com** (for print support); **journalsonlinesupport-usa@elsevier.com** (for online support).

Reprints. For copies of 100 or more of articles in this publication, please contact the Commercial Reprints Department, Elsevier Inc., 360 Park Avenue South, New York, NY 10010-1710. Tel.: 212-633-3812; Fax: 212-462-1935; E-mail: reprints@elsevier.com.

Clinics in Chest Medicine is covered in *MEDLINE/PubMed (Index Medicus), Current Contents/Clinical Medicine, EMBASE/Excerpta Medica, Science Citation Index,* and *ISI/BIOMED.*

Printed and bound by CPI Group (UK) Ltd, Croydon, CR0 4YY

Transferred to digital print 2012

Contributors

GUEST EDITORS

CARRIE A. REDLICH, MD, MPH
Program Director, Yale Occupational and
Environmental Medicine, Professor of
Medicine, Occupational and Environmental
Medicine Program and Section of Pulmonary
and Critical Care Medicine, Yale University
School of Medicine, New Haven, Connecticut

PAUL D. BLANC, MD, MSPH
Professor in Residence, Division of
Occupational and Environmental Medicine,
UCSF School of Medicine, San Francisco,
California

MRIDU GULATI, MD, MPH
Assistant Professor, Section of Pulmonary and
Critical Care Medicine, and Yale Occupational
and Environmental Medicine Program,
Yale School of Medicine, New Haven,
Connecticut

WARE G. KUSCHNER, MD
Associate Professor of Medicine, Division of
Pulmonary and Critical Care Medicine,
Veterans Affairs Palo Alto Health Care System,
Stanford University School of Medicine,
Palo Alto, California

AUTHORS

SHAMBHU ARYAL, MD
Division of Pulmonary, Critical Care, and Sleep
Medicine, University of Kentucky College of
Medicine, Lexington, Kentucky

JEFFREY S. BIRKNER, PhD, CIH
V.P. Technical Services, Moldex-Metric, Culver
City, California

CHRIS CARLSTEN, MD, MPH
Director, Air Pollution Exposure Laboratory
(APEL), Vancouver Coastal Health Research
Institute; Associate Professor and Chair in
Occupational and Environmental Lung
Disease, University of British Columbia;
Director of Occupational Lung Disease Clinic,
The Lung Centre, Vancouver General Hospital,
Vancouver, British Columbia, Canada

HOWARD J. COHEN, PhD, CIH
Associate Clinical Professor/Lecturer, Yale
University School of Medicine, Guilford,
Connecticut

ENRIQUE DIAZ-GUZMAN, MD
Division of Pulmonary, Critical Care, and Sleep
Medicine, University of Kentucky College of
Medicine, Lexington, Kentucky

R. WILLIAM FIELD, PhD, MS
Professor, Department of Occupational and
Environmental Health, Department of
Epidemiology, College of Public Health,
University of Iowa, Iowa City, Iowa

**DAVID FISHWICK, MBChB, FRCP,
FFOM (Hon), MD**
Consultant Respiratory Physician and Honorary
Professor of Occupational and Environmental
Respiratory Disease, Centre for Workplace
Health, Sheffield Teaching Hospitals NHS Trust,
Health and Safety Laboratory and the University
of Sheffield, Harpur Hill, Buxton, Derbyshire,
United Kingdom

MRIDU GULATI, MD, MPH
Assistant Professor, Section of Pulmonary and
Critical Care Medicine, and Yale Occupational
and Environmental Medicine Program, Yale
School of Medicine, New Haven, Connecticut

LAWRENCE A. HO, MD
Fellow in Pulmonary and Critical Care
Medicine, Division of Pulmonary and Critical
Care Medicine, Veterans Affairs Palo Alto
Health Care System, Stanford University
School of Medicine, Palo Alto, California

WARE G. KUSCHNER, MD
Associate Professor of Medicine, Division of
Pulmonary and Critical Care Medicine,
Veterans Affairs Palo Alto Health Care System,
Stanford University School of Medicine,
Palo Alto, California

A. SCOTT LANEY, PhD
Research Epidemiologist, Division of
Respiratory Disease Studies, National Institute
for Occupational Safety and Health, Centers
for Disease Control and Prevention,
Morgantown, West Virginia

DAVID M. MANNINO, MD
Division of Pulmonary, Critical Care, and Sleep
Medicine, University of Kentucky College of
Medicine; Department of Preventive Medicine
and Environmental Health, University of
Kentucky College of Public Health,
Lexington, Kentucky

ANNA-CARIN OLIN, PhD, MD
Associate Professor, Senior Consultant,
Occupational and Environmental Medicine,
Sahlgrenska Academy, Gothenburg University,
Göteborg, Sweden

CECILE S. ROSE, MD, MPH
Professor of Medicine, Director, Occupational
and Environmental Medicine Clinic Program,
Division of Environmental and Occupational
Health Sciences, National Jewish Health,
Denver, Colorado; Division of Pulmonary
Sciences and Critical Care, Colorado School of
Public Health, University of Colorado Denver,
Aurora, Colorado

MAOR SAULER, MD
Postdoctoral Fellow, Section of Pulmonary and
Critical Care Medicine, Yale School of
Medicine, New Haven, Connecticut

FRANCESCO SAVA, MD, MSc, FRCPC
Air Pollution Exposure Laboratory (APEL),
Vancouver Coastal Health Research Institute,
University of British Columbia; The Lung
Centre, Vancouver General Hospital,
Vancouver, British Columbia, Canada

DENNIS SHUSTERMAN, MD, MPH
Professor of Clinical Medicine, Emeritus,
Division of Occupational and Environmental
Medicine, University of California,
San Francisco, San Francisco, California

AKSHAY SOOD, MD, MPH
Associate Professor, Department of Medicine,
School of Medicine, Health Sciences Center,
University of New Mexico, Albuquerque,
New Mexico

ANTHONY M. SZEMA, MD
Assistant Professor of Medicine and Surgery,
Chief, Allergy Section, Veterans Affairs Medical
Center, Northport, New York; Department of
Medicine, Stony Brook University School of
Medicine, Stony Brook, New York

ANN Y. TENG, DO
Clinical Fellow, Occupational Environmental
Medicine, Yale School of Medicine,
New Haven, Connecticut

DAVID N. WEISSMAN, MD
Director, Division of Respiratory Disease
Studies, National Institute for Occupational
Safety and Health, Centers for Disease Control
and Prevention, and Adjunct Professor,
West Virginia University, Morgantown,
West Virginia

BRIAN L. WITHERS, DO
Occupational Medicine Resident, Department
of Occupational and Environmental Health,
Occupational Medicine, Heartland Center
for Occupational Health and Safety, College
of Public Health, University of Iowa,
Iowa City, Iowa

CHRISTINE WON, MD, MS
Assistant Professor, Pulmonary and Critical
Care Medicine, Yale School of Medicine,
New Haven, Connecticut

YU A. ZHAO, MD, MS
Clinical Fellow, Division of Occupational and
Environmental Medicine, University of
California, San Francisco, San Francisco,
California

Contents

> Asthma and extrinsic allergic alveolitis (EAA) remain prevalent respiratory diseases and the cause of a significant disease burden. This article reviews the recent occupational and environmental causes described for these conditions. Even over the limited time spam addressed by this article, novel agents and new data relating to already suggested causes have been described. Various types of work tasks or exposures are described that appear to cause both asthma and EAA. Isocyanates, the best example of dual potential to cause asthma and EAA are discussed, as is the new understanding of the role metal-working fluids play when causing respiratory diseases.

> A task force of the American Thoracic Society has defined work-exacerbated asthma (WEA) as the worsening of asthma caused by conditions at work. Occupational asthma (OA) is asthma that is initiated by occupational exposures in people without prior asthma. In contrast, WEA is asthma (*already present or coincident [new onset]*) that is worsened because of conditions at work. This difference is critical because asthma is a common disease (present in approximately 7% of working adults). Among working adults with asthma, approximately 20% may have WEA. WEA has potential implications regarding asthma morbidity, health care use, and the economy.

> Chronic obstructive pulmonary disease represents a major cause of morbidity and mortality in industrialized and nonindustrialized countries. Although tobacco use remains the main factor associated with development of the disease, occupational risk factors represent an important and preventable cause. The most common occupationally related factors include exposure to organic dusts, metallic fumes, and a variety of other mineral gases and/or vapors. This article summarizes the literature on the subject and provides an update of the most recent advances in the field.

> The nose and upper airways form the initial area of impact for air pollutants and allergens. The development of nasal allergies in the workplace (occupational rhinitis) may herald subsequent development of occupational asthma. Exposure controls, periodic surveillance, and early intervention may circumvent work-related airways disease and prevent unnecessary worker impairment and disability.

Almost 3 billion people worldwide burn solid fuels indoors. Despite the large population at risk worldwide, the effect of exposure to indoor solid fuel smoke has not been adequately studied. Indoor air pollution from solid fuel use is strongly associated with chronic obstructive pulmonary disease, acute respiratory tract infections, and lung cancer, and weakly associated with asthma, tuberculosis, and interstitial lung disease. Tobacco use further potentiates the development of respiratory disease among subjects exposed to solid fuel smoke. There is a need to perform additional interventional studies in this field.

With the introduction of new materials and changes in manufacturing practices, occupational health investigators continue to uncover associations between novel exposures and chronic forms of diffuse parenchymal lung disease and terminal airways disease. To discern exposure–disease relationships, clinicians must maintain a high index of suspicion for the potential toxicity of occupational and environmental exposures. This article details several newly recognized chronic parenchymal and terminal airways. Diseases related to exposure to indium, nylon flock, diacetyl used in the flavorings industry, nanoparticles, and the World Trade Center disaster are reviewed. Also reviewed are methods in worker surveillance and the potential use of biomarkers in the evaluation of exposure–disease relationships.

Because tobacco smoking is a potent carcinogen, secondary causes of lung cancer are often diminished in perceived importance. The goal of this review is to describe the occurrence and recent findings of the 27 agents currently listed by the International Agency for Research on Cancer (IARC) as lung carcinogens. The IARC's updated assessments of lung carcinogens provide a long-overdue resource for consensus opinions on the carcinogenic potential of various agents. Supplementary new information, with a focus on analytic epidemiologic studies that has become available since IARC's most recent evaluation, are also discussed.

Military personnel can be exposed to toxicants and conditions that can contribute to lung diseases. This article describes what is known about these exposures and diseases, focusing on the Iraq and Afghanistan wars. Adverse lung health outcomes have been reported in US military personnel deployed to Iraq and/or Afghanistan. Most studies to date have been hindered by limited deployment-specific exposure assessment, lack of baseline lung health information, and variable medical evaluations and case definitions. Further research is warranted. Medical surveillance has been recommended for returning troops, but the challenges are substantial.

Lawrence A. Ho and Ware G. Kuschner

Many home-based and leisure activities can generate hazardous respirable exposures. Routine domestic activities and a variety of hobbies, avocations, and leisure pursuits have been associated with a spectrum of respiratory tract disorders. Indoor environments present a special risk for high-intensity exposures and adverse health effects. There are important knowledge gaps regarding the prevalence of specific health hazards within and across communities, exposure-response effects, population and individual susceptibilities, best management strategies, the adverse health effects of mixed exposures, and long-term clinical outcomes following exposures. The home environment presents special health risks that should be part of the health assessment.

Ann Y. Teng and Christine Won

This article illustrates the impact of obstructive sleep apnea (OSA) on the work force and emphasizes that there are public health risks and significant societal financial losses in untreated OSA. Specifics of OSA impact on individuals are discussed with regard to veterans, first responders, farmers, and pilots, specially focusing on commercial vehicle drivers. The pathophysiology of OSA and the consequence of impairment and disability due to OSA on work capacity are introduced. Federal guidelines for occupational-specific recommendations are presented. The health care provider's role in identifying and incorporating effective screening and treatment strategies for workers with sleep apnea is emphasized.

A. Scott Laney and David N. Weissman

The purpose of this article is to provide an update on selected issues of current interest and recent developments related to 3 types of inorganic mineral dust exposures causing classic forms of pneumoconiosis: coal mine dust, crystalline silica, and asbestos. Common themes include new imaging modalities, emerging exposures, and evolving appreciation of additional adverse health effects associated with exposure to these inorganic mineral dusts.

Francesco Sava and Chris Carlsten

There is new evidence for ambient air pollution (AAP) leading to an increased incidence of respiratory diseases in adults. Research has demonstrated that co-exposures have the potential to dramatically augment the effects of AAP and lower the threshold of effect of a given pollutant. Interactions between genes related to oxidative stress and AAP seem to significantly alter the effect of AAP on an individual and population basis. A better definition of vulnerable populations may bolster local or regional efforts to remediate AAP. Advances in genetic research tools have the potential to identify candidate genes that can guide further research.

Anna-Carin Olin

Sensitive methods to detect airways inflammation caused by exposures associated with adverse respiratory effects are crucial, as is the identification of individuals with early-stage disease. In this review, the use of induced sputum and sampling of the fraction of nitric oxide to identify airways inflammation associated with occupational exposures is discussed. In addition, a new method to assess airways inflammation in small airways (sampling and analyses of particles in exhaled air) is introduced.

Respiratory protection is used as a method of protecting individuals from inhaling harmful airborne contaminants and in some cases to supply them with breathable air in oxygen-deficient environments. This article focuses on the use and types of personal respiratory protection (respirators) worn by individuals at workplaces where airborne hazardous contaminants may exist. Respirators are increasingly also being used in nonindustrial settings such as health care facilities, as concerns regarding infectious epidemics and terrorist threats grow. Pulmonologists and other clinicians should understand fundamental issues regarding respiratory protection against airborne contaminants and the use of respirators.

CLINICS IN CHEST MEDICINE

DOWNLOAD
Free App!

Review Articles
THE CLINICS

NOW AVAILABLE FOR YOUR iPhone and iPad

CLINICS IN CHEST MEDICINE

Preface

Lung diseases associated with occupational and environmental exposures subsume a wide spectrum of conditions. These include asthma, chronic obstructive pulmonary disease (COPD), parenchymal lung diseases, and lung cancer, but there are other less common but noteworthy entities as well, as the recent outbreak of diacetyl-associated bronchiolitis obliterans has taught us. The most recent issue of *Clinics in Chest Medicine* that was devoted exclusively to the topic of Occupational and Environmental Lung Disease was published ten years ago. The past decade has seen a marked increase in our appreciation of the breadth and depth of respiratory tract morbidities that can be linked to an ever-expanding list of workplace and environmental hazardous exposures. New knowledge touches on emerging lung diseases, novel exposure scenarios for well-established pathologies, evolving risk factor characterization pointing to previously under-recognized associations, and fresh insights into pathophysiological mechanisms of occupational and environmental respiratory disease. Clinicians, researchers, and policy makers need to be updated on the ever-changing landscape of occupationally and environmentally associated lung diseases. Far from being esoteric or of historical interest only, this is a relevant and even cutting edge topic area, as the articles in this issue of *Clinics in Chest Medicine* demonstrate. Moreover, the failure to appropriately recognize work and environmental factors in disease hinders proper diagnosis, management, and, vitally, the appropriate protection of others also at risk.

The first four articles in this volume highlight new developments in occupational and environmental asthma and hypersensitivity pneumonitis (a topic area characterized by a continuing emergence of novel factors), COPD (until recently not well-appreciated as being associated with occupational or environmental exposures beyond cigarette smoking), and upper airway conditions (which are too often excluded from consideration of occupational respiratory tract diseases). In the first article, Dr Fishwick details a number of recently recognized occupational and environmental causes of asthma, including newly appreciated plant, animal, and chemical allergens. He also tackles mixed exposures and selected high-risk occupations. This article also addresses recently recognized exposures and settings associated with extrinsic allergic alveolitis, a topic that has warranted better integration with asthma-causing agents given many similar exposure scenarios (for example certain organic materials and isocyanates). Dr Szema reviews the recent literature on a common but only more recently appreciated occupational scenario for respiratory morbidity, work-exacerbated asthma, that is, "ordinary" asthma (as opposed to classic work-caused asthma) that is exacerbated by various work exposures. In his update on occupational COPD, Dr Mannino summarizes recent studies, including from the United States and internationally, confirming that a substantial proportion of COPD (15% or more) is attributable to occupational exposures. His review also highlights progress that has been made identifying epidemiological associations with specific causative agents, such as organic dusts, metallic fumes, and mineral dusts. Dr Shusterman provides an update of work-related rhinitis and upper airway conditions, which are an important cause of morbidity in their own right but can also progress to asthma.

Several articles address important new and/or newly recognized occupational and environmental exposures and associated respiratory diseases. Drs Gulati and Sauler review data on emerging parenchymal and terminal airways diseases that have been documented among workers exposed to indium (a metal used in flat-panel displays), diacetyl (important as a food flavorant), nylon and other synthetics (in the form of "flock" or short-cut fibers), and the after-affects of acute inhalational exposures to the World Trade Center disaster. Dr Rose provides a timely unique synthesis of what is known about inhalational exposures and lung diseases associated with military service, focusing primarily on the U.S. military personnel who were deployed to Iraq and Afghanistan, among whom a number of inhalational exposures and adverse lung health outcomes have recently been reported. Dr Sood provides a useful update on indoor fuel exposures and the substantial burden of associated lung diseases (including risk of infectious and obstructive adverse outcomes) in both developing and developed countries. Drs Ho and Kuschner summarize the diverse array of potential hazardous exposures and associated respiratory morbidity that might be linked to all too common home and leisure activities, including cooking, cleaning, hobbies and indoor sports. The review by Drs Won and Teng addresses the impact

Clin Chest Med 33 (2012) xi–xii
http://dx.doi.org/10.1016/j.ccm.2012.09.006

of an increasingly common disease, obstructive sleep apnea, on workers and their ability to work. There have also been important new developments in our understanding of the classic pneumoconioses, the health effects of ambient air pollution, and occupational and environmental causes of lung cancer, each of which is well addressed in a series of separate articles in this volume of *Clinics in Chest Medicine*. The review of occupation and lung cancer is particularly timely given the recent classification of diesel exhaust as a human lung carcinogen by the International Agency for Research on Cancer (IARC). We do not neglect additional cutting edge diagnostic and research tools, as covered by Dr Olin in her erudite review of non-invasive diagnostic and research approaches to detect airways inflammation and disease, including the use of induced sputum and exhaled breath analysis. Finally, Drs Cohen and Birkner provide a practical summary for clinicians of personal respiratory protection (respirators) used in hospitals and industrial settings.

The unifying principle of all of these articles is that taking a thorough yet targeted occupational and environmental history is the key that unlocks the puzzle of occupational and environmental respiratory disease. We hope that the articles contained in this edition of *Clinics in Chest Medicine* will increase awareness of the changing realities of occupational and environmental exposures, their substantial contribution to airways, parenchymal, and malignant lung diseases, and, ultimately to encourage each reader to ask their patients what they do for a living, as well as what their unsalaried endeavors and avocations at home may be.

We are grateful to all of the authors for their outstanding and thoughtful contributions to this issue of *Clinics in Chest Medicine*.

Carrie A. Redlich, MD, MPH
Occupational and Environmental Medicine
Program and Section of Pulmonary
and Critical Care Medicine
Yale University School of Medicine
135 College Street
New Haven, CT 06510, USA

Paul D. Blanc, MD, MSPH
Division of Occupational and
Environmental Medicine
UCSF School of Medicine
350 Parnassus Avenue, Suite 609
San Francisco, CA 94117, USA

Mridu Gulati, MD, MPH
Section of Pulmonary and Critical Care Medicine
Yale University School of Medicine
15 York Street
New Haven, CT 06510, USA

Ware G. Kuschner, MD
Division of Pulmonary and Critical Care Medicine
Stanford University School of Medicine
VA Palo Alto Health Care System
3801 Miranda Avenue
Palo Alto, CA 94304, USA

E-mail addresses:
carrie.redlich@yale.edu (C.A. Redlich)
paul.blanc@ucsf.edu (P.D. Blanc)
mridu.gulati@yale.edu (M. Gulati)
kuschner@stanford.edu (W.G. Kuschner)

New Occupational and Environmental Causes of Asthma and Extrinsic Allergic Alveolitis

David Fishwick, MBChB, FRCP, MD

KEYWORDS

- Asthma • Extrinsic allergic alveolitis • Hypersensitivity pneumonitis • Antigen • Allergen
- Respiratory • Occupational • Environmental

KEY POINTS

- Asthma and extrinsic allergic alveolitis (EAA) remain prevalent respiratory diseases, and remain the cause of a significant disease burden.
- Both conditions have strong causative links to the environment.
- This article reviews the recent occupational and environmental causes described for these 2 conditions.

INTRODUCTION

Asthma remains a highly prevalent childhood and adult disease. Although research activity over recent years has contributed greatly to the understanding of this condition, and in particular asthma of childhood origin and its natural history, important causes of later-onset asthma caused by factors encountered at work, or in the wider environment, and the outcomes of this subset of disease, are less well researched. Missing the links between exposure to antigenic or irritant substances and the development of asthma is potentially disastrous for affected workers and their similarly exposed colleagues who may be at risk of further incident disease. There are parallel implications for other potentially work-related causes of immune-mediated respiratory conditions, in particular extrinsic allergic alveolitis (EAA, also known as hypersensitivity pneumonitis).

This review summarizes the recent biomedical literature relating to specific, as well as more general, aspects of selected agents that have been shown to be associated with asthma or EAA, including exposures that have been found capable of eliciting both responses. The general subject of occupational asthma has been extensively reviewed elsewhere,[1,2] including a major textbook on this topic.[3] The emphasis here is on *newly* appreciated causes of disease or emerging insights into mechanisms of initiation and progression.

By its nature, the literature on emerging hazards is largely made up of a potpourri of case reports or small case series that document interesting presentations of disease or workplace investigations, consequent upon an initial suspicion that a new exposure scenario or a novel agent may be responsible for causing respiratory illness. Consistent with the focus on new and emerging

The content of this publication, including any opinions and/or conclusions expressed, are those of the author alone and do not necessarily reflect HSE policy.
Centre for Workplace Health, Health and Safety Laboratories, The University of Sheffield, Harpur Hill, Buxton, Derbyshire SK17 3JN, UK
E-mail address: d.fishwick@sheffield.ac.uk

Clin Chest Med 33 (2012) 605–616
http://dx.doi.org/10.1016/j.ccm.2012.07.002

data, this review is limited primarily to citations appearing from 2007 onward. To be as broad as possible, however, and recognizing that relevant exposure conditions are frequently encountered internationally, information from abstracts in English summarizing non–English language publications has been included.

It is evident, appraising the breadth of the recent literature, that asthma and EAA remain enigmatic diseases. Articles identified for this review deal not only with new at-risk exposed populations, but also novel causes of asthma and alveolitis. Recent data also suggest that a number of allergens are being characterized and newly incorporated in clinical testing. Indeed, for associations that may appear to be well understood, the recent literature demonstrates the relative naivety of our understanding of the mechanistic role played by occupational and environmental exposures. Hamlet summarized the situation well: "There are more things in heaven and earth, Horatio, than are *dreamt of* in your philosophy!"

ASTHMA OVERVIEW

In an attempt to stratify the asthma literature into clearly definable subcategories of disease, the recent literature is categorized into 3 sections, first dealing primarily high molecular weight asthma-causing sensitizers; second, low molecular weight allergens; and third, occupational and environmental mixed low and high molecular weight potential exposures. The low molecular weight literature generally relates to chemical exposures (which can be synthetic or naturally occurring), whereas reports of high molecular weight substances generally focus on agents of biologic origin, as these are *a priori* more likely to be of high molecular weight.

ASTHMA: HIGH MOLECULAR WEIGHT AGENTS

A fascinating miscellany of evidence has emerged in relation to sensitization to high molecular weight agents, including exposures as diverse as *Ascaris lumbricoides tropomyosin* to laxative allergy and on through to risks posed by exposure in an insect-breeding facility.

The potential to develop TH2-type responses to *A lumbricoides tropomyosin* was recently identified,[4] given its central role in the development of immunity to parasites. This allergen was found to bind specific immunoglobulin (Ig)E, and induce mediator release from effector cells. This effect was found to be cross-reactive to mite tropomyosins. Whether this mechanism and allergen are indeed important in the pathogenesis of environmental asthma in tropical regions remains to be seen. Similarly in terms of environmental factors, the role of an array of olive pollens has been reexamined as a major contributor to allergic diseases in Mediterranean areas.[5] Specifically, at least 20 proteins with allergic activity have been demonstrated in olive pollen, and 10 of these have been characterized (Ole e 1 to Ole e 10). Response to Ole e 1, considered the most important of these allergens, is now identified to have a significant genetic influence. The authors postulate that exposure to high doses of olive pollen allergen in a specific genetic context can trigger different allergic conditions, including asthma.

Such "environmental" allergens can also be relevant to occupational settings. For example, allergy to *Sinapis alba* pollen (white mustard), an entomophilic species included in the Brassicaceae family, associated with allergic symptoms and in certain cases positive nasal challenge, has been recently described in a small group of olive farmers.[6] Twelve orchard workers with a combination of rhinitis and (or) asthma were investigated with skin prick tests, alongside air monitoring to assess levels of exposure. The clinical relevance of the allergy, identified in all workers by the presence of specific IgE, was confirmed with a positive nasal challenge test, and levels of exposure to *S alba* pollen were identified to be high in work environments, with peaks of 1801 grains/m^3 detected. These levels were shown to be higher than background environmental levels.

Table grape workers also appear to be at risk of the potential for the 2-spotted spider mite to cause sensitization and allergy end points. A South African group[6] has reported specific sensitization to the mite *Tetranychus urticae*, and present data to support the clinical relevance of this sensitization. A further novel, predominantly indoor-encountered allergen has recently been described. Nakazawa and colleagues[7] report sensitivity to Asian ladybugs (*Harmonia axyridis*), introduced between 1916 and 1990 to the United States. Given that these beetles do not tolerate cold, they migrate indoors during winter months and are consequently a potential source of indoor allergen (of course, which can additionally include indoor occupational settings). Testing of 20 individuals with allergic symptoms living in Asian ladybug-infested accommodation confirmed positive specific IgE in a high proportion, and a lesser proportion of those with asthma. Interestingly, cross reactivity to *Blatella germanica* was found only among those with additional exposure to cockroaches.

Soybean exposure continues to interest the research community. Cummings and colleagues[8] have recently described results of a further study of workers exposed to the products of soy bean processing. Of interest, both soy-specific IgE and IgG were raised in exposed workers in comparison with controls, and it was specifically the IgE response that was associated with a threefold greater risk of current asthma, or asthmalike symptoms. Work from South African soybean processors[9] produced consistent findings, and identified that the strongest predictor of work-related nasal symptoms was sensitization, as judged by specific IgE, to soybean. Recent further work in soy flake–processing workers[10] has bettered the understanding of the specific immune response to soybean. Data from 135 such workers demonstrated that the prominent proteins that bound soy IgE were the high molecular weight storage proteins, β-conglycinin (Gly m 5) and Glycinin (Gly m 6). In contrast, no specific IgE reactivity could be identified to lower molecular weight allergens.

Coffee exposure, and in particular exposure to the contaminant *Neurospora sitophila*, has been described as a recent cause of occupational asthma in 2 separate case reports.[11,12] The latter identified exposure to *Chrysonilia sitophila*, the asexual state of *N sitophila*, as the likely cause of asthma in a 43-year-old man exposed to coffee beans contaminated with a powder containing this agent. Serial peak expiratory flow (PEF) recordings identified an immediate response following a workplace challenge (a 20% fall) and specific IgE was identified to an isolate of *C sitophila*, biotinylated with a prewashed streptavidin ImmunoCAP. The exact nature of the wider range of coffee antigens capable of causing asthma has been long debated[13] and is not yet resolved

Various other likely high molecular weight allergens recently described as causing asthma specifically include *Plantago ovata* seed, as part of a laxative preparation, in health care workers,[14] *Artemia* fish fry feed in aquaculture,[15] konjac glucomannan in a food worker,[16] and gum arabic.[17] The latter as a cause of allergic disease, reported by a Finnish group, is supported by the identification of 4 cases (from 11 workers studied) who had developed occupational asthma as a result of exposure in the food industry. Gum arabic, a complex mix of glycoproteins and polysaccharides, is used as a food stabilizer and should be considered as a potential cause of asthma and rhinitis in exposed workers with allergic symptoms.

ASTHMA: LOW MOLECULAR WEIGHT AGENTS AND CHEMICAL IRRITANTS

Cleaning agents continue to attract the limelight and underscore that allergic sensitization with an amnestic response, irritant-induced new-onset disease, and aggravation of preexisting asthma can all occur in association with this broad group of materials. Evidence of sensitization to chloramine T, used as a disinfectant, was recently described in a nurse working with this agent, in addition to glutaraldehyde.[18] The individual reported asthma symptoms following exposure to both these agents in the endoscopy suite, but subsequent specific inhalation challenge (SIC) testing confirmed a negative challenge to glutaraldehyde but a positive dual reaction following inhalation of 0.5% solution of chloramine T. The wider issue of the role of cleaning agents as causes of asthma was also recently reviewed by Zock and colleagues,[19] who concluded that recent publications have strengthened the evidence linking cleaning agent exposures and specifically the development of asthma. This link appears to hold for both asthma caused by, and aggravated by, cleaning agent exposures. The authors postulate that cleaning sprays, chlorine bleach, and other disinfectants may be the most likely candidates.[19]

There are no recent data to assist differentiation in relation to causative mechanisms of cleaning product–associated asthma. It is equally plausible that low molecular weight chemicals in cleaning agents may exert a primary irritant effect, rather than that mediated either via haptenation, and thus IgE, mechanism, or indeed other as yet uncharacterized mechanisms (for example, adjuvant effects facilitating sensitization to other exposures).

Health care workers exposed to the antibiotic group of cephalosporins have also recently been identified[20] to display evidence of sensitization, as judged by specific IgE, to various cephalosporin-human serum albumin (HSA) conjugates. Using both exposed workers and a nonexposed control group, relatively high (but variable agent to agent) levels of sensitization were identified; 17.4% for any cephalosporin, 10.4% for cefotiam, 6.8% for ceftriaxone, and 3.7% for ceftizoxime. Overall, these levels were higher than those identified using skin prick testing. Of interest, a previous history of atopic dermatitis appeared to be a risk factor for the presence of IgE to the cefotiam-HSA conjugate, at least suggesting that a dermal route of sensitization may be important. This assertion is important to unravel in more detail, given the importance of developing effective simple preventive strategies for exposed workers.

A Spanish observational study[21] has further added to the evidence base relating to the propensity for acrylates to cause both allergic skin problems and asthma. Acrylates in this context were used to sculpt artificial nails, and the investigators reported a case series of 15 female patients who had presented over a prolonged period to their institution. Most patients were beauticians, although one client was included in the series, and exhibited a very wide range (1–15 years) of latent period of exposure during which the investigators postulated that sensitization had occurred. All had certain features of dermatitis, and 3 (including the client, interestingly) had a diagnosis of asthma. Patch testing identified that the most frequent allergens were ethylene glycol dimethacrylate (13/15, 86.7%), hydroxyethyl methacrylate (13/15, 86.7%), triethylene glycol dimethacrylate (7/15, 46.7%), 2-hydroxypropyl methacrylate (5/15, 33.3%), and methyl methacrylate (5/15, 33.3%). The investigators concluded that acrylate monomers are important, primarily skin sensitizers, although no challenge data were presented in the cases where asthma was thought to be causally related to exposures.

Metabisulphite, a low molecular weight agent previously intermittently associated with the development of allergic disease, was implicated again as the likely cause of asthma in a Dublin Bay prawns fisherman.[22] The investigators describe long-term exposure to these creatures and the development of work-related respiratory symptoms. An added complication appeared to be the breakdown of ventilation systems used aboard a trawler designed to reduce these exposures. No tests of immunologic response or SIC were performed, although negative skin tests to standard allergens were reported.

Asthma related to a further low molecular weight agent was described following exposure to an electrostatic powder paint containing 2.5% to 10.0% triglycidyl isocyanurate (TGIC) in a 28-year-old worker coating aluminum frames.[23] Serial peak-flow measurements noted increased diurnal variation on work days (up to 46%) and nonspecific bronchial reactivity varied between periods of work and rest, and an isolated late reaction (20% fall in forced expiratory volume in 1 second) was observed following SIC, this response not being seen following work days. Attempts were also made to assess for evidence of immunologic response to TGIC, but no evidence of specific IgE was detected by enzyme-linked immunosorbent assay, and no IgE-binding bands were found by immunoblot analysis of patient and control serum.

ASTHMA ASSOCIATED WITH COMPLEX, MIXED EXPOSURES

Various recent studies have addressed workplaces with the potential for complex and mixed exposures, a summary of which is included here to provide the reader with a flavor of these reports.

In addition, studies relating to potential environmental causes, by definition inherently complex and mixed, will also be dealt with where appropriate.

Job tasks with wood exposure continue to attract attention. Burton and colleagues[24] describe a case series of occupational asthma related to medium-density fiberboard exposures (a mix of soft and hard woods bound using a resin and formaldehyde), supported variably by work-related changes in PEF and SIC testing. Schlünssen and colleagues[25] remind us of the limitations of immunologic testing in this group of workers, with specific reference to limitations of pine and beech sensitization testing.

Harris-Roberts and colleagues[26] also identified a rather unusual workplace as being associated with occupational asthma. This group identified occupational asthma as a consequence of working with multiple, presumably, high and low molecular weight allergens in an insect-breeding facility, including locust and mealworms. Work with fish has also been described recently as a cause of asthma in South African saltwater fish–processing workers[27] and fish-farm workers exposed to turbot.[28]

Patiwael and colleagues[29] have returned to follow up their cohort of workers exposed to Bell pepper pollens. Originally fully investigated in 1999 when a high level of sensitization was found, this group of workers was reevaluated using a questionnaire and further skin prick testing. Over the follow-up period, cumulative incidences for sensitization respectively to bell pepper pollen, work-related rhinitis, and asthma symptoms were found to be 9%, 19%, and 8%. The presence of atopy and, interestingly, smoking were identified as risk factors for developing work-related symptoms.

Occupational groups commonly reported to surveillance schemes with occupational lung diseases and particularly asthma, and indeed identified in large epidemiologic studies as having levels of self-reported asthma include bakers, cleaners, and health care workers. The debate relating to the exact causative agent or agents responsible for baker's asthma continues to simmer. Rye allergens have long been assumed to play a role in the development of this disease in addition to the established role of wheat flour. Letrán and colleagues[30] reported 2 isolated cases of asthma where rye was thought to be central to causation. Both had evidence of asthma and rhinoconjunctivitis, and both had positive SIC to rye, but not to wheat flour alone. Immunoblotting suggested that rye flour enzymatic inhibitors might be responsible. Wheat lipid transfer protein was also recently described as a further putative allergen responsible for baker's asthma.[31]

Two recent articles deal with allergy to lupin, a diverse and beautiful species, mostly comprising herbaceous perennial plants and shrubs with a characteristic leaf shape. The yellow legume seeds of lupins, commonly called lupin beans, are edible and popular. The first of the 2 articles explores allergic sensitization at work.[32] A cross-sectional study of a food-processing company, with workers exposed to lupin, identified high levels of specific sensitization (21%), the latter clearly linked to allergic symptoms of rhinitis and asthma. Although only small numbers were challenged, one worker had a dual response following SIC.

The second article[33] provocatively, yet perhaps aptly, titled "Lupin allergy: a hidden killer at home, a menace at work," reminds us that allergy to such plants is only relatively recently appreciated, the consequences poorly understood, and that exposure at work and at home can cause the typical allergic combinations of asthma and rhinoconjunctivitis. Possible cross-reactivity to peanut allergy is also discussed, and the investigators believe that heightening awareness of this novel allergen is key to preventing future cases of allergic disease. On balance, these probably represent primarily proteinaceous high molecular weight interactions.

Environmental, as opposed to occupational, exposures are also of interest in this context. In reality, these "real life" environmental exposures are a complex, poorly characterized mix of varying antigens and irritants. As these are difficult to characterize accurately, they are dealt with in this section. The urban environment has again been placed into focus in relation to causation of asthma and allergy, with 2 recent publications relating to the contribution made by horse allergens, perhaps more typically associated with rural environments. Long understood to be allergenic to humans, the role of horse allergen has been assessed by 2 publications from the same Italian group. By assessing a large number of consecutive patients from an outpatient clinic environment, Liccardi and colleagues[34] identified approximately 3.5% of all those with positive skin prick tests to common allergens to be sensitized to horse dander sensitization. Interestingly, no patients were sensitized solely to horse dander, although only a minority of those sensitized reported regular horse contact. The clinical significance of these findings is less clear, given the lack of contact to horses for most of those sensitized, although most did complain of a combination of respiratory and rhinitic symptoms.

Similarly, work from the same group, published in 2011, looked further afield in Italy,[35] collecting data from more than 3000 patients recruited from similar centers. Slightly higher levels of sensitization to horse dander were seen, with approximately 5.4% of those with a positive skin prick test to any tested allergen having evidence of horse sensitization. A similar mix of self-reported horse exposure was seen. It remains to be determined whether the development of such sensitization is of clinical relevance for those patients living in a predominant urban environment without regular horse contact.

Various other indoor allergens have attracted new interest in the recently published evidence base, and include further evidence relating to cockroach sensitization in children, silverfish allergen, and the role of mouse allergen. A recent Italian study,[36] designed primary to assess point prevalence of sensitization to German cockroaches, identified that high levels of sensitization were seen in older children to *Blattella germanica* (BG). The number of other positive skin prick tests also increased the likelihood of BG sensitization. The investigators also estimated a high population attributable risk of approximately 20% for the effects of BG sensitization on the development of rhinoconjunctivitis.

Less familiar perhaps as a potential important indoor allergen, Barletta and colleagues[37] described the potential for sensitization to silverfish (*Lepisma saccharina*), one of the most primitive living insects commonly identified in the indoor environment. The investigators are currently developing an extract, so that future studies can incorporate allergen testing to this insect. Lep s 1 has been cloned and characterized as a silverfish tropomyosin and is likely to be the basis of future allergen assessments.

The role of mouse allergen is highlighted by 2 publications. The first, published in 2006,[38] studied US-based schoolchildren with a combination of questionnaire and assessments of indoor exposure to mouse allergen, Mus m 1. Twenty-six percent of the studied children were found to be sensitized to mouse, and interestingly there appeared to be a relationship within the sensitized group between levels of Mus m 1 exposure and reported asthma symptoms and reliever use. These effects withstood the typical corrections applied for confounding and bias. The investigators' conclusions at that time were consistent with the conclusions of a subsequent overview article published in 2009,[39] that exposure to mouse allergen is associated with substantial asthma morbidity, including hospitalizations, and that pest management is recommended for sensitized patients with asthma.

Recent Finnish work[40] identified certain HLA associations with the development of sensitization to cow allergens, part of a group of allergens in the family of lipocalin proteins. The HLA-DR/DQ geno-types of 40 Bos d 2-sensitized individuals were analyzed, and compared with a larger group of unrelated Finnish participants. Various HLA class II alleles were found to be overrepresented in those sensitized.

EAA OVERVIEW

Despite its recognition for many decades, new and novel causes of EAA continue to surface in the peer-reviewed literature. Broadly speaking, causes identified in this review fall into 2 categories: first, a traditional, or, in a sense, anticipatable group of causes, largely microbiological in nature, and second, a rather more unusual or less intuitive group of possible causes. Paralleling the recent literature relating to asthma, most of the recent articles identified deal with small numbers of cases or isolated case reports. Consequently, criticism can always be leveled at the diagnostic rigor with which a diagnosis is made or how effectively differential or alternate diagnoses have been excluded. Nevertheless, the inherently fascinating nature of these observations is now detailed, dealing first with the classical, or anticipatable, causes of this condition.

EAA ATTRIBUTABLE TO CLASSICAL OR ANTICIPATABLE CAUSES

Duvet exposure has previously been associated with the development of EAA, and a Japanese case report again highlights this risk. Nishikawa and colleagues[41] describe a case of shortness of breath, cough, and fever in a 44-year-old duvet manufacturer, typified by ground glass opacities on HRCT, coupled with a positive lymphocyte proliferation test to pigeon serum. Clinical improvement occurred on removal from occupational exposures.

Other various fungal or related microbiological exposures thought to be causative of EAA include *Thermoactinomyces vulgaris* exposure from a dehumidifier (Otsuka and colleagues,[42] with supportive biopsy and precipitating antibodies), *Aspergillus niger* in a greenhouse worker working cultivating roses (Hamaguchi and colleagues,[43] with supportive biopsy and precipitating antibodies), and air conditioner exposures (Ishikawa and colleagues,[44] with supportive biopsy and challenge, but negative precipitating antibodies).

Thermoactinomyces were also implicated in a further cases of EAA related to sugar cane exposure in Nicaraguan workers.[45] This Italian contribution describes the consequences of bagasse exposure in a group of exposed workers, with precipitin response to *Thermoactinomyces*

sacchari and *T vulgaris* being related to the presence of reported respiratory symptoms. No further clinical characterization was undertaken, given the epidemiologic and workplace-based nature of the study.

Work in food preparation continues to carry a significant risk of EAA. Further case reports support exposure to Shiitake mushroom and dry sausage mold as causative. Kai and colleagues,[46] a Japanese group, describe a case of Shiitake mushroom chronic EAA in an elderly man with long-standing cough and breathlessness, although no biopsy evidence was given to support the assumption. An associated literature review identified a further 5 previous Japanese cases caused by the same agent. Guillot and colleagues[47] add to the gastronomic causes of EAA by describing 3 cases of EAA associated with occupational dry sausage mold exposure. Each case exhibited typical HRCT features and, although no biopsy data were included, each case was supported by positive precipitating antibodies to an extract of the sausage (containing, among presumably a complex mix of potential antigens, penicillium), and improved clinical state following cessation of exposure. Similarly, a recent Spanish[48] article described 5 cases of "Chacinero's lung," 3 with an acute form, and 2 with a subacute form. Bronchoalveolar lavage (BAL) in 3 patients showed significant lymphocytosis (17%, 40%, and 40%), with a CD4/CD8 ratio of less than 0.6. Specific IgG to *Penicillium frequentans* and *Aspergillus fumigatus* were positive in 3. No biopsy data were recorded.

The use of musical instruments play their part in the cause of EAA. Two case reports identify playing trombone (trombone player's lung[49]) and saxophone[50] as being significantly bad for your health. The unfortunate saxophonist was a 48-year-old patient being investigated for interstitial lung disease, during which an open biopsy was performed, revealing a nonspecific interstitial pneumonitis appearance. A lymphocytic BAL led to further assessment of the saxophone itself, played for a hobby. Two fungi were isolated from this, *Ulocladium botrytis* and *Phoma* sp, against which the patient's serum had developed antibody responses. The investigators raise the wider and unknown issue of how commonplace colonization is in these, and related, instruments. The 35-year-old saxophonist was a professional musician who complained of a very long-standing, unabating nonproductive cough. HRCT showed evidence of a mosaic pattern on the expiratory views, and the diagnosis was suspected after improvement following a period of not playing the offending instrument, the interior of which revealed a biofilm with fungal elements, and isolation of

Mycobacterium chelonae/abscessus group, *Fusarium* sp, as well as scanty *Stenotrophomonas maltophilia* and *Escherichia coli.* The cough improved following regular cleaning.

Selected indoor water-related pursuits also appear to have adverse health consequences. Engelhart and colleagues[51] describe a case of EAA in a child, highly likely to be related to exposure to fungal contaminants of indoor hydroponic cultivation. Supported by precipitins to *Aureobasidum pullulans*, a lymphocytic BAL and consistent biopsy, this case occurred in a 14-year-old girl. She improved markedly when the offending plants were removed from the home. Exposure to microbiological contaminants of poorly maintained hot tubs continues to be identified as a cause of EAA. First described more than a decade ago (for example, see Kahana and colleagues[52]), a Canadian group[53] recently described a further 2 cases of this condition, one of which presented acutely, whereas the other presented as a more chronic process. Even though the exact cause probably varies among cases, nontuberculous mycobacterium have been frequently implicated.

It appears that poorly maintained hot tubs not only carry a risk of EAA, as described by Huhulescu and colleagues.[54] This Austrian group describes a fatal *Pseudomonas* pneumonia in a previously fit 49-year-old woman. This event occurred shortly after returning from a spa weekend; water samples from the hot tub revealing 37,000 colony-forming units of *Pseudomonas aeruginosa* per 100 mL. The investigators postulated that a massive biofilm had been produced in the bath circulation system as a consequence of substandard maintenance.

Other perhaps classical exposures recently associated with EAA also include steam iron exposure, previously described and accepted as a cause[55]; cork exposure[56] causing the EAA called suberosis, this recent case based on BAL results and a supportive biopsy; exposure to *Trichoderma viride* from a contaminated ultrasonic humidifier,[57] confirmed by immunologic responses and improvement following removal of exposure; and work in citrus farming.[58] The latter report was of a cluster of 3 farmers with EAA confirmed by a combination of clinical features, including symptom improvement on removal from exposure and challenge testing. *Aspergillus* and *Penicillium* species were postulated by the investigators to have relevance, although testing in the patients revealed mixed results.

EAA FROM LESS ANTICIPATABLE CAUSES

Perhaps of rather more interest are a group of articles dealing with likely diagnoses of EAA caused by agents that are less intuitively likely to be associated with this condition. Agents and exposure types in this group included zinc fume, paints, the hydrofluorocarbon 1,1,1,2-tetrafluoroethane, and the enzyme phytase. Further evidence is also included in this group relating to the previously described respiratory problems in yacht manufacturers.

Miyazaki and colleagues[59] described a respiratory problem in a 55-year-old welder after having inhaled the products of a galvanizing process on mild steel, with an array of HRCT findings that the investigators concluded were consistent with EAA, including diffuse centrilobular nodules, panlobular ground-glass opacity, and interlobular septal thickening. The patient underwent BAL, which was lymphocytic in nature, again interpreted as supportive of an EAA, as opposed to an alternate diagnosis, although lack of a definitive biopsy does leave unclear the nature of the actual pathology. Additionally, the potential for mixed exposures in welding is always present.

Other rather unusual exposures reported to cause EAA include 1,1,1,2-tetrafluoroethane[60] in the context of using this agent as a coolant for a hair-removal diode laser. The young woman exposed became unwell, complaining of shortness of breath, with an associated fever. HRCT showed diffuse centrilobular opacities, and biopsy noted eosinophil infiltration, which recurred following SIC to this agent. Although the investigators report this as EAA, the presence of an eosinophilic response suggest that a wider set of differential diagnoses should perhaps be considered.

Phytase enzyme used as an additive to cattle feed has also been highlighted in a recent publication as a potential contributor to EAA. The former case diagnosis[61] was supported by restrictive lung physiology, typical radiology, lymphocytosis in bronchoalveolar lavage fluid, and a positive exposure test at work. Occupational contact dermatitis and allergic rhinoconjunctivitis has also recently been attributed to lactase exposure.[62]

The yacht and luxury boat-manufacturing story continues with this American group reporting a further case of possible EAA associated with this type of work. Volkman and colleagues[63] report a 46-year-old woman with a short history of dyspnea, chest tightness, and cough with marked work effect. Her radiograph revealed pulmonary infiltrates, not responding to standard treatment for infection. Symptoms and signs improved on removal from the workplace, and the authors postulated that dimethyl phthalate and styrene were among the most likely candidate causes for this response.

ASTHMA AND EAA "CROSS-OVERS"

Various publications describe exposures that are described as causing asthma and EAA. Before reviewing these articles, it is reasonable to assume that very little is understood about the potential for single agents (or indeed single workplace exposures or work tasks) to cause the 2 separate disease manifestations in the forms of asthma and EAA. It is at least plausible that, in addition to the development of asthma or EAA attributable to exposures to different causative agents within a complex mix, that a single exposure may cause a single disease, the extremes of the clinical spectrum of which may have either asthma or EAA features. The latter will be better understood only with improved phenotyping of affected workers, better understanding of basic mechanisms, and, ultimately, developing better clinical case definitions.

Isocyanate exposure is perhaps the best example of this potential dual role. Already well-described to cause asthma, a Swiss group, Bieler and colleagues,[64] identified paint exposure as a possible cause of EAA in a worker exposed to 1,6-Hexamethylene diisocyanate (HDI) in the form of hardeners. The lung disease was characterized by rapidly progressive breathlessness, leading to respiratory failure. No biopsy was undertaken, presumably given the severity of the illness, but air sampling and urine biomarker estimates implied HDI exposure, and subsequent patch testing confirmed a delayed hypersensitivity to HDI. The investigators were keen to stress the speculative nature of these findings, but these are at least consistent with other case reports supporting the ability of isocyanates to cause EAA, including a further recent report implicating low-level exposure to diisocyanates in a secretary.[65] This latter case, from Germany, was of EAA in a secretary employed at a car-body paint facility. Although not biopsied, lung function, HRCT appearances, and the presence of IgG to diisocyanate human serum albumin conjugates were concluded as supportive evidence. The patient improved following cessation of exposure, measured to be generally below current exposure limits.

A group of other nonisocyanate exposures described as causing both conditions is now considered. A research letter by a Canadian group,[66] expert in the assessment of occupational lung disease, displayed the results for 2 challenges, 1 performed on a malt-exposed worker where the likely diagnosis was asthma owing to sensitization by an IgE mechanism, and 1 on a malt worker suspected of having developed EAA. Various outcomes differ between the challenges, the former showing a biphasic response, the latter a fall in FVC and diffusing capacity. Body temperature did not elevate in the former, but did on the final exposure day for the latter case. Interestingly, although the latter worker, suspected of EAA, developed a peripheral blood neutrophilia, the former patient, suspected of asthma, did not show any increase in the proportion of sputum eosinophils. This latter finding aside, the investigators postulate that asthma and EAA are perhaps 2 discrete and separate outcomes that were caused by an identical exposure.

Similarly, chicory exposure is the focus of recent publications that proposed its involvement in the development of typical type I allergic-mediated sensitization causing asthma and rhinoconjunctivitis and also its involvement in causing EAA. Pirson and colleagues[67] described rhinoconjunctivitis and asthma in a worker from an insulin-producing facility, using chicory roots as a substrate. An immediate response was seen to SIC, and the worker also had evidence of type I–mediated sensitization with positive skin prick tests and specific IgE to chicory. Chicory leaf handling was also recently described[68] as a cause of presumed EAA, supported by a typical clinical features and positive specific IgG, although the actual causative agent appears not to be the chicory itself, but a fungal contaminant, *Fusarium* sp.

Similarly again, exposure to onion as part of a more general inhaled spice exposure was investigated by a South African group.[69] Detailed investigations were undertaken on 3 workers heavily exposed to spice dusts, all of whom had developed asthma. Specific IgE was measured to a range of common inhalant, food, and spice allergens. In addition, basophil stimulation was used to potentially assess non-IgE–mediated responses. Specific allergens were also identified using an immunoblotting technique. Of interest, dry powdered garlic and onion demonstrated greater IgE binding than seen from the raw plant. Onion exposure (as part of a task of onion and potato sorting) has also been recently described as a risk for developing EAA. This German paper[70] described a case report of an onion and potato sorter who developed EAA characterized by pulmonary infiltrates, a lymphocytic BAL, and specific IgG presence to *Penicillium* sp and *Fusarium solani*. Again, it was the fungal contaminant rather than any onion-derived epitope that appears to have been responsible.

Exposure to esparto grass is also worthy of discussion here. Ruiz-Hornillos and colleagues[71] describe a case of occupational asthma attributed to esparto exposure. Esparto is a gramineous plant with an interesting array of potential uses, including use as a fabric and fence-building material. This Spanish group described a 58-year-old man who developed work-related asthma symptoms and a correlated effect in serial PEF measures. Changes in PEF values appeared to relate to esparto use and there was evidence of sensitization as judged by a positive skin prick test to esparto. Potential cross-reactivity to proteins from *Aspergillus fumigatus* was also identified. Enríquez and colleagues[72] also recently reported a further case of occupational asthma related to esparto grass usage, on this occasion in a 30-year-old man. Following 12 years of work with esparto fibers, he presented with a 3-year history of work-related cough, shortness of breath, and wheeze. There were no systemic features or fever to suggest an alternate diagnosis of EAA. Peripheral eosinophilia and a positive skin prick test to esparto were noted, and serial PEF noted a work effect. A sample of esparto cultured a *Mucor* sp. The result of subsequent skin prick testing with *Mucor* extract was positive and specific IgE against *Mucor racemosus* was detected. A SIC challenge was positive (early reaction only) when tipping esparto between trays. In contradistinction to these recent asthma data, historically, esparto exposure has also been described as causing EAA (for example, by Flandes and colleagues[73]), although no other recent papers were identified relating to this for the purposes of this review. Flandes and colleagues[73] described a 25-year-old plasterer, exposed to esparto fibers as they were added to plaster to alter its consistency and strength. Supported by consistent symptoms, restrictive physiology, reduced diffusing capacity, computed tomography ground-glass changes, a lymphocytic BAL, and supportive biopsy, they concluded this case related to EAA from esparto exposure, but actually caused by exposure to *Aspergillus fumigatus*.

Excluding isocyanates, to date in this review, therefore, exposures linked to asthma and EAA appear actually to be caused by separate agents within a complex mix of exposures, rather than a body of evidence supporting a single exposure causing 2 diseases. The dual responses to malt is the exception, at least in principle, suggesting that a single exposure may lead to differing outcomes, although the exact nature of the challenge material used, and its potential contaminants, is not provided.

Finally, pertaining to the example of metal-working fluid lung diseases, the largest outbreak of this to occur in the United Kingdom was published by Robertson and colleagues[74] in 2007, and carefully reviewed recently also from the perspective of clinical features[75] and demography.[76] The article by Robertson and colleagues[74] described the clinical approach to investigating a large outbreak of respiratory illness in a group of motor vehicle manufacturing workers exposed to potentially contaminated metal-working fluids. Workers were investigated in a phased manner, to limit more detailed investigations on those least likely to have developed either EAA or asthma as a result of their exposures. Of the entire work force, 87 persons (10.4%) were diagnosed as having either asthma (n = 74) or EAA (n = 19). Seven workers were diagnosed as suffering from humidifier fever. The approach taken by the study team was to identify case definitions for each condition a priori. No discussion was entertained relating to potential overlap of these conditions, and case definitions used were based on previous work. Nevertheless, a definite cause, or group of causes, has not yet been consistently identified from outbreaks of respiratory disease related to such exposures, and it remains to be proven as to whether a single contaminant can be responsible for both asthma and EAA, whether separate individual exposures account for each separate outcome, or whether in fact a single disease entity is responsible, behaving in some workers like occupational asthma, and in others like EAA.

CONCLUDING REMARKS

The recent evidence base offers insights into a vast array of complex and difficult occupational and environmental causes of lung disease. Despite their complexity, the lungs remain vulnerable to such insults from a wide variety of sources. Hamlet may well still reign true here when he lays out such mysteries for us all to solve, but the continuing research in this field from a diverse group of interested authors is beginning to unravel some. Perhaps these Shakespearean words are more appropriate: "Their understanding begins to swell, and the approaching tide will shortly fill the reasonable shores that now lie foul and muddy?"[77]

REFERENCES

1. Fishwick D, Barber CM, Bradshaw LM, et al. Standards of care for occupational asthma. Thorax 2012;67(3):278–80 [Epub 2011 Dec 9].
2. Malo JL, Vandenplas O. Definitions and classification of work-related asthma. Immunol Allergy Clin North Am 2011;31(4):645–62.
3. Bernstein IL. Asthma in the workplace. In: Bernstein DI, Chan-Yeung M, Malo JL, et al, editors. 3rd edition. Boca Raton (FL): CRC Press; 2006. ISBN 0824729773, 9780824729776.
4. Acevedo N, Erler A, Briza P, et al. Allergenicity of *Ascaris lumbricoides tropomyosin* and IgE

sensitization among asthmatic patients in a tropical environment. Int Arch Allergy Immunol 2011; 154(3):195–206 [Epub 2010 Sep 21].

5. Cárdaba B, Llanes E, Chacártegui M, et al. Modulation of allergic response by gene-environment interaction: olive pollen allergy. J Investig Allergol Clin Immunol 2007;17(Suppl 1):31–5.

6. Jeebhay MF, Baatjies R, Chang YS, et al. Risk factors for allergy due to the two-spotted spider mite (*Tetranychus urticae*) among table grape farm workers. Int Arch Allergy Immunol 2007;144(2): 143–9 [Epub 2007 May 25].

7. Nakazawa T, Satinover SM, Naccara L, et al. Asian ladybugs (*Harmonia axyridis*): a new seasonal indoor allergen. J Allergy Clin Immunol 2007; 119(2):421–7.

8. Cummings KJ, Gaughan DM, Kullman GJ, et al. Adverse respiratory outcomes associated with occupational exposures at a soy processing plant. Eur Respir J 2010;36(5):1007–15 [Epub 2010 Apr 22].

9. Harris-Roberts J, Robinson E, Fishwick D, et al. Sensitization and symptoms associated with soybean exposure in processing plants in South Africa. Am J Ind Med 2012;55(5):458–64.

10. Green BJ, Cummings KJ, Rittenour WR, et al. Occupational sensitization to soy allergens in workers at a processing facility. Clin Exp Allergy 2011;41(7): 1022–30.

11. Heffler E, Nebiolo F, Pizzimenti S, et al. Occupational asthma caused by *Neurospora sitophila* sensitization in a coffee dispenser service operator. Ann Allergy Asthma Immunol 2009;102(2):168–9.

12. Francuz B, Yera H, Geraut L, et al. Occupational asthma induced by in a worker exposed to coffee grounds. Clin Vaccine Immunol 2010;17(10):1645–6 [Epub 2010 Aug 4].

13. Osterman K, Zetterström O, Johansson SG. Coffee worker's allergy. Allergy 1982;37(5):313–22.

14. Bernedo N, García M, Gastaminza G, et al. Allergy to laxative compound (*Plantago ovata* seed) among health care professionals. J Investig Allergol Clin Immunol 2008;18(3):181–9.

15. Granslo JT, Van Do T, Aasen TB, et al. Occupational allergy to *Artemia* fish fry feed in aquaculture. Occup Med (Lond) 2009;59(4):243–8 [Epub 2009 Apr 1].

16. Bernstein JA, Crandall MS, Floyd R. Respiratory sensitization of a food manufacturing worker to konjac glucomannan. J Asthma 2007;44(8):675–80.

17. Viinanen A, Salokannel M, Lammintausta K. Gum arabic as a cause of occupational allergy. J Allergy (Cairo) 2011;2011:841508 [Epub 2011 May 19].

18. Sartorelli P, Paolucci V, Rendo S, et al. Asthma induced by chloramine T in nurses: case report. Med Lav 2010;101(2):134–8.

19. Zock JP, Vizcaya D, Le Moual N. Update on asthma and cleaners. Curr Opin Allergy Clin Immunol 2010; 10(2):114–20.

20. Kim JE, Kim SH, Jin HJ, et al. IgE Sensitization to cephalosporins in health care workers. Allergy Asthma Immunol Res 2012;4(2):85–91.

21. Roche E, de la Cuadra J, Alegre V. Sensitization to acrylates caused by artificial acrylic nails: review of 15 cases. Actas Dermosifiliogr 2008;99(10):788–94.

22. Pougnet R, Loddé B, Lucas D, et al. A case of occupational asthma from metabisulphite in a fisherman. Int Marit Health 2010;62(3):180–4.

23. Sastre J, Carnes J, García del Potro M, et al. Occupational asthma caused by triglycidyl isocyanurate. Int Arch Occup Environ Health 2011;84(5):547–9 [Epub 2010 Aug 18].

24. Burton C, Bradshaw L, Agius R, et al. Medium-density fibreboard and occupational asthma. A case series. Occup Med (Lond) 2011;61(5):357–63.

25. Schlünssen V, Kespohl S, Jacobsen G, et al. Immunoglobulin E-mediated sensitization to pine and beech dust in relation to wood dust exposure levels and respiratory symptoms in the furniture industry. Scand J Work Environ Health 2011;37(2):159–67.

26. Harris-Roberts J, Fishwick D, Tate P, et al. Respiratory symptoms in insect breeders. Occup Med (Lond) 2011;61(5):370–3.

27. Jeebhay MF, Robins TG, Miller ME, et al. Occupational allergy and asthma among salt water fish processing workers. Am J Ind Med 2008;51(12): 899–910.

28. Pérez Carral C, Martín-Lázaro J, Ledesma A, et al. Occupational asthma caused by turbot allergy in 3 fish-farm workers. J Investig Allergol Clin Immunol 2010;20(4):349–51.

29. Patiwael JA, Jong NW, Burdorf A, et al. Occupational allergy to bell pepper pollen in greenhouses in the Netherlands, an 8-year follow-up study. Allergy 2010;65(11):1423–9.

30. Letrán A, Palacín A, Barranco P, et al. Rye flour allergens: an emerging role in baker's asthma. Am J Ind Med 2008;51(5):324–8.

31. Palacin A, Quirce S, Armentia A, et al. Wheat lipid transfer protein is a major allergen associated with baker's asthma. J Allergy Clin Immunol 2007; 120(5):1132–8 [Epub 2007 Aug 22].

32. Campbell CP, Jackson AS, Johnson AR, et al. Occupational sensitization to lupin in the workplace: occupational asthma, rhinitis, and work-aggravated asthma. J Allergy Clin Immunol 2007;119(5):1133–9 [Epub 2007 Mar 26].

33. Campbell CP, Yates DH. Lupin allergy: a hidden killer at home, a menace at work; occupational disease due to lupin allergy. Clin Exp Allergy 2010; 40(10):1467–72.

34. Liccardi G, Salzillo A, Dente B, et al. Horse allergens: an underestimated risk for allergic sensitization in an urban atopic population without occupational exposure. Respir Med 2009;103(3): 414–20 [Epub 2008 Nov 8].

35. Liccardi G, D'Amato G, Antonicelli L, et al, Allergy Study Group of the Italian Society of Respiratory Medicine (SIMeR). Sensitization to horse allergens in Italy: a multicentre study in urban atopic subjects without occupational exposure. Int Arch Allergy Immunol 2011;155(4):412–7 [Epub 2011 Feb 22].

36. La Grutta S, Cibella F, Passalacqua G, et al. Association of *Blattella germanica* sensitization with atopic diseases in pediatric allergic patients. Pediatr Allergy Immunol 2011;22(5):521–7.

37. Barletta B, Di Felice G, Pini C. Biochemical and molecular biological aspects of silverfish allergens. Protein Pept Lett 2007;14(10):970–4.

38. Matsui EC, Eggleston PA, Buckley TJ, et al. Household mouse allergen exposure and asthma morbidity in inner-city preschool children. Ann Allergy Asthma Immunol 2006;97(4):514–20.

39. Matsui EC. Role of mouse allergens in allergic disease. Curr Allergy Asthma Rep 2009;9(5):370–5.

40. Kauppinen A, Peräsaari J, Taivainen A, et al. Association of HLA class II alleles with sensitization to cow dander Bos d 2, an important occupational allergen. Immunobiology 2012;217(1):8–12 [Epub 2011 Sep 8].

41. Nishikawa E, Taooka Y, Tsubata Y, et al. A case of acute hypersensitivity pneumonia in a worker at a feather duvet factory. Nihon Kokyuki Gakkai Zasshi 2011;49(2):93–6.

42. Otsuka M, Akiyama T, Saikai T, et al. A case of hypersensitivity pneumonitis due to the contamination of a dehumidifier by *Thermoactinomyces vulgaris*. Nihon Kokyuki Gakkai Zasshi 2008;46(1):39–43.

43. Hamaguchi R, Saito H, Kegasawa K, et al. A case of hypersensitivity pneumonitis resulting from inhalation of *Aspergillus niger* in a greenhouse worker who raised roses. Nihon Kokyuki Gakkai Zasshi 2009;47(3):205–11.

44. Ishikawa R, Kamiya H, Ikushima S, et al. A patient with acute hypersensitivity pneumonitis with a diagnosis of air-conditioner lung, who responded to therapy. Nihon Kokyuki Gakkai Zasshi 2010;48(2):134–9 [in Japanese].

45. Romeo L, Dalle Molle K, Zanoni G, et al. Respiratory health effects and immunological response to *Thermoactinomyces* among sugar cane workers in Nicaragua. Int J Occup Environ Health 2009;15(3):249–54.

46. Kai N, Ishii H, Iwata A, et al. Chronic hypersensitivity pneumonitis induced by Shiitake mushroom cultivation: case report and review of literature. Nihon Kokyuki Gakkai Zasshi 2008;46(5):411–5.

47. Guillot M, Bertoletti L, Deygas N, et al. Dry sausage mould hypersensitivity pneumonitis: three cases. Rev Mal Respir 2008;25(5):596–600.

48. Morell F, Cruz MJ, Gómez FP, et al. Chacinero's lung—hypersensitivity pneumonitis due to dry sausage dust. Scand J Work Environ Health 2011;37(4):349–56.

49. Metersky ML, Bean SB, Meyer JD, et al. Trombone player's lung: a probable new cause of hypersensitivity pneumonitis. Chest 2010;138(3):754–6.

50. Metzger F, Haccuria A, Reboux G, et al. Hypersensitivity pneumonitis due to molds in a saxophone player. Chest 2010;138(3):724–6.

51. Engelhart S, Rietschel E, Exner M, et al. Childhood hypersensitivity pneumonitis associated with fungal contamination of indoor hydroponics. Int J Hyg Environ Health 2009;212(1):18–20 [Epub 2008 Mar 28].

52. Kahana LM, Kay JM, Yakrus MA, et al. *Mycobacterium avium* complex infection in an immunocompetent young adult related to hot tub exposure. Chest 1997;111(1):242–5.

53. Verma G, Jamieson F, Chedore P, et al. Hot tub lung mimicking classic acute and chronic hypersensitivity pneumonitis: two case reports. Can Respir J 2007;14(6):354–6.

54. Huhulescu S, Simon M, Lubnow M, et al. Fatal *Pseudomonas aeruginosa* pneumonia in a previously healthy woman was most likely associated with a contaminated hot tub. Infection 2011;39(3):265–9 [Epub 2011 Apr 1].

55. Sogo A, Morell F, Muñoz X. Hypersensitivity pneumonitis associated with the use of a steam iron. Arch Bronconeumol 2009;45(5):258–9 [Epub 2009 Mar 27].

56. Villar A, Muñoz X, Cruz MJ, et al. Hypersensitivity pneumonitis caused by *Mucor* species in a cork worker. Arch Bronconeumol 2009;45(8):405–7 [Epub 2009 Apr 18].

57. Enríquez-Matas A, Quirce S, Cubero N, et al. Hypersensitivity pneumonitis caused by *Trichoderma viride*. Arch Bronconeumol 2009;45(6):304–5 [Epub 2009 May 12].

58. Yasui H, Matsui T, Yokomura K, et al. Three cases of hypersensitivity pneumonitis in citrus farmers. Nihon Kokyuki Gakkai Zasshi 2010;48(2):172–7 [in Japanese].

59. Miyazaki H, Hirata T, Shimane S, et al. A case of hypersensitivity pneumonitis caused by zinc fume. Nihon Kokyuki Gakkai Zasshi 2006;44(12):985–9 [in Japanese].

60. Ishiguro T, Yasui M, Nakade Y, et al. Extrinsic allergic alveolitis with eosinophil infiltration induced by 1,1,1,2-tetrafluoroethane (HFC-134a): a case report. Intern Med 2007;46(17):1455–7 [Epub 2007 Sep 3].

61. van Heemst RC, Sander I, Rooyackers J, et al. Hypersensitivity pneumonitis caused by occupational exposure to phytase. Eur Respir J 2009;33(6):1507–9.

62. Laukkanen A, Ruoppi P, Remes S, et al. Lactase-induced occupational protein contact dermatitis and allergic rhinoconjunctivitis. Contact Dermatitis 2007;57(2):89–93.

63. Volkman KK, Merrick JG, Zacharisen MC. Yacht-maker's lung: a case of hypersensitivity pneumonitis in yacht manufacturing. WMJ 2006;105(7):47–50.

64. Bieler G, Thorn D, Huynh CK, et al. Acute life-threatening extrinsic allergic alveolitis in a paint controller. Occup Med (Lond) 2011;61(6):440–2 [Epub 2011 Aug 8].

65. Schreiber J, Knolle J, Sennekamp J, et al. Sub-acute occupational hypersensitivity pneumonitis due to low-level exposure to diisocyanates in a secretary. Eur Respir J 2008;32(3):807–11.

66. Miedinger D, Malo JL, Cartier A, et al. Malt can cause both occupational asthma and allergic alveolitis. Allergy 2009;64(8):1228–9 [Epub 2009 Mar 27].

67. Pirson F, Detry B, Pilette C. Occupational rhinoconjunctivitis and asthma caused by chicory and oral allergy syndrome associated with bet v 1-related protein. J Investig Allergol Clin Immunol 2009; 19(4):306–10.

68. Colin G, Lelong J, Tillie-Leblond I, et al. Hypersensitivity pneumonitis in a chicory worker. Rev Mal Respir 2007;24(9):1139–42.

69. van der Walt A, Lopata AL, Nieuwenhuizen NE, et al. Work-related allergy and asthma in spice mill workers. The impact of processing dried spices on IgE reactivity patterns. Int Arch Allergy Immunol 2010;152(3):271–8 [Epub 2010 Feb 12].

70. Merget R, Sander I, Rozynek P, et al. Occupational hypersensitivity pneumonitis due to molds in an onion and potato sorter. Am J Ind Med 2008;51(2):117–9.

71. Ruiz-Hornillos FJ, De Barrio Fernández M, Molina PT, et al. Occupational asthma due to esparto hypersensitivity in a building worker. Allergy Asthma Proc 2007;28(5):571–3.

72. Enríquez A, Fernández C, Jiménez A, et al. Occupational asthma induced by *Mucor* species contaminating esparto fibers. J Investig Allergol Clin Immunol 2011;21(3):251–2.

73. Flandes J, Heili S, Gómez Seco J, et al. Hypersensitivity pneumonitis caused by esparto dust in a young plaster worker: a case report and review of the literature. Respiration 2004;71(4):421–3.

74. Robertson W, Robertson AS, Burge CB, et al. Clinical investigation of an outbreak of alveolitis and asthma in a car engine manufacturing plant. Thorax 2007;62(11):981–90 [Epub 2007 May 15].

75. Rosenman KD. Asthma, hypersensitivity pneumonitis and other respiratory diseases caused by metalworking fluids. Curr Opin Allergy Clin Immunol 2009;9(2):97–102.

76. Burton CM, Crook B, Scaife H, et al. Systematic review of respiratory outbreaks associated with exposure to water-based metalworking fluids. Ann Occup Hyg 2012;56(4):374–88 [Epub 2012 Jan 20].

77. The Tempest. William Shakespeare. The Arden Shakespeare, Third Series. ISBN 978-1-903436-08-0.

Work-Exacerbated Asthma

Anthony M. Szema, MD[a,b,]*

KEYWORDS

- Work-exacerbated asthma • Allergy • Occupational exposures • Chemical irritants
- Work-related asthma

KEY POINTS

- A spectrum of workplace exposures can result in work-exacerbated asthma (WEA), including exposures to chemical, smoke, paints, solvents, cleaning agents, allergens, cold temperature, and exercise.
- Patients with WEA are more symptomatic, use more health care resources and have a lower quality of life than those with asthma exacerbations unrelated to work.
- Materials safety data sheets (MSDSs) may identify agents that may exacerbate asthma in the workplace.
- The NIOSH Pocket Guide to Chemical Hazards may help identify potential triggers of WEA.
- The Americans with Disabilities Act mandates that employers adjust for reasonable accommodations for disabilities, including asthma.

GENERAL PRINCIPLES

A spectrum of workplace exposures can result in work-exacerbated asthma (WEA). These exposures include chemical irritants, paints, solvents,[1] and cleaning agents.[2–4] Additional potentially hazardous exposures include dust, indoor and outdoor aeroallergens (sources include molds, cats, trees, grasses, weeds), cold temperature, emotional stress, and exercise.[5]

Patients with WEA are more symptomatic, use more health care resources, and report a lower quality of life compared with those who have asthma exacerbations unrelated to work. Patients with WEA resemble patients with occupational asthma (OA) with respect to asthma severity; medication requirements; and socioeconomic factors, including unemployment and loss of income from work.[6–8]

Evidence-based reports regarding the prevention of WEA and its natural history are limited, although common management strategies include (1) avoidance of common triggers (ie, primary prevention), (2) diagnosing early in the course of the disease by assessing the temporal relationship between asthma exacerbations and work (ie, secondary prevention), and (3) eliminating exposures once the diagnosis is confirmed (ie, tertiary prevention). Eliminating the source of the exposure is important. Examples of such interventions include installing pigeon guards on windowsills to prevent bird-dropping contamination of indoor air, improved heating ventilation and air conditioning (HVAC) filtration systems, and using high-efficiency particulate air filters to remove airborne particles. Depending on the work setting, respirators may be beneficial. However, the World Trade Center disaster showed that in a setting where job duties require intense physical exertion, workers may remove their masks in response to a sensation of suffocation while working.[9,10] In other settings, personal respiratory protection may be practical

Disclosure: Dr Szema's research is funded by Merck (through the Naussau Health Care Foundation), Garnett McKeen Laboratory, and The New York State Center for Biotechnology.
a Department of Medicine, Allergy Section, Veterans Affairs Medical Center, Northport, NY 11768, USA;
b Department of Medicine, Stony Brook University School of Medicine, Stony Brook, NY 11794-8161, USA
* Department of Medicine, Stony Brook University School of Medicine, Stony Brook, NY 11794-8161.
E-mail address: anthony.szema@stonybrookmedicine.edu

Clin Chest Med 33 (2012) 617–624
http://dx.doi.org/10.1016/j.ccm.2012.08.004
0272-5231/12/$ – see front matter Published by Elsevier Inc.

and well accepted (eg, respirators for spray painters).[11-13]

Materials safety data sheets (MSDSs) may identify agents that exacerbate asthma in the workplace. MSDSs may be incomplete or inaccurate and, therefore, should be viewed as just one tool for exploring potentially relevant workplace exposures. The *NIOSH Pocket Guide to Chemical Hazards* and Web-based searches are additional sources for identifying the potential respiratory effects of agents encountered in the workplace.

The Americans with Disabilities Act mandates that employers adjust for reasonable accommodations for disabilities, including asthma.[14] Although a complete review of the legal obligations of employers for promoting workplace safety is beyond the purview of this article, it merits emphasis that a diagnosis of WEA has vocational and socioeconomic consequences in addition to medical implications.

More research is needed to understand dose-response relationships, to identify causal agents in complex environments, and to model these situations. For example, some soldiers in Iraq and Afghanistan who have developed respiratory complaints have been exposed to burning trash, improvised explosive devices, indoor and outdoor aeroallergens, and dust storms.[15-18] Another complex setting is exposure to multiple cleaning agents in the context of domestic chores and janitorial services.[4,19] In these complex exposure settings, it is difficult to establish clear causal relationships between a specific airborne exposure and respiratory health effects, including asthma. These types of complex exposures are difficult and perhaps impossible to study in an experimental model.

CASE DEFINITION OF WEA

In 2011, the American Thoracic Society Ad Hoc Committee on Work-Exacerbated Asthma published the following case definition of WEA:

1. Worker has pre-existing or concurrent asthma. Pre-existing asthma is defined as asthma that was present before the worker entered the worksite of interest, or asthma predated changes in exposures at an existing job due to the introduction of new processes or materials, which trigger asthma. Concurrent asthma or co-incident asthma is defined as asthma with onset while employed in a worksite of interest, but not due to exposures in that worksite.

2. *Temporally-related asthma exacerbations at work, with exacerbations based on self-reports of symptoms or medication use at work, or based on peak expiratory flow rates.*

3. *Conditions exist at work that can exacerbate asthma.*

4. OA (asthma caused by work) is unlikely.[20]

PREVALENCE OF WEA

The prevalence of asthma varies depending on the population studied. In one study, 23% of adult patients with asthma in a health maintenance organization (HMO) had WEA.[6] Another study showed 14% of members in an HMO with self-reported peak expiratory flow rates had WEA.[21] In the European Community Respiratory Health Survey, 4% of workers had WEA; this was associated with low schooling and socioeconomic status.[22] In an analysis of 12 published reports, the prevalence of WEA ranged from 13% (in an analysis that included all adults with asthma) to 58% (in an analysis of working adults with asthma) with a median of 21%.[20]

JOBS ASSOCIATED WITH WEA

Jobs with exposures associated with WEA include those with secondhand tobacco smoke exposure (eg, hospitality workers), dust exposure, HVAC maintenance professionals, poultry workers, and firefighters (although asthma is an exclusion criterion for hiring in some jurisdictions).[23-25] Other occupations at an increased risk for WEA include medical technicians (exposed to latex or larger proteins, such as psyllium dispensed by nurses), farmers, welders, cleaners, bleachers, bakers, spray painters, cabinetmakers, and carpenters.[26,27]

A spectrum of organic and inorganic exposures can cause exacerbations of asthma, including work with animals (animal dander); work near incinerators producing high concentrations of ambient airborne pollutants (**Fig. 1**); pollen, natural disasters, such as active volcanoes; mold related to water accumulation (**Fig. 2**); tobacco smoke; and hairdressers' aerosolized products.[28-35]

Ragweed and particulate matter air pollution may trigger asthma among workers who work outdoors, such as landscapers, even in those not allergically sensitized.[36] **Table 1** shows high-risk occupations for WEA. Many cases of WEA may be attributed to irritant exposure. Among these are ethanol, paints, solvents, calcium oxide, acids, ammonia, cigarette smoke, glutaraldehyde (eg, technicians who clean endoscopes), and welders exposed to fumes.

In an analysis of 5600 health care providers, 3650 replied to a questionnaire about their occupation, asthma diagnosis, variability of asthma symptoms at and away from work, and exposure to individual cleaning substances. WEA was

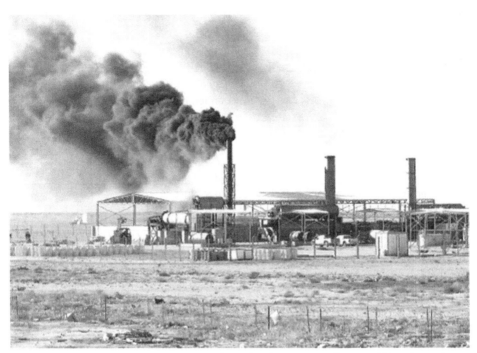

Fig. 1. Incinerator in Fallujah, Iraq, 2008. Photograph used with permission from a soldier who wishes to remain anonymous. This incinerator is a source of particulate matter air pollution, which can exacerbate a soldier's asthma.

defined as a categorical variable with 4 mutually exclusive categories: work-related asthma symptoms (WRAS), WEA, OA, and none. Multivariable logistic regression analysis was used to evaluate the association between self-reported use of cleaning substances and asthma outcomes among health care providers. Prevalence of WRAS, WEA, and OA were 3.3%, 1.1%, and 0.8%, respectively. Women had higher prevalence estimates than men. The odds increased in a dose-dependent manner for exposure in the longest job to cleaning agents and disinfectants,

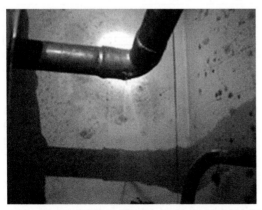

Fig. 2. Black mold (*Epicoccum* by culture) on wall of furnace room after water pipe burst from a water heater.

respectively. For exposure in any job, the odds of WRAS were significantly elevated for both factor 1 exposures (bleach, cleaners/abrasives, toilet cleaners, detergents, and ammonia) and factor 2 exposures (glutaraldehyde/ortho-phtaldehyde, chloramines, and ethylene oxide). Risk for WEA was observed for exposure to bleach, factor 2, and formalin/formaldehyde. Exposure to chloramines was associated with nearly fivefold elevated odds of OA. These investigators determined that health care providers are at risk of developing work-related asthma (WRA) from exposure to cleaning substances.[19]

Another study examined the frequency of claims for OA and WEA allowed by the compensation board in Ontario, Canada for which industry was coded as *health care* between 1998 and 2002. Five claims were allowed for sensitizer OA, 2 for natural rubber latex (NRL), and 3 for glutaraldehyde/photographic chemicals. The 2 NRL cases occurred in nurses who had worked for more than 10 years before the date of the accident. There were 115 allowed claims for WEA; health care was the most frequent industry for WEA. Compared with the rest of the province, claims in health care made up a significantly greater proportion of WEA claims (17.8%) than OA (5.1%) (odds ratio, 4.1). The WEA claims rate was 2.1 times greater than that in the rest of the workforce. WEA claims occurred in many jobs (eg, clerk) other than classic health care jobs, such as nurses, and were

Table 1
High-risk occupations for work-exacerbated asthma

Occupation	Things that can Cause or Worsen Asthma
Autobody workers	Acrylate in resins, glues, sealants, adhesives
Animal handlers, veterinarians, animal researchers, farmers	Dander, hair, scales, fur, saliva, and body wastes
Bakers, grain workers, farmers	Cereal grains, flour, amylase, enzymes, tobacco
Carpet makers	Gums
Dental hygienists	Latex gloves, material for filings, impressions, disinfectants
Forestry workers, carpenters, sawmill workers, cabinetmakers, woodworkers	Wood dust
Firefighters	Smoke
Hairdressers	Bleach, dye
Health care professionals	Latex gloves, formaldehyde, glutaraldehyde, antibiotics, detergent enzymes
Janitors, cleaning staff	Disinfectants, detergent enzymes, mixtures of chemicals (eg, mixing bleach and ammonia), fragrances
Jewelry, alloy, and catalyst makers	Platinum
Landscapers, gardeners, other outdoor workers	Cold air, humidity, mold, pollens, smog pollution, exercise
Manicurists	Acrylate in artificial nails
Office workers	Mold, fungus, dust
Pharmaceutical workers	Antibiotics, psyllium, enzymes
Printing industry	Gum arabic, reactive dyes, acrylates
Seafood processors who work with lobster, crab, shrimp, clam, oyster, scallop, squid, mussel, whelk, sea urchins, sea cucumber	Proteins in the shellfish
Shellac handlers	Amines
Teachers	Viral or other kinds of lung infections, mold, dust
Waiters, bar staff	Secondhand smoke
Welders, refiners, metal platers	Metals, nickel sulfate, solder fluxes
Spray painters, autobody shop painters, insulation installers, plastics, foam, and foundry industry workers	Diisocyanates (chemicals found in polyurethane products like flexible and rigid foams); molded parts; coatings, such as paints and varnishes; building insulation materials
Textile workers	Dyes
Users of plastics, epoxy resins	Chemicals, such as anhydrides

From The Canadian Lung Association (www.lung.ca/diseases-maladies/asthma-asthme/work-travail/who-qui_e.php); with permission.

associated with a variety of agents: construction dust, secondhand smoke, paint fumes. These investigators concluded that WEA occurs frequently in this professional sector. Those affected and attributed agents include many not typically expected in health care.[37]

WEA shares many features with asthma unrelated to work and with OA, but important differences exist. At an HMO in Massachusetts, patients with WEA were more likely to be men and to be affected by asthma symptoms on more days during the past week than other adults with asthma. Nevertheless, the 2 types of patients with asthma were similar in age, race/ethnicity, education, annual income level, cigarette smoking, severity of asthma, and number of treatments for acute asthma attacks and number of workdays missed because of asthma in the previous year.[6] Patients with WEA from the workers' compensation system in Washington were more likely to be women than patients with OA. In this analysis, the median age of workers with WEA and OA was similar. The patients with WEA were less likely than their counterparts with OA to have received treatment from a specialist or to have completed pulmonary function and allergy tests.[38,39]

In Quebec, WEA often led to workers leaving their jobs after diagnosis. WRA can have an adverse impact on patients' working life and income. Spirometry, methacholine challenge results, sputum cell counts, and symptom frequency were compared between when patients were diagnosed and at follow-up. The patients with OA and WEA were similar, with improvement in respiratory symptoms and little change in other clinical features by follow-up. In another study comparing 115 patients with WEA with 82 patients with OA, atopy was more common among the patients with OA (87%) than the patients with WEA (74%). The 2 types of WRA were similar in other clinical and functional features, except for differences in specific inhalation challenge findings that were used to delineate OA from WEA.[40]

WORK-RELATED RHINITIS AND WEA

Some patients are affected by both work-related rhinitis and WEA. Work-related rhinitis includes work-exacerbated rhinitis and occupational rhinoconjunctivitis. Implicated substances leading to occupational rhinitis include (1) high-molecular-weight proteins and (2) low-molecular-weight chemicals. The diagnosis of work-related rhinitis is established based on occupational history and documentation of immunoglobulin E (IgE)–mediated sensitization to the causative agent, if possible. The treatment of occupational rhinoconjunctivitis includes elimination or reduction of exposure to causative agents combined with pharmacotherapy, which is similar to other causes of rhinitis. Allergen immunotherapy is one option.[41]

In one study, 105 out of 363 patients with clinical WEA who demonstrated nonspecific bronchial hyperresponsiveness to histamine, but a negative response to a specific inhalation challenge with the suspected occupational agents, were considered as having WEA. Their characteristics were compared with those of 172 patients with OA ascertained by a positive response to a specific inhalation challenge. A high proportion of patients with WEA (83%) and OA (90%) reported at least one nasal symptom at work. Symptoms of (1) sneezing/itching or (2) rhinorrhea were more frequent in patients with OA (78% for sneezing/itching and 70% for rhinorrhea) than in those with WEA (61% for sneezing/itching and 57% for

rhinorrhea), whereas postnasal discharge was more common in WEA (30%) than in OA (18%). Nasal symptoms were less severe in WEA (median [25th–75th percentiles] global severity score: 4 [2–6]) as compared with OA (median global severity score: 5 [4–7]). Nasal symptoms preceded less frequently those of asthma in patients with WEA (17%) than in patients with OA (43%). Nasal symptoms are highly prevalent in patients with WEA, although their clinical pattern differs from that found in OA.[42]

PREVENTION AND MANAGEMENT

Early in the course of disease, identification and mitigation of triggers is crucial. Reviewing MSDSs may help in addition to reviewing processes at work. Environmental controls including ensuring adequate ventilation and air filtration, and the use of personal respirators, are cornerstones of prevention. Medical surveillance may identify early cases of WEA. Work rotation, and even worker's compensation policies may influence the motivation of workers to seek treatment. The American with Disabilities Act mandates that employers make reasonable accommodations for individuals with disabilities such as asthma.

The Ontario Work-Related Asthma Surveillance System: Physician Reporting (OWRAS) Network was established in 2007 to estimate the prevalence of WRA in Ontario and to test the feasibility of collecting data for cases of WRA from physicians voluntarily. More than 300 respirologists, occupational medicine physicians, allergists, and primary care providers in Ontario were invited to participate in monthly reporting of WRA cases by telephone, postal service, or e-mail. Since 2007, 49 physicians have registered with the OWRAS Network and, to date, have reported 34 cases of OA and 49 cases of WEA. Highly reactive chemicals were the most frequently reported suspected causative agent of the 108 suspected exposures reported. Despite the challenge of enlisting a representative sample of physicians in Ontario willing to report, the OWRAS Network has shown that it is feasible to implement a voluntary reporting system for WRA; however, its long-term sustainability is unknown.[43]

Reducing exposure to relevant workplace triggers (ie, prevention) is a cornerstone to disease management. Medication management is similar to that of asthma unrelated to work. A summary flow chart (**Fig. 3**) reviews the American College of Chest Physicians' recommendations for clinical evaluation and management of WEA.

Consider diagnosis in all patients with:
WRA symptoms, new asthma, and/or worsening asthma symptoms

Confirm Asthma and Onset
Medical history–childhood asthma, allergies
Symptoms – onset / nature / timing
Spirometry - bronchodilator response and/or
airway reactivity–methacholine challenge
Medications

Asthma

No Asthma

Assess Exposures /Factors that Cause or Exacerbate Asthma
Occupational history
Allergens, irritants
Exertion, cold, infections
Type of work process / setting
Ventilation / use of respiratory protection
Obtain MSDSs
Co-workers – symptoms
Magnitude / timing of exposures
Environmental history
Pets, hobbies, home exposures, ambient air pollution
Atopy / allergies

Evaluate other causes of asthma-like symptoms*
Vocal cord dysfunction
Upper respiratory tract irritation
Hypersensitivity pneumonitis
Rhinosinusitis
Psychogenic factors
These conditions can co-exist with asthma

Assess Relationship of Asthma to Work**
Symptoms – onset / timing /severity related to work, other environments
Physiology
PEFRs, spirometry, methacholine responsiveness, SIC – changes related to work
Immunologic tests (IgE antibodies, skin prick)
** *The more positive findings the more certain the relationship to work*
Best to complete evaluation and/or refer to specialist before removing patient from work

Work-related Asthma

Asthma but _not_ Work-related Asthma

Decide if primary Occupational Asthma (Sensitizer or Irritant) based on above
Yes   No

Occupational Asthma

Work-exacerbated Asthma

Management OA
A) Sensitizer
Avoid sensitizer exposures
Consider reduction exposure and/or immunotherapy in selected situations
Surveillance of exposed workers
B) Irritant
Reduce irritant exposures
Both:
Optimize medical treatment asthma
Monitor patient - Job change if severe/worse asthma
Assist with compensation
Consider prevention for other exposed workers

Management WEA
Optimize medical treatment asthma
Reduce workplace and non-work triggers
Monitor patient - job change if severe / worse asthma
Consider compensation
Consider prevention for other exposed workers

Fig. 3. Summary flow chart of clinical evaluation and management of WRA. PEFRs, peak expiratory flow rate; SIC, Specific Inhalational Challenge; WRA, Work Related Asthma. (*From* Tarlo SM, Balmes J, Balkissoon R, et al. Diagnosis and management of work-related asthma: American College of Chest Physicians Consensus Statement. Chest 2008;134:1S–41S; with permission.)

SUMMARY AND FUTURE RESEARCH

WEA is defined as preexisting asthma exacerbated by conditions at work, making it different from OA, which is caused by work. Jobs associated with WEA may entail exposure to secondhand smoke, dust, and cleaning agents, especially in health care and office workers. Work-related rhinitis and conjunctivitis may be concurrent. Prevention and management principles are based on identifying triggers, removing exposure, cleaning the work environment, and medications. Future research is needed to help understand dose-response relationships and causal agents in complex environments.

ACKNOWLEDGMENTS

The author would like to acknowledge medical student Edward Forsyth for his assistance.

REFERENCES

1. Kurt E, Demir AU, Cadirci O, et al. Occupational exposures as risk factors for asthma and allergic diseases in a Turkish population. Int Arch Occup Environ Health 2011;84:45–52.
2. Omland O, Hjort C, Pedersen OF, et al. New-onset asthma and the effect of environment and occupation among farming and nonfarming rural subjects. J Allergy Clin Immunol 2011;128:761–5.
3. Lieberman JA, Sicherer SH. The diagnosis of food allergy. Am J Rhinol Allergy 2010;24:439–43.
4. Quirce S, Barranco P. Cleaning agents and asthma. J Investig Allergol Clin Immunol 2010;20:542–50 [quiz: 542–50].
5. Henneberger PK. Work-exacerbated asthma. Curr Opin Allergy Clin Immunol 2007;7:146–51.
6. Henneberger PK, Derk SJ, Sama SR, et al. The frequency of workplace exacerbation among health maintenance organisation members with asthma. Occup Environ Med 2006;63:551–7.
7. Larbanois A, Jamart J, Delwiche JP, et al. Socioeconomic outcome of subjects experiencing asthma symptoms at work. Eur Respir J 2002;19:1107–13.
8. Henneberger PK, Hoffman CD, Magid DJ, et al. Work-related exacerbation of asthma. Int J Occup Environ Health 2002;8:291–6.
9. Antao VC, Pallos LL, Shim YK, et al. Respiratory protective equipment, mask use, and respiratory outcomes among World Trade Center rescue and recovery workers. Am J Ind Med 2011;54:897–905.
10. Wheeler K, McKelvey W, Thorpe L, et al. Asthma diagnosed after 11 September 2001 among rescue and recovery workers: findings from the World Trade Center Health Registry. Environ Health Perspect 2007;115:1584–90.
11. Liu Y, Stowe MH, Bello D, et al. Respiratory protection from isocyanate exposure in the autobody repair and refinishing industry. J Occup Environ Hyg 2006;3:234–49.
12. Sparer J, Stowe MH, Bello D, et al. Isocyanate exposures in autobody shop work: the SPRAY study. J Occup Environ Hyg 2004;1:570–81.
13. Cullen MR, Redlich CA, Beckett WS, et al. Feasibility study of respiratory questionnaire and peak flow recordings in autobody shop workers exposed to isocyanate-containing spray paint: observations and limitations. Occup Med (Lond) 1996;46:197–204.
14. Portman C. Determining a qualifying disability under the ADA: case study–mild asthma and indoor air quality. AAOHN J 1994;42:230–5.
15. Szema AM, Schmidt MP, Lanzirotti A, et al. Titanium and iron in lung of a soldier with nonspecific interstitial pneumonitis and bronchiolitis after returning from Iraq. J Occup Environ Med 2012;54:1–2.
16. Szema AM, Salihi W, Savary K, et al. Respiratory symptoms necessitating spirometry among soldiers with Iraq/Afghanistan war lung injury. J Occup Environ Med 2011;53:961–5.
17. Szema AM, Peters MC, Weissinger KM, et al. New-onset asthma among soldiers serving in Iraq and Afghanistan. Allergy Asthma Proc 2010;31:67–71.
18. King MS, Eisenberg R, Newman JH, et al. Constrictive bronchiolitis in soldiers returning from Iraq and Afghanistan. N Engl J Med 2011;365:222–30.
19. Arif AA, Delclos GL. Association between cleaning-related chemicals and work-related asthma and asthma symptoms among healthcare professionals. Occup Environ Med 2012;69:35–40.
20. Henneberger PK, Redlich CA, Callahan DB, et al. An official American Thoracic Society statement: work-exacerbated asthma. Am J Respir Crit Care Med 2011;184:368–78.
21. Bolen AR, Henneberger PK, Liang X, et al. The validation of work-related self-reported asthma exacerbation. Occup Environ Med 2007;64:343–8.
22. Caldeira RD, Bettiol H, Barbieri MA, et al. Prevalence and risk factors for work related asthma in young adults. Occup Environ Med 2006;63:694–9.
23. Szema AM, Khedkar M, Maloney PF, et al. Clinical deterioration in pediatric asthmatic patients after September 11, 2001. J Allergy Clin Immunol 2004;113:420–6.
24. Landrigan PJ, Lioy PJ, Thurston G, et al. Health and environmental consequences of the world trade center disaster. Environ Health Perspect 2004;112:731–9.
25. Endres M, Kullmann L, Simon G, et al. Rehabilitation of hemiplegic leg amputees. Orv Hetil 1987;128:2741–3 [in Hungarian].
26. Blanc PD, Ellbjar S, Janson C, et al. Asthma-related work disability in Sweden. The impact of workplace exposures. Am J Respir Crit Care Med 1999;160:2028–33.

27. Bernedo N, Garcia M, Gastaminza G, et al. Allergy to laxative compound (Plantago ovata seed) among health care professionals. J Investig Allergol Clin Immunol 2008;18:181–9.

28. Erwin EA, Woodfolk JA, Custis N, et al. Animal danders. Immunol Allergy Clin North Am 2003;23: 469–81.

29. Terzano C, Di Stefano F, Conti V, et al. Air pollution ultrafine particles: toxicity beyond the lung. Eur Rev Med Pharmacol Sci 2010;14:809–21.

30. van der Walt A, Lopata AL, Nieuwenhuizen NE, et al. Work-related allergy and asthma in spice mill workers - the impact of processing dried spices on IgE reactivity patterns. Int Arch Allergy Immunol 2010;152:271–8.

31. Carlsen HK, Gislason T, Benediktsdottir B, et al. A survey of early health effects of the Eyjafjallajokull 2010 eruption in Iceland: a population-based study. BMJ Open 2012;2:e000343.

32. Dahlman-Hoglund A, Renstrom A, Larsson PH, et al. Salmon allergen exposure, occupational asthma, and respiratory symptoms among salmon processing workers. Am J Ind Med 2012;55:624–30.

33. Jarvholm B, Reuterwall C, Bystedt J. Mortality attributable to occupational exposure in Sweden. Scand J Work Environ Health 2012;3284. [Epub ahead of print].

34. Remen T, Acouetey DS, Paris C, et al. Diet, occupational exposure and early asthma incidence among bakers, pastry makers and hairdressers. BMC Public Health 2012;12:387.

35. Bernstein RS, Sorenson WG, Garabrant D, et al. Exposures to respirable, airborne Penicillium from a contaminated ventilation system: clinical, environmental and epidemiological aspects. Am Ind Hyg Assoc J 1983;44:161–9.

36. Wiszniewska M, Palczynski C, Krawczyk-Szulc P, et al. Occupational allergy to Limonium sinuatum: a case report. Int J Occup Med Environ Health 2011;24:304–7.

37. Liss GM, Buyantseva L, Luce CE, et al. Work-related asthma in health care in Ontario. Am J Ind Med 2011;54:278–84.

38. Anderson NJ, Reeb-Whitaker CK, Bonauto DK, et al. Work-related asthma in Washington State. J Asthma 2011;48:773–82.

39. Curwick CC, Bonauto DK, Adams DA. Use of objective testing in the diagnosis of work-related asthma by physician specialty. Ann Allergy Asthma Immunol 2006;97:546–50.

40. Singh T, Bello B, Jeebhay MF. Risk factors associated with asthma phenotypes in dental healthcare workers. Am J Ind Med 2012 Apr 2. [Epub ahead of print].

41. Sublett JW, Bernstein DI. Occupational rhinitis. Immunol Allergy Clin North Am 2011;31:787–96, vii.

42. Vandenplas O, Van Brussel P, D'Alpaos V, et al. Rhinitis in subjects with work-exacerbated asthma. Respir Med 2010;104:497–503.

43. To T, Tarlo SM, McLimont S, et al. Feasibility of a provincial voluntary reporting system for work-related asthma in Ontario. Can Respir J 2011;18:275–7.

Occupational Chronic Obstructive Pulmonary Disease
An Update

Enrique Diaz-Guzman, MD[a], Shambhu Aryal, MD[a],
David M. Mannino, MD[a,b],*

KEYWORDS

- COPD • Chronic bronchitis • Emphysema • Occupation

KEY POINTS

- Chronic obstructive pulmonary disease (COPD) represents a major cause of morbidity and mortality in industrialized and nonindustrialized countries.
- Occupational risk factors represent an important and preventable cause of COPD.
- The most common occupationally related factors include exposure to organic dusts, metallic fumes, and a variety of other mineral gases and/or vapors.
- This article summarizes the literature on the subject and provides an update of the most recent advances in the field.

INTRODUCTION

Chronic obstructive pulmonary disease (COPD), one of the most prevalent health care problems in the world, constitutes a major cause of morbidity and mortality in developed and developing countries and accounts for over 120,000 deaths per year in the United States, representing the third leading cause of mortality.[1,2] COPD is estimated to be responsible for the death of 250 people per hour worldwide with the annual deaths from the disease surpassing lung cancer and breast cancer combined.[2] The global economic burden of the disease is large and, according to the World Health Organization (WHO), is projected to rank fifth in burden of disease caused worldwide by year 2020.[3]

Tobacco use remains the main risk factor for development of COPD; nevertheless, this disease also develops in never smokers.[4] Occupational risk factors have been well described in previous reports in the literature and represent important and preventable causes of COPD. For example, data from the Third National Health and Nutrition Examination Survey (NHANES), estimated that 19% of all cases of COPD (31% among never smokers) were attributed to occupational factors.[5] Similarly, a study performed by the WHO in 2000, estimated that selected occupational risk factors were responsible worldwide for 13% of COPD and 11% of asthma.[6]

A systematic review published by the American Thoracic Society (ATS) in 2003 estimated a 15% population attributable risk (PAR) for the work-related burden of COPD.[7] Several subsequent reports provide further evidence of the occupational burden of COPD. This article summarizes

Disclosures: EDG and SA have nothing to disclose. DM has served as a consultant for Boehringer Ingelheim, Pfizer, GlaxoSmithKline, Astra-Zeneca, Novartis, Nycomed, Merck, and Forest; and has received research grants from Astra-Zeneca, GlaxoSmithKline, Novartis, Boehringer-Ingelheim, Forest, and Pfizer; and serves on the Board of Directors for the COPD Foundation.
a Division of Pulmonary, Critical Care, and Sleep Medicine, University of Kentucky College of Medicine, 740 South Limestone Street, L543, Lexington, KY 40536, USA; b Department of Preventive Medicine and Environmental Health, University of Kentucky College of Public Health, 111 Washington Avenue, Lexington, KY 40536, USA
* Corresponding author.
E-mail address: dmannino@uky.edu

Clin Chest Med 33 (2012) 625–636
http://dx.doi.org/10.1016/j.ccm.2012.07.004
0272-5231/12/$ – see front matter © 2012 Elsevier Inc. All rights reserved.

the previous studies of occupationally related COPD, including systematic reviews and selected original reports, and provides an update of the most recent advances in the field.

HISTORICAL BACKGROUND AND TERMINOLOGY

The association between dust exposure and development of chronic bronchitis dates back to the nineteenth century when this was reported among workers laboring in various trades characterized by heavy organic dust exposure (eg, coffee workers, malt workers, flax seed workers, rag paper makers, and grain millers).[8] Although the pathology of lung disorders caused by inorganic dust exposure was also demonstrated in the nineteenth century (especially among miners) and the term pneumoconiosis was introduced to describe such fibrotic interstitial lung disease, it was only later that airway disease due to inorganic and coal dust exposure was recognized. Thus, between 1940 and 1960, several reports described a link between the presence of irreversible airflow obstruction in patients with chronic bronchitis, which was observed among mine workers heavily exposed to inorganic dust and fumes.[9]

Despite more than a century elapsing between the original descriptions of occupationally related dust exposure and development of chronic bronchitis, the term occupational COPD has not been used frequently in the literature. Moreover, the clinical spectrum of occupational exposures and obstructive lung disorders is wide, with many airway disorders overlapping or evolving into fixed airway obstruction.

COPD is defined by the Global Initiative on Chronic Obstructive Lung Disease (GOLD) and the ATS-European Respiratory Society guidelines[10,11] as a disease characterized by airflow limitation that is not fully reversible and is progressive and associated with an abnormal inflammatory response of the lungs to noxious particles or gases.[12] In addition to airflow obstruction, COPD traditionally comprises two overlapping clinical entities with different pathologic characteristics: emphysema and chronic bronchitis. Recent data, however, have emphasized the phenotypic complexity of disease and the importance of factors such as inflammation and polymorbidity.[13]

Occupational Asthma and COPD

Asthma is defined as a chronic inflammatory disorder of the airways characterized by recurrent episodes of coughing, wheezing, dyspnea, and the presence of reversible airflow obstruction. Work-related asthma represents a subset of patients in which asthma either develops de novo or is exacerbated in occupational environments.[7] According to a review of the literature published by the ATS, the occupational burden of asthma is significant in the general population, with a population-attributable risk of 15%.[7] Additionally, recent studies that followed the ATS review have reaffirmed that a substantial proportion of the new adult onset asthma cases can be attributed to occupational exposures. Even though long-standing asthma is believed to progress to poorly reversible obstruction consistent with COPD, the contribution of occupational asthma to the overall prevalence of COPD is not well studied.[14] In contrast to occupational asthma, occupational COPD is complicated by frequent concomitant tobacco use and the long time between exposure and development of airflow limitation. Thus, the term occupational COPD is infrequently used in clinical practice.[15]

Other Work-related Obstructive Airway Disorders

In addition to asthma, chronic bronchitis, and emphysema, work-related exposures can be associated with other obstructive airway disorders that do not meet standard criteria for COPD. For example, occupational exposure to organic dusts has been associated with variable airflow limitation and acute (as opposed to chronic) bronchitis. Examples of organic dust airway disease with an acute response pattern include exposure to cotton, flax, hemp, jute, sisal, and several organic grains.[16] Nonetheless, these same exposures can lead to a stage of disease more akin to COPD than asthma. Byssinosis, an occupational lung disease resulting from chronic exposure to cotton dust, is characterized by episodes of dyspnea, productive cough, and chest tightness accompanied by a reduction in forced expiratory volume in 1 second (FEV_1). Prolonged exposure, however, results in frequent and severe symptoms and functional changes that are indistinguishable from COPD.[17] In addition, severe and progressive airflow limitation and obliterative bronchiolitis has been reported in association with diacetyl exposure among workers of flavoring plants and microwave popcorn plants.[18] These examples suggest that many workers may be at risk for development of a wide spectrum of airway disorders that can lead into fixed and potentially severe obstructive airway limitation, not all of which may be labeled as COPD.

EPIDEMIOLOGIC EVIDENCE

Ascertaining the true incidence and prevalence of occupational COPD can be difficult owing to multiple factors: (1) a large proportion of patients with a diagnosis of COPD who have experienced occupational exposures share other risk factors, such as concomitant tobacco use; (2) COPD is multifactorial, so a clear single cause-and-effect relationship may not be established; (3) there are no pathognomonic features of occupational COPD that allow it to be distinguishable as a subcategory of COPD; and (4) there has been significant heterogeneity in the definitions of COPD that have been applied during the last 20 years, complicating comparisons among different prevalence estimates for various populations at risk.

There is substantial scientific and epidemiologic evidence to support the association between work-related exposure to dust, noxious gases, or fumes and development of COPD. For example, longitudinal studies involving coal miners, hardrock miners, tunnel workers, and concrete manufacturing workers have found that exposures are associated with a progressive annual decline of lung function measured by spirometry (mean decrease in FEV_1 across studies of 7–8 mL/year) even after adjustment for cigarette smoking.[7] Although a mean decrement of 8 mL/year may seem minimal, over a 40-year career this translates to a mean loss of greater than 300 mL (with a higher upper range within the CI of that estimated mean). This is a supplemental deficit in addition to that attributable to aging, smoking, and other factors. Furthermore, other evidence suggests that in some cases the cumulative effect of dust exposure may exceed that from cigarette smoking in the absence of dust exposure. For example, a study that included 100 tunnel workers found that the decrease in FEV_1 associated with cumulative exposure to respirable dust was greater among nonsmoking tunnel workers (50–60 mL/year) compared with nonexposed smokers (35 mL/year).[19]

A large number of cross-sectional and longitudinal community-based studies have reported an increased risk for symptoms or lung-function decrements consistent with COPD among occupationally exposed workers. Although the major limitations of these studies are the potential for exposure misclassification and variations in the definition of COPD, they do provide evidence to support the association between occupational exposures and the risk of developing COPD.

Two major studies performed in the United States, including more than 17,000 subjects, provide the largest North American cross-sectional cohorts evaluating occupational exposures and COPD. Korn and colleagues[20] studied a random sample of 8515 subjects from six major metropolitan areas in the United States and analyzed the self-reported occupational exposure to dust, gas, or fumes. After adjusting for smoking and other risk factors for airflow limitation, the investigators found that subjects with reported occupational exposure had a higher prevalence of symptoms (chronic cough, wheezing, and dyspnea). In addition, occupational exposure was associated with a higher prevalence of COPD defined by the presence of a FEV_1 to forced vital capacity (FVC) ratio of less than 0.6. (odds ratio [OR] = 1.53, 95% CI = 1.17–2.08). More recently, Hnizdo and colleagues[5] analyzed data from 9823 subjects included in the NHANES III study in the United States and concluded that approximately 19% of all cases of COPD were attributable to multiple occupational exposures (31% among never smokers).

Large community-based studies describing the relation between occupation and COPD have also been performed in other countries. For example, in a cross-sectional study from China that included 3606 adults (40–69 years of age), dust exposure was associated with an increased risk for chronic respiratory symptoms (OR 1.30, CI 1.09–1.48) and a decline in FEV_1 and FEV_1/ FVC ratio after adjustment for smoking status.[21] Similarly, another cross-sectional study in Netherlands included 1906 subjects and found that organic dust exposure was associated with a higher risk for asthma (OR 1.48, 95% CI 0.95–2.30) and lower FEV_1 (−59 mL, 95% CI [−114 to −4]). Mineral exposure in this study was associated with increased risk for chronic bronchitis symptoms (OR 2.22, 95% CI 1.16–4.23) and lower FEV_1/FVC ratio (−1.1%, 95% CI −1.8 to −0.3). A prospective longitudinal study in Italy evaluated 2734 males as part of a surveillance program and found that self-reported occupational exposures to dust, vapor, or fumes, was associated with an increased risk of COPD (OR 2.62, 95% CI 2.02–3.41).[22]

Occupational Contribution to the Burden of COPD

The overall work-related burden of COPD at a population level has been well studied in the last decade. The systematic analysis reported in the 2002 ATS statement on COPD has already been described. Blanc and Toren later performed follow-up review studies published over the ensuing years until their 2007 publication, including earlier data omitted from the ATS analysis.[23] They found that among eight studies yielding 11 risk estimates additional to ATS review, the median PAR for occupationally related COPD was 15% (range 0%–37%). The previous ATS PAR estimate had been 18% based on six lung function-based studies. For chronic bronchitis, also based on eight estimates, the median PAR value was also 15% (range 0%–35%), matching the previous estimate of 15%, reflecting eight earlier studies.

After that review, Weinmann and colleagues[24] published a case-control study involving 388 workers in a northwest metropolitan area of the United States and estimated the occupational PAR for COPD to be 43%. More recently, Blanc[25] summarized the two previous systematic analyses and supplemented that with the findings of seven additional population-based studies on occupational COPD (including the Weinmann and colleagues[24] study), and again concluded that a PAR of 15% is a reasonable estimate for the occupational burden of COPD.

Relevant findings continue to emerge on the population-based occupational risk for COPD. A recent prospective cohort study by Mehta and colleagues[26] evaluated the incidence of COPD in 4267 Swiss workers exposed to biologic dusts, mineral dusts, gases and/or fumes, and vapors and found an increased risk (twofold to fivefold) of COPD (GOLD stage II) and high level of occupational exposures. The PAR of stage II COPD was between 31% and 32% for biologic dusts among smokers, and ranged between 43% and 56% for non-smokers, depending on type and level of exposure.

The findings of selected population-based studies evaluating the risk of COPD associated with occupation and published in the last decade (eg, since the initial ATS statement) are summarized in **Table 1** and illustrated in **Fig. 1**.

SPECIFIC CATEGORIES OF OCCUPATIONAL EXPOSURES

The association between exposure to specific chemical agents, noxious gases, dust, and vapors and development of chronic bronchitis in humans has been widely demonstrated in the literature. Various occupations that result in organic and inorganic compound exposures have been associated with development of chronic bronchitis and potentially fixed irreversible airflow obstruction. These are summarized by category below.

Organic Dusts

Organic dusts are a major cause of respiratory disorders in agricultural industry. Bacterial and fungal contamination (associated with endotoxin, mycotoxin, and other components) are likely to be responsible for at least part of observed organic dust airway effects. Such exposures occur in association with silage, grain dust, straw, wood chips, and animal confinement buildings.[32]

Organic dust exposure resulting from agricultural work has been associated with development of COPD in multiple studies. For example, Dalphin and colleagues[33] studied the effects of organic dust exposure in 250 dairy farmers from a province in France and found an increased prevalence of chronic bronchitis and worse pulmonary function compared with matched controls. Eduard and colleagues[34] compared the likelihood of chronic bronchitis and COPD among crop farmers and live-stock farmers. Livestock farmers were more likely to suffer from both those conditions, with an odds ratio for chronic bronchitis of 1.9 (95% CI: 1.4–2.6), and for COPD of 1.4 (95% CI: 1.1–1.7). Importantly, the investigators evaluated the effects of exposure to biologic agents and found that exposure to most agents predicted respiratory morbidity, with a significant reduction in FEV_1 (−41 mL; 95% CI: −75 to −7), although the effects of specific substances could not be assessed. Monso and colleagues[35] studied 105 nonsmoking animal farmers working inside confined buildings and found a prevalence of COPD of 17%; the investigators describe a dose-related relationship between dust and endotoxin exposure, with the highest prevalence of COPD among subjects with highest exposures. Finally, an analysis of the NHANES III study found that proportional mortality ratios for crop farm workers and livestock farm workers had significantly higher mortality associated with respiratory conditions; in addition, landscape, horticultural, and forestry workers had elevated mortality for COPD.[36]

Industrial exposure to wood particles represents another important organic dust exposure occupational risk for COPD. Wood is processed in many industries, including sawmills processing fresh wood, ply wood mills, and furniture factories or smaller workshops using dry wood only. A review that included 10 cross-sectional studies found significant associations between exposure to wood dust and lung function decline, including a direct response rate between decline in FEV_1 and the diffusing capacity for carbon monoxide and years of employment, and an increased risk for airflow obstruction (defined as FEV_1/FVC <0.70). The risk seems to be independent of type of wood (hardwood or softwood).[37] Other major organic dust exposure sources beyond primary agricultural work and the forestry and wood industry include grain handling and flour milling, and cotton and other primary textile processing.

Metallic Fumes and Dusts

Industrial exposures to metals have been associated with development of airflow obstruction.

Osmium is a highly volatile and highly toxic compound that may result in severe lung injury when inhaled, although human exposures have been limited.[38] Vanadium, another metallic compound associated with lung inflammation, is released into the environment during oil and coal combustion and from metallurgic work. Occupational exposure can result from petrochemical, mining, and steel industries.[39] A study that included 79 employees at a factory making vanadium pentoxide found an increase in incidence of chronic bronchitis symptoms.[40]

Cadmium is a by-product of zinc production and is used industrially in electroplating and battery production. Common occupational exposures to cadmium may result from heavy metal mining, metallurgy, welding and sheet metal work, fossil fuel combustion, exposure to fertilizers, and from iron, steel, and cement production. In the industry, cadmium exposure results from inhalation of toxic fumes, although tobacco smoking is the most important single source of cadmium exposure in the general population.[41] Cadmium is capable of inducing alveolar cell damage in vitro, affecting several levels of cellular function, including repair of DNA, cellular enzyme activity and membrane structure, and alpha1-antitrypsin inhibitory capacity. Experimental emphysema can be induced in animals by administration of cadmium chloride, and several reports suggest that work exposure to cadmium can lead to the development of emphysema.[42,43] Although cadmium exposure may be associated with COPD in highly exposed workers, an analysis of the NHANES III study by Mannino and colleagues[44] found that urinary cadmium levels were not elevated among never smokers with COPD (although very few people in this study were likely to have had occupational cadmium exposure).

Industrial aluminum exposure has been related to development of asthma and reduction of FEV_1 after long-term exposure. For example, a study of workers laboring in a Dutch aluminum production plant, showed that long exposure time was associated with low FEV_1 percentage predicted at 5-years follow-up, even after removal from the exposure. The mechanism of this effect is not established and may reflect other exposures encountered in this industry.[45] Finally, metal smelting activities have also been related with worsening annual decline of FEV1, suggesting that exposure to dusts and fumes arising from this activity may result in an increased risk for COPD.[46]

Mineral and Other Mixed Dusts and Fumes

Mining and quarrying were the first occupations associated with significant reductions in lung function and development of irreversible airflow obstruction and severe parenchymal lung abnormalities (pneumoconiosis). These exposures can subsume inorganic (eg, silica) and organic (eg, coal dust) materials, as well as complex mixtures of gases and particulates (eg, diesel exhaust). Studies of mining cohorts have shown that cumulative dust exposure is an independent predictor of chronic bronchitis and airflow obstruction, and that correlates to the degree of emphysema independent of cigarette smoking among coal miners and hard-rock miners.[47–50] Kuempel and colleagues[51] studied autopsy findings of 616 coal miners and quantitatively estimated cumulative exposures to respirable coal dust using survey data from the US Bureau of Mines. In this study, the highest emphysema index was found in miners with history of smoking. However, for the individuals who never smoked, the severity of emphysema for miners was almost six times that of nonminers. Besides coal mining, several other mineral mining activities (eg, gold, iron, copper; generally characterized by silica exposure) and quarrying industries (eg, talc, potash, slate, kaolin) have been reported to carry increased risk for chronic bronchitis.[15] Occupational diesel engine exhaust exposure has been associated with an increased risk of COPD. Underground mining is one important source of exposures. Other occupations associated with routine diesel exhaust inhalation include transportation, construction, and maintenance. Data from the NHANES III study showed that the risk for COPD is elevated among workers (never smokers) likely to be exposed to diesel gases and fumes; for example, construction (OR 3.5; 95% CI 0.9–14.0) and transportation and trucking (OR 2.0; 95% CI 0.3–15.0). The risk is also elevated for occupations such as vehicle mechanics, transportation, construction workers, and motor vehicle operators.[49] Similarly, a more recent case-control study in the United States found that workers with diesel exhaust exposure had an increased risk for COPD (OR, 1.9; 95% CI 1.3–3.0), and the risk was higher among never smokers (OR 6.4, 95% CI 1.3–31.6).[26]

Also relevant to mixed exposure, studies done in rescue workers, residents, clean-up workers, and other volunteers exposed to a massive dust cloud resulting from the World Trade Center attack, have found evidence of bronchial hyperreactivity, bronchial wall thickening on CT scans, and a significant reduction in 1-year decline in FVC and FEV_1. A pathologic study of 12 local residents exposed to World Trade Center dust, gas, and fumes reported presence of emphysematous changes and small airway abnormalities and macrophages had particles containing silica, aluminum, titanium dioxide,

Table 1
List of population studies of occupational exposure and risk of COPD

Reference	Type of Study	Population Type	Sample Size	Exposure Assessment	Diagnosis	Outcomes	Comments
Matheson et al,[27] 2005	Cross-sectional cohort	Population study in Australia	1232	Self-report and coding of occupation	FEV_1/FVC <0.70 with symptoms (dyspnea and chronic bronchitis) or DLCO <0.80	OR 2.70 (1.39–5.23) for biologic dust	No significant increased risks were found for mineral dust (OR 1.13; 95% CI 0.57–2.27) or gases and fumes (OR 1.63; 95% CI 0.83–3.22)
Jaen et al,[28] 2006	Cross-sectional cohort	Urban industrial area of Spain	497	Self-report	FEV_1 <80% and FEV_1/FVC <0.7 (before bronchodilator)	FEV_1 −80 mL (95% CI 186–26); FEV_1/FVC 1.7%, (CI 3.3–0.2)	Textile industry was most common exposure
Boggia et al,[22] 2008	Prospective	Population study in Italy	2734 males	Expert review of job classification and exposures	FEV_1<80% and FEV_1/FVC <0.7 with symptoms (ATS diagnosis criteria)	OR 2.62 (2.02–3.41)	Workers involved in a national health surveillance program Study included only male workers
Weinmann et al,[24] 2008	Case control	Northwest urban and nonurban areas of US	388 cases and 356 controls	Self-reported exposure plus expert review	FEV_1/FVC < LLN and use of a validated algorithm	Diesel exhaust (OR 1.9, 95% CI 1.3–3.0), mineral dust (OR 1.7, 95% CI 1.1–2.7), irritant gases and vapors (OR 1.6, 5% CI 1.2–2.2)	PAR of 24% (95% CI 5–39) overall, 19% (95% CI 0–37) for ever smokers 43% (95% CI 0–68) for never-smokers

Study	Study type	Location	Sample size	Exposure assessment	COPD definition	Results	Comments
Blanc et al,[29] 2009	Case control	Northern area of US	1202 cases and 302 controls	Self-reported exposure	$FEV_1/FVC <0.7$ and health care use	OR 2.11, 95% CI 1.6–2.8	PAR 13%–33% Smoking and exposure to vapors, gas, dust, or fumes exponentially increased the risk (OR 14.1, 95% CI 9.3–21.2)
Melville et al,[30] 2010	Cross-sectional Cohort	Northern United Kingdom	845	Self-reported exposure	After bronchodilator $FEV_1<80\%$ of the predicted value and an $FEV_1/FVC <0.7$	OR 3.53 95% CI 1.58–7.89	PAR 50%
Govender et al,[31] 2011	Case control	South Africa	110	Self-reported plus expert review	$FEV_1 < 80\%$ and $FEV_1/FVC <0.7$ (before bronchodilator)	High-dust exposure-y and high-chemical, gas, and fumes exposure-y 5.9 (95% CI 2.6–13.2) and 3.6 (95% CI 1.6–7.9)	PAR 25% for self-reported high exposures
Mehta et al,[26] 2012	Prospective cohort	Population study in Switzerland	4267	Self-reported	Before bronchodilator GOLD and LLN criteria	Increase 2–5 times incidence-risk ratio for COPD (GOLD stage ≥II) at high-level exposure	PAR 31%–32% for smokers and 43%–56% for nonsmokers

Abbreviations: DCLO, diffusing capacity for carbon monoxide; LLN, lower limit of normal.

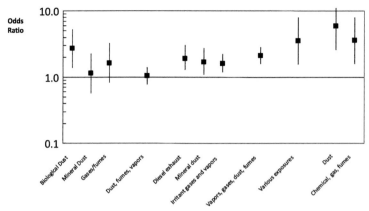

Fig. 1. Risk of occupational exposure for COPD from selected recent studies. (*Data from* Refs.[22,24,27,29–31])

talc, and metals.[52] These findings suggest that a person with massive dust exposure associated with building and construction site debris (largely, but not wholly, inorganic in nature), may have an increased risk for future development of COPD.[53]

ESTABLISHING THE ASSOCIATION BETWEEN OCCUPATION AND COPD

The diagnosis of occupational COPD is infrequently made in clinical practice. Thus, the clinician must be attentive to all potential occupational causes in patients diagnosed with irreversible airflow obstruction, particularly among never smokers or those with no history of atopy or asthma. The most important tool to help identify the cause in these patients is to perform a thorough occupational exposure history, which should include a list of previous jobs, a description of the job activities and potential exposures, and a detailed analysis of the extent and duration of the potential exposure. In addition, the clinician should inquire about the current and past use of protective equipment (ie, masks and respirators) and attempt to obtain a description of the relevant ventilation system of the workplace.[46,54]

Induced sputum facilitated by inhalation of hypertonic saline solution generated by a nebulizer has been used to support the diagnosis of dust burden in exposed workers as a marker of risk and a tool in attribution. Fireman and colleagues[55] analyzed induced sputum samples and bronchoalveolar lavage samples obtained from 14 workers exposed to silica and hard metals. The investigators found that mineralogical analysis of induced sputum was comparable to that of bronchoalveolar lavage samples, and concluded that induced sputum analysis represents a biologic monitoring method to detect dust burden in

healthy workers exposed to hazardous dusts. Lerman and colleagues,[56] in a study related to Fireman and colleagues,[55] investigation, found a correlation between the distribution of particle size in induced sputum and pulmonary function tests among 54 foundry workers, of whom 34 had been exposed to a variety of metals. The investigators found that particle size correlated with lung function decline and helped differentiate between exposed and nonexposed workers.

Currently, however, there is no clinically established method of laboratory-based confirmatory exposure quantification. The diagnosis of occupational COPD relies on clinical history of significant occupational exposure to gases, dusts, fumes, or vapors, and the presence of irreversible airflow obstruction and/or the presence of emphysema on imaging studies of the chest.

PROGNOSIS

Given the difficulties of establishing the diagnosis of occupational COPD, few studies have been able to address the prognosis of this group of patients. Nevertheless, some studies suggest that patients with occupational exposures who are diagnosed with occupational lung diseases other than COPD may have a worse prognosis and excess mortality. For example, a study that analyzed risk of mortality by occupation over a 22-year period in England and Wales, found that mortality was highest among coal miners with diagnoses of COPD or coal worker's pneumoconiosis. The largest component of excess mortality in this study was from diseases caused by exposure to dusts and fumes and, in particular, from COPD caused by coal mine dust, silica dust, and metal fumes.[57] More recently, Jarvholm and colleagues[58] used population-based case referent studies from Sweden and estimated that the number of work-related COPD deaths was much higher than asthma (about 90 vs 4 cases), and that COPD had an attributable fraction of 15% for work-related deaths from respiratory conditions. Similarly, a study by Attfield and Kuempel[59] investigated the causes of mortality in a cohort of coal miners from the United States. The investigators used *International Classification of Diseases* codes to define presence of chronic bronchitis and/or emphysema.[60] Although most subjects had a history of smoking (80%), the investigators found that mortality from COPD was associated with cumulative dust exposure with a relative risk of 1.0065 per mg-year/m3 (CI 1.0017–1.0054), although the association of cumulative dust exposure and mortality from emphysema as underlying or contributing cause was not statistically significant.

MANAGEMENT AND PREVENTION

There is minimal literature on the management and prevention of occupational COPD and currently there are no published guidelines. This is in contrast to the management of occupational asthma, for which clear guidelines have been published.[61] Nevertheless, effective management should focus on medical treatment of already prevalent COPD as well as efforts to prevent and/or limit ongoing or further damage via reduction of exposure.

There is no evidence to suggest that the clinical treatment of established COPD secondary to occupational exposures should be in any way different from that of COPD due to cigarette smoking. A detailed discussion of this treatment is beyond the scope of this article. However, smoking cessation is of paramount importance because this is frequently a coexisting risk factor in many patients. Moreover, several studies of occupational risk for COPD suggest that smoking risk is at least an addition to that of concomitant work-related factors. Although it has not been studied, it is also reasonable to presume that other risk factors for COPD (eg, secondhand cigarette smoke, biomass combustion byproduct exposure) should also be addressed with patients at combined occupational risk. Similar to other work-related diseases, prevention is the primary tool for decreasing the incidence of morbidity and disability from occupational COPD. Prevention must involve cooperation between employers, workers, and their representatives, regulators, and medical personnel.[62] For health care providers, detailed history of occupational exposure is obviously important. However, it is also important to identify whether the patient has been adequately trained in the dangers of these exposures, early identification of symptoms, alternatives to the exposure, and the management options available. Preventative measures are generally classified into three types: primary, secondary and tertiary.

Primary prevention is designed to abate hazards before any damage or injury has occurred. In case of respiratory tract irritants, different strategies are available to reduce exposures. These strategies in the order of decreasing effectiveness but increasing ease of implementation include: (1) elimination (eg, substitute alternate materials), (2) engineering controls (eg, exhaust ventilation or process enclosure), (3) administrative controls (eg, transfer to another job or change in work practices), and (4) personal protective equipment (eg, masks or respirators).[63] In many cases, personal protective equipment may be the only option, but it is the strategy with the most equivocal protection. This is because the effective use of personal protective equipment requires that the appropriate equipment be selected, properly fit-tested, maintained, and worn when there is potential for exposure. The failure to properly carry out any one of these essential tasks may cause failure of personal protective equipment to prevent exposure.

In many cases of occupational COPD, people have no reasonable alternatives to their job and may discount the severity and degree of exposures for fear of loss of employment. Moreover, unlike workers with sensitizer-induced asthma, workers with occupational COPD may continue to work in their usual jobs if their exposure to the inciting agent is diminished.[63] Consequently, secondary and tertiary prevention measures are also of great importance.

Secondary prevention addresses early detection of preclinical changes so that morbidity can be prevented by means of timely intervention. Examples include worker education and training in work processes, safety equipment, and procedures, as well as some of the primary prevention strategies. Medical surveillance programs are a type of secondary prevention. Any diagnosis of occupational COPD must be considered a sentinel event; other exposed workers are at risk and need to be identified promptly. A general approach to surveillance programs includes medical screening of coworkers, as well as exposure monitoring.[64] For medical surveillance of COPD, short symptom questionnaires can be administered before employment and repeated annually. They should include items such as improvement in respiratory symptoms on week-ends and holidays.[63] In addition, spirometry can be performed on an annual basis and compared with baseline spirometry testing at the time of hire, as well as to normal population-based predicted rates of decline. Action prompted by an accelerated decline that had not yet reached a point of frank obstruction would be paradigmatic of secondary prevention. Review of peak expiratory flow rate records over several weeks can also detect workers at risk for developing irritant-induced COPD.[63]

Tertiary prevention applies to individuals who have already been diagnosed with occupational COPD. It includes institution of appropriate health care and an effort to prevent permanent disease by early removal from, or reduction of, exposure.[62] Furthermore, early recognition of the disease and early removal from, or reduction of, exposure, makes it more likely that the patient will have a slower progression of COPD.

Although there is lack of intervention studies in occupational COPD, data from certain other occupational or environmental lung diseases could be extrapolated to this condition. In occupational asthma for example, elimination of exposure has been shown to be associated with improvement in the health of already-diagnosed cases of work-related asthma in a plant where use of diisocyanates was halted.[62] Similarly, reduction in air pollution during the Beijing Olympics and Summer Olympic games in Atlanta was associated with reduced incidence of asthma exacerbations.[65,66] In Dublin, there was a 15.5% reduction in respiratory deaths after ban on coal sales related to improvement in air pollution.[66] Similarly, intervention studies for indoor air pollution from bio-mass fuels in areas where they are heavily used have shown that improved stoves result in significant reduction in respiratory symptoms and a significantly lower decrease in FEV_1.[65]

SUMMARY

COPD is a leading cause of morbidity and mortality globally. The contribution of occupational exposures to dust, vapors, gas, and fumes remains an important factor in the development and progression of COPD in both smokers and nonsmokers. Indeed, a recent editorial stated that sufficient data have accumulated to support a causal association between occupational factors and COPD.[67] Prevention strategies targeting occupational exposures to respiratory irritants will become increasingly important in the prevention of COPD.

REFERENCES

1. Decramer M, Sibille Y. European conference on chronic respiratory disease. Lancet 2011;377(9760):104–6.

2. WHO. World health statistics. 2008. Available at: http://www.whoint/whosis/whostat/EN_WHS08_Full.pdf. Accessed January 31, 2011.

3. Murray CJ, Lopez AD. Alternative projections of mortality and disability by cause 1990–2020: Global Burden of Disease Study. Lancet 1997;349(9064):1498–504.

4. Lamprecht B, McBurnie MA, Vollmer WM, et al. COPD in never smokers: results from the population-based burden of obstructive lung disease study. Chest 2011;139(4):752–63.

5. Hnizdo E, Sullivan PA, Bang KM, et al. Association between chronic obstructive pulmonary disease and employment by industry and occupation in the US population: a study of data from the Third National Health and Nutrition Examination Survey. Am J Epidemiol 2002;156(8):738–46.

6. Fingerhut M, Nelson DI, Driscoll T, et al. The contribution of occupational risks to the global burden of disease: summary and next steps. Med Lav 2006;97(2):313–21.

7. Balmes J, Becklake M, Blanc P, et al. American Thoracic Society Statement: occupational contribution to the burden of airway disease. Am J Respir Crit Care Med 2003;167(5):787–97.

8. Rom WN, Markowitz S. Environmental and occupational medicine. 4th edition. Philadelphia: Wolters Kluwer/Lippincott Williams & Wilkins; 2007.

9. Trupin L, Earnest G, San Pedro M, et al. The occupational burden of chronic obstructive pulmonary disease. Eur Respir J 2003;22(3):462–9.

10. Pauwels RA, Buist AS, Calverley PM, et al. Global strategy for the diagnosis, management, and prevention of chronic obstructive pulmonary disease. NHLBI/WHO Global Initiative for Chronic Obstructive Lung Disease (GOLD) Workshop summary. Am J Respir Crit Care Med 2001;163(5):1256–76.

11. Celli BR, MacNee W. Standards for the diagnosis and treatment of patients with COPD: a summary of the ATS/ERS position paper. Eur Respir J 2004;23(6):932–46.

12. Barnes PJ, Kleinert S. COPD—a neglected disease. Lancet 2004;364(9434):564–5.

13. Agusti A, Sobradillo P, Celli B. Addressing the complexity of chronic obstructive pulmonary disease: from phenotypes and biomarkers to scale-free networks, systems biology, and P4 medicine. Am J Respir Crit Care Med 2011;183(9):1129–37.

14. Toren K, Ekerljung L, Kim JL, et al. Adult-onset asthma in west Sweden—incidence, sex differences and impact of occupational exposures. Respir Med 2011;105(11):1622–8.

15. Becklake MR. Chronic airflow limitation: its relationship to work in dusty occupations. Chest 1985;88(4):608–17.

16. Eisner MD, Anthonisen N, Coultas D, et al. An official American Thoracic Society public policy

statement: novel risk factors and the global burden of chronic obstructive pulmonary disease. Am J Respir Crit Care Med 2010;182(5):693–718.

17. Khan AJ, Nanchal R. Cotton dust lung diseases. Curr Opin Pulm Med 2007;13(2):137–41.

18. Kanwal R. Bronchiolitis obliterans in workers exposed to flavoring chemicals. Curr Opin Pulm Med 2008;14(2):141–6.

19. Ulvestad B, Bakke B, Eduard W, et al. Cumulative exposure to dust causes accelerated decline in lung function in tunnel workers. Occup Environ Med 2001;58(10):663–9.

20. Korn RJ, Dockery DW, Speizer FE, et al. Occupational exposures and chronic respiratory symptoms. A population-based study. Am Rev Respir Dis 1987;136(2):298–304.

21. Xu X, Christiani DC, Dockery DW, et al. Exposure-response relationships between occupational exposures and chronic respiratory illness: a community-based study. Am Rev Respir Dis 1992;146(2):413–8.

22. Boggia B, Farinaro E, Grieco L, et al. Burden of smoking and occupational exposure on etiology of chronic obstructive pulmonary disease in workers of Southern Italy. J Occup Environ Med 2008;50(3):366–70.

23. Blanc PD, Torén K. Occupation in chronic obstructive pulmonary disease and chronic bronchitis: an update. Int J Tuberc Lung Dis 2007;11(3):251–7 [Review].

24. Weinmann S, Vollmer WM, Breen V, et al. COPD and occupational exposures: a case-control study. J Occup Environ Med 2008;50(5):561–9.

25. Blanc PD. Occupation and COPD: a brief review. J Asthma 2012;49(1):2–4.

26. Mehta AJ, Miedinger D, Keidel D, et al. Occupational exposure to dusts, gases, and fumes and incidence of chronic obstructive pulmonary disease in the Swiss Cohort Study on Air Pollution and Lung and Heart Diseases in Adults. Am J Respir Crit Care Med 2012;185:1292–300.

27. Matheson MC, Benke G, Raven J, et al. Biological dust exposure in the workplace is a risk factor for chronic obstructive pulmonary disease. Thorax 2005;60(8):645–51.

28. Jaen A, Zock JP, Kogevinas M, et al. Occupation, smoking, and chronic obstructive respiratory disorders: a cross sectional study in an industrial area of Catalonia, Spain. Environ Health 2006;5:2.

29. Blanc PD, Iribarren C, Trupin L, et al. Occupational exposures and the risk of COPD: dusty trades revisited. Thorax 2009;64(1):6–12.

30. Melville AM, Pless-Mulloli T, Afolabi OA, et al. COPD prevalence and its association with occupational exposures in a general population. Eur Respir J 2010;36(3):488–93.

31. Govender N, Lalloo UG, Naidoo RN. Occupational exposures and chronic obstructive pulmonary disease: a hospital based case-control study. Thorax 2011;66(7):597–601.

32. Spurzem JR, Romberger DJ, Von Essen SG. Agricultural lung disease. Clin Chest Med 2002;23(4):795–810.

33. Dalphin JC, Bildstein F, Pernet D, et al. Prevalence of chronic bronchitis and respiratory function in a group of dairy farmers in the French Doubs province. Chest 1989;95(6):1244–7.

34. Eduard W, Pearce N, Douwes J. Chronic bronchitis, COPD, and lung function in farmers: the role of biological agents. Chest 2009;136(3):716–25.

35. Monso E, Riu E, Radon K, et al. Chronic obstructive pulmonary disease in never-smoking animal farmers working inside confinement buildings. Am J Ind Med 2004;46(4):357–62.

36. Greskevitch M, Kullman G, Bang KM, et al. Respiratory disease in agricultural workers: mortality and morbidity statistics. J Agromedicine 2007;12(3):5–10.

37. Jacobsen G, Schaumburg I, Sigsgaard T, et al. Non-malignant respiratory diseases and occupational exposure to wood dust. Part II. Dry wood industry. Ann Agric Environ Med 2010;17(1):29–44.

38. Luttrell W, Giles C. Toxic tips: osmium tetroxide. Journal of Chemical Health and Safety 2007;14(5):40–1.

39. Rondini EA, Walters DM, Bauer AK. Vanadium pentoxide induces pulmonary inflammation and tumor promotion in a strain-dependent manner. Part Fibre Toxicol 2010;7:9.

40. Kiviluoto M. Observations on the lungs of vanadium workers. Br J Ind Med 1980;37(4):363–6.

41. Bernard A. Cadmium & its adverse effects on human health. Indian J Med Res 2008;128(4):557–64.

42. Rubio ML, Sanchez-Cifuentes MV, Peces-Barba G, et al. Intrapulmonary gas mixing in panacinar- and centriacinar-induced emphysema in rats. Am J Respir Crit Care Med 1998;157(1):237–45.

43. Davison AG, Fayers PM, Taylor AJ, et al. Cadmium fume inhalation and emphysema. Lancet 1988;1(8587):663–7.

44. Mannino DM, Holguin F, Greves HM, et al. Urinary cadmium levels predict lower lung function in current and former smokers: data from the Third National Health and Nutrition Examination Survey. Thorax 2004;59(3):194–8.

45. Sorgdrager B, de Looff AJ, Pal TM, et al. Factors affecting FEV1 in workers with potroom asthma after their removal from exposure. Int Arch Occup Environ Health 2001;74(1):55–8.

46. Balmes JR. Occupational contribution to the burden of chronic obstructive pulmonary disease. J Occup Environ Med 2005;47(2):154–60.

47. Becklake MR, Irwig L, Kielkowski D, et al. The predictors of emphysema in South African gold miners. Am Rev Respir Dis 1987;135(6):1234–41.

48. Hnizdo E, Sluis-Cremer GK. Silica exposure, silicosis, and lung cancer: a mortality study of South African gold miners. Br J Ind Med 1991;48(1):53–60.

49. Cockcroft A, Seal RM, Wagner JC, et al. Post-mortem study of emphysema in coalworkers and non-coalworkers. Lancet 1982;2(8298):600–3.

50. Santo Tomas LH. Emphysema and chronic obstructive pulmonary disease in coal miners. Curr Opin Pulm Med 2011;17(2):123–5.

51. Kuempel ED, Wheeler MW, Smith RJ, et al. Contributions of dust exposure and cigarette smoking to emphysema severity in coal miners in the United States. Am J Respir Crit Care Med 2009;180(3): 257–64.

52. Caplan-Shaw CE, Yee H, Rogers L, et al. Lung pathologic findings in a local residential and working community exposed to World Trade Center dust, gas, and fumes. J Occup Environ Med 2011;53(9): 981–91.

53. Rom WN, Reibman J, Rogers L, et al. Emerging exposures and respiratory health: World Trade Center dust. Proc Am Thorac Soc 2010;7(2):142–5.

54. Felton JS. The heritage of Bernardino Ramazzini. Occup Med (Lond) 1997;47(3):167–79.

55. Fireman E, Greif J, Schwarz Y, et al. Assessment of hazardous dust exposure by BAL and induced sputum. Chest 1999;115(6):1720–8.

56. Lerman Y, Schwarz Y, Kaufman G, et al. Case series: use of induced sputum in the evaluation of occupational lung diseases. Arch Environ Health 2003; 58(5):284–9.

57. Coggon D, Harris EC, Brown T, et al. Work-related mortality in England and Wales, 1979–2000. Occup Environ Med 2010;67(12):816–22.

58. Jarvholm B, Reuterwall C, Bystedt J. Mortality attributable to occupational exposure in Sweden. Scand J Work Environ Health 2012. http://dx.doi.org/10.5271/sjweh.3284. [Epub ahead of print].

59. Attfield MD, Kuempel ED. Mortality among U.S. underground coal miners: a 23-year follow-up. Am J Ind Med 2008;51(4):231–45.

60. National Center for Health Statistics, CDC. ICD-9-CM guidelines, conversion table, and addenda. Classification of diseases, functioning, and disability. Retrieved: January 24, 2010.

61. Baur X, Sigsgaard T, Aasen TB, et al. Guidelines for the management of work-related asthma. Eur Respir J 2012;39(3):529–45.

62. Venables KM. Prevention of occupational asthma. Eur Respir J 1994;7(4):768–78.

63. Balmes JR. Occupational airways diseases from chronic low-level exposures to irritants. Clin Chest Med 2002;23(4):727–35, vi.

64. Tarlo SM, Boulet LP, Cartier A, et al. Canadian Thoracic Society guidelines for occupational asthma. Can Respir J 1998;5(4):289–300.

65. Laumbach RJ, Kipen HM. Respiratory health effects of air pollution: update on biomass smoke and traffic pollution. J Allergy Clin Immunol 2012;129(1):3–11 [quiz: 12–3].

66. Friedman MS, Powell KE, Hutwagner L, et al. Impact of changes in transportation and commuting behaviors during the 1996 Summer Olympic Games in Atlanta on air quality and childhood asthma. JAMA 2001;285(7):897–905.

67. Naidoo RN. Occupation exposures and chronic obstructive pulmonary disease: incontrovertible evidence for causality? Am J Respir Crit Care Med 2012;185:1252–3.

Occupational Rhinitis and Other Work-Related Upper Respiratory Tract Conditions

Yu A. Zhao, MD, MS, Dennis Shusterman, MD, MPH*

KEYWORDS

- Occupational rhinitis • Occupational asthma • Sinusitis • Sinonasal cancer • Olfactory dysfunction
- Vocal cord dysfunction • Sensory irritation • Allergy

KEY POINTS

- The upper airway serves as an air conditioner, filter, and sensory monitor.
- Irritants and allergens can impact the upper airway.
- According to the "unified airway" hypothesis, the development of occupational allergic rhinitis may herald the onset of occupational asthma, and airway irritant exposures may also contribute to both conditions.
- Other occupational upper airway conditions include sinusitis, nasal erosions, sinonasal cancer, olfactory dysfunction, and vocal cord dysfunction.

INTRODUCTION

The upper airway acts as a sentinel for the respiratory tract, alerting individuals to the physical and chemical qualities of inspired air. It also acts as a filter and air conditioner, and plays an important role in communication. Common occupational upper airway conditions include rhinitis, sinusitis, laryngitis, and vocal cord dysfunction (VCD). Less common are nasal erosions, sinonasal neoplasms, and chemically induced olfactory dysfunction. Etiologic agents range from those specific to occupational settings (eg, chromic acid in the case of nasal erosions) to more ubiquitous environmental agents, such as office dust, cold air, or second-hand tobacco smoke. The epidemiology, pathophysiology, diagnosis, and treatment of occupational upper airway conditions, in particular occupational rhinitis, are reviewed in this article.

ANATOMY OF THE UPPER AIRWAY

The upper airway refers to the airway above the vocal folds, including nasal cavities, nasopharynx, oropharynx, and hypopharynx. Along with the oral cavity, the oropharynx and hypopharynx (and glottis) are sometimes referred to as the "aerodigestive tract."[1] The cofunctionalities of breathing and swallowing dictate that the area be heavily innervated and endowed with a variety of reflex responses.

Anatomically, the lateral walls of the nasal cavity are invested with turbinates or concha (literally, "shells"), the functional consequence of which is to increase the surface area of contact between the mucosa and inspired air. The histology of the nasal cavity has evolved to meet the functional requirements of heat and humidity transfer; biochemical metabolism of inhaled substances; and mucociliary transport of particulate matter to the

Disclosures: None (for both authors).
Conflicts of Interest: None (for both authors).
Division of Occupational and Environmental Medicine, University of California, San Francisco, Campus Box 0843, San Francisco, CA 94143, USA
* Corresponding author. Upper Airway Biology Laboratory, 1301 South 46th Street, Building 112, Richmond, CA 94804.
E-mail address: dshusterman@sfghoem.ucsf.edu

chestmed.theclinics.com

oropharynx (from which it is either swallowed or expectorated). Posterior to the resilient squamous and transitional epithelium of the anterior nares lies a pseudostratified columnar epithelium consisting of ciliated columnar, goblet, and basal cells, and submucous glands.[2]

PHYSIOLOGIC FUNCTIONS
Air Conditioning, Filtration, and Scrubbing

The nose serves as the main portal of entry for the respiratory tract, filtering, scrubbing, physically conditioning inspired air; signaling the quality of the surrounding atmosphere; and playing a role in communication (hearing and phonation). Under most climatic conditions, inspired air is heated and humidified in the upper airway, thereby reducing any thermal or osmotic stress on the tracheobronchial tree.[3]

Filtration of large particles is accomplished mechanically (by nasal vibrissae) and by the process of impaction (whereby particles collide with the turbinates, and are subsequently cleared by the mucociliary apparatus).[4] Finer particles, however, are more likely to evade this clearance system and reach the lower respiratory tract (**Fig. 1**). In the case of inhaled droplets carrying infectious agents, the mucosa produces specific and nonspecific defenses, the former including secretory IgA and the latter including lactoferrin and lysozyme.[5]

Water-soluble irritants, including such gases and vapors as ammonia, organic acids, aldehydes, and chlorine, readily dissolve in mucous membrane water, providing for immediate sensory impact and mass removal.[6] This effect (scrubbing) protects the lower respiratory tract during nasal breathing and incidentally reinforces the sensations of eye,

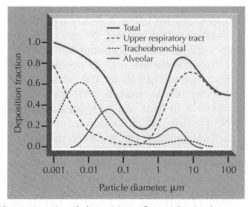

Fig. 1. Fractional deposition of particles in the upper respiratory tract, tracheobronchial tree, and alveolar region of the lung as a function of particle size. (*From* Shusterman D. Toxicology of nasal irritants. Curr Allergy Asthma Rep 2003;3(3):258–65; with permission.)

nose, and throat irritation, which can serve as a warning to reduce exposure (**Fig. 2**).

In contrast to the lower airway, patency in the upper airway is controlled through vascular engorgement rather than smooth muscle tone. Underlying this vasoactivity is an elaborate network of arterioles, capacitance vessels, and arteriovenous shunts located beneath the mucosal surface.[7] Controlling nasal patency (and secretory responses) is a variety of endogenous mediators derived from immune effector cells and mucosal nerves.[8,9]

Sensation and Reflexes

The sentinel function of the nose is achieved through the sense of smell and nasal irritant perception (chemesthesis). These senses are mediated by cranial nerve I (olfactory nerve) and cranial nerve V (trigeminal nerve), respectively (**Fig. 3**). Just as the appreciation of flavor involves a seamless combination of taste and smell, the appreciation of inhaled compounds involves smell and trigeminal stimulation. It is not unusual for an individual to describe "a pungent odor," and in the process integrate information from two separate cranial nerves.[10]

Peripherally, the terminal branches of the trigeminal nerve include small diameter nociceptive neurons (C- and Aδ-fibers) invested with a variety of nociceptive (pain-perceiving) ion channels.[11] The C-fiber population also elaborates vasoactive neuropeptides, which in turn can be released as part of nociceptive reflexes.[12] Similar neurophysiology applies to the glossopharyngeal and vagal nerves (cranial nerves IX and X), which convey the sense of irritation for the hypopharynx and larynx. A recent development has been the identification of specialized receptor cells (solitary chemoreceptors cells) in the human nose, carrying transduction mechanisms for bitter taste and selected airborne irritants, further linking chemical exposures to airway inflammation.[13]

Reflexes in the upper airway include sneezing, secretion, and nasal obstruction. Upper respiratory tract nerves also participate in the laryngeal adductor reflex, cough, and bronchospasm.[14] Along with cold, dry air, chemical irritants can trigger upper respiratory tract symptoms that are virtually indistinguishable from those of allergic rhinitis, leading to inevitable diagnostic confusion (see later).

PATHOPHYSIOLOGY
Irritation

Upper airway irritation can be defined variously as stimulation of nociceptors (resulting in sensations

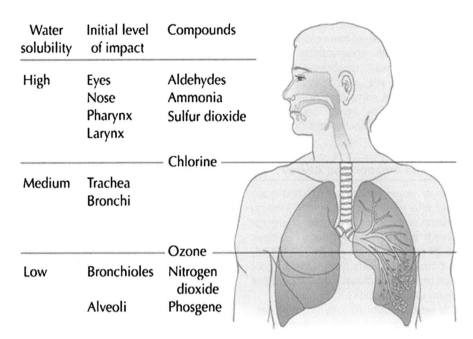

Water solubility	Initial level of impact	Compounds
High	Eyes Nose Pharynx Larynx	Aldehydes Ammonia Sulfur dioxide
		——— Chlorine ———
Medium	Trachea Bronchi	
		——— Ozone ———
Low	Bronchioles Alveoli	Nitrogen dioxide Phosgene

Fig. 2. Water solubility and site of initial impact of airborne irritants. (*From* Shusterman D. Toxicology of nasal irritants. Curr Allergy Asthma Rep 2003;3(3):258–65; with permission.)

of burning, stinging, or tingling); reflex vascular and secretory changes triggered by nerve stimulation; chemically induced tissue damage; or some combination of these.[15] Irritation of the combined mucosal distribution of the trigeminal nerve (eye, nose, and throat) has been termed "sensory irritation," which is also a principal constituent of nonspecific building-related illness (or sick building syndrome).[16] Because of their acute (and reversible) nature and the frequent lack of corresponding physical signs, sensory irritation complaints can be a source of frustration to clinicians and patients. Potential upper airway irritants

commonly found in indoor environments include combustion products (from cigarette smoke); volatile organic compounds (from building materials, furnishings, cleaning products, or microbial overgrowth); and reactive chemicals found in household and commercial cleaning products (eg, chlorine and ammonia).[17]

Allergy

In contrast to nonspecific irritation, allergic reactions involve hypersensitivity to specific substances (allergens). Irritation can occur on first exposure, whereas hypersensitivity requires a period of asymptomatic exposure during which time cellular or humoral responses develop to the specific allergen. Immediate hypersensitivity refers to a range of IgE-mediated responses, including rhinitis, conjunctivitis, asthma, urticaria, angioedema, and anaphylaxis. Airborne allergens encountered in workplace settings include macromolecules (chiefly proteins) and low-molecular-weight chemical allergens (the mechanism of response to which is less fully understood than for high-molecular-weight allergens).

Cranial nerve I

Cranial nerve V

Fig. 3. Innervation of the nasal cavity. Cranial nerve I, olfactory nerve; cranial nerve V, trigeminal nerve. (*From* Shusterman D. The upper airway, including olfaction, as mediator of symptoms. Environ Health Perspect 2002;110(Suppl 4):649–53; with permission.)

"Unified Airway" Hypothesis

IgE-mediated hypersensitivity can involve the upper airway (rhinitis) or the lower airway (asthma). The onset of occupational allergic rhinitis often precedes that of asthma in a given individual, particularly if the sensitizer is a high-molecular-weight antigen.[18,19] Multiple epidemiologic, physiologic, and biochemical observations support a so-called unified airway hypothesis, in which rhinitis and asthma are pathophysiologically linked.[20–22] Furthermore, some investigators have linked skin exposure with airway sensitization, particularly in the case of diisocyanates (a component of polyurethanes).[23]

Interplay Between Irritation and Allergy

Augmentation of upper airway allergy has been demonstrated with several air pollutants. Priming (increased nasal response to allergen challenge after exposure to an irritant air pollutant) has been shown, for example, after ozone exposure.[24,25] Adjuvancy (or boosting of underlying sensitization) has also been shown with diesel exhaust particles and sidestream tobacco smoke.[26–28]

In terms of susceptibility to irritants, the presence of pre-existing allergic inflammation seems to confer greater upper airway sensitivity to air pollutants, including subjective irritation and objective airway obstruction.[29,30] Given the rising prevalence of atopy and allergies in the general population, and the ubiquitous nature of indoor and outdoor air pollutants, interactions between irritants, allergens, and atopy likely play an important role in promoting allergic and irritant rhinitis.

The pathophysiology of rhinitis explains the two main determinants of occupational rhinitis that have been identified in the epidemiology literature: exposure to the causative agents and a history of atopy. Atopy, typically defined as reactivity to common environmental allergens, increases the risk of occupational allergic rhinitis caused by large-molecular-weight allergens, but is not a risk factor for most low-molecular-weight allergens, such as isocyanates.[29] Smoking has not consistently been identified as a risk factor for occupational rhinitis.[29]

UPPER AIRWAY DISORDERS
Occupational Rhinitis

Occupational rhinitis has, until recently, lacked standardization in its clinical definition. In 2009, however, a task force of the European Academy of Allergy and Clinical Immunology proposed a working definition closely resembling that of occupational asthma:

Occupational rhinitis is an inflammatory disease of the nose, which is characterized by intermittent or persistent symptoms (ie, nasal congestion, sneezing, rhinorrea, itching), and/or variable nasal airflow limitation and/or hypersecretion due to causes and conditions attributable to a particular work environment and not to stimuli encountered outside the workplace.[31]

The task force further specified:

Work-related rhinitis may be distinguished into: (1) occupational rhinitis that is due to causes and conditions attributable to a particular work environment (2) work exacerbated rhinitis that is pre-existing or concurrent rhinitis exacerbated by workplace exposures.[31]

Irritant rhinitis

Several different industrial chemicals and manufacturing processes have been associated with irritant rhinitis or sinusitis in workers (**Table 1**). Among these are woodworking; spice grinding; exposure to fuel oil ash, nickel fumes, or dicumylperoxide in industry; and use of glutaraldehyde in medical sterilization.[32–37] Work processes that have occasionally proved problematic to office workers include use of photocopiers, laser printers, and carbonless copy paper.[38,39] Symptoms of irritant rhinitis can include nasal stinging or burning, rhinorrhea, congestion, postnasal drip, sinus headache, and epistaxis.

In polluted urban areas, outdoor workers may be more highly exposed to ambient air pollution than are indoor workers. Several studies have documented the effects of photochemical air pollutants on the upper respiratory tract. Two such studies were performed in a heavily polluted portion of Mexico City, where ozone levels are far in excess of US (and Mexican) standards. These studies compared urban residents with residents of an unpolluted locale, and examined visitors to the city who came from more rural areas. The results were dramatic: permanent residents showed squamous metaplasia, loss of normal cilia, vascular congestion, and glandular atrophy on nasal biopsy, whereas short-term visitors developed epithelial desquamation and neutrophilic inflammation that took more than 2 weeks to resolve after returning to their home towns.[40,41]

Irritant-induced rhinitis has been observed after one-time, high-level exposures to airborne irritants, similar to irritant-induced asthma (or reactive airways dysfunction syndrome).[42] Meggs[43] has coined the term "reactive upper airways dysfunction syndrome" to describe acute onset, irritant-induced rhinitis. Biopsies of the nasal mucosa among individuals acutely exposed to irritants reportedly have shown epithelial desquamation, defective epithelial cell junctions, and increased numbers of nerve fibers, although

Table 1
Selected occupations and associated irritants

Occupation	Irritant
Agricultural workers	Ammonia, nitrogen dioxide, hydrogen sulfide
Custodians	Ammonia, bleach (hypochlorite), chloramines, other cleaning products
Firefighters	Smoke, hazardous materials releases
Food service workers	Cooking vapors, cigarette smoke
Health professionals	Glutaraldehyde, formaldehyde
Laboratory workers	Solvent vapors, inorganic acid vapors or mists
Military personnel	Zinc chloride smoke
Power plant and oil refinery workers	Sulfur dioxide
Printers, painters	Solvent vapors
Pulp mill workers	Chlorine, chlorine dioxide, hydrogen sulfide
Railroad personnel, miners, truck drivers	Diesel exhaust
Refrigeration workers (commercial)	Ammonia
Roofers, pavers	Asphalt vapors, PAHs[a]
Swimming pool service workers	Chlorine, hydrogen chloride, nitrogen trichloride
Teachers and office workers	Cleaning products, printers, copiers
Waste water treatment workers	Chlorine, hydrogen sulfide
Welders	Metallic oxide fumes, nitrogen oxides, ozone
Woodworkers	Wood dust

[a] Polycyclic aromatic hydrocarbons (also skin and lung carcinogen).

patients and control subjects did not differ in staining for neuropeptides.[44]

Nasal septal perforation
Nasal septal perforation is an unusual outcome associated with protracted and high-level exposure to chromates (as in the electroplating industry).[45,46] Chromates (Cr^{6+} compounds) are also of concern with respect to carcinogenesis in the upper and lower respiratory tract (see later). Differential diagnostic considerations in such cases should include such nonoccupational causes as Wegener granulomatosis and recreational drug use (ie, cocaine).

Occupational allergic rhinitis
Allergens responsible for occupational allergic rhinitis are essentially the same as those seen in occupational asthma (ie, various high- and low-molecular-weight sensitizers; **Table 2**). The development of rhinitis may presage the development of asthma; hence, early recognition of occupational allergic rhinitis and timely removal from exposure may interrupt disease progression. Differentiating allergic from irritant rhinitis in the occupational setting may be challenging, however, for a variety of reasons: (1) presenting symptoms (eg, rhinorrhea and nasal obstruction) overlap between the two conditions; (2) there is a paucity of Food and Drug Administration–approved reagents for skin testing or serum immunoassays for specific

Table 2
Selected occupational allergens: rhinitis & asthma

Allergen	Occupation
High molecular weight	
Natural rubber latex	Healthcare workers
Psyllium	Pharmacists, nurses
Animal proteins	Animal handlers, veterinarians
α-Amylase, grain and flour dust	Bakers, grain workers
Insects and mites	Bakers, farm, animal workers
Gum arabic	Printers, food workers
Mold spores	Various
Pollens	Landscapers, florists
Fish, seafood proteins	Fish and seafood workers
Low molecular weight	
Abeitic acid (rosin, pine resin, colophony, solder)	Solderers, gluers
Plicatic acid (Western red cedar), other wood dusts	Wood workers, carpenters
Anhydrides	Plastics workers
Diisocyanates (MDI, TDI, HDI)	Car painters, boat builders, spray foam, construction and shipping workers

occupational allergens; and (3) some substances (eg, formaldehyde, glutaradehyde) can act as both sensitizers and irritants.[31]

Symptomatically, occupational allergic rhinitis commonly presents with nasal pruritus and sneezing, in addition to the less specific symptoms of hypersecretion and obstruction. Reflex secretion or nasal obstruction in response to nonspecific physical and chemical stimuli (termed "nasal hyperreactivity") can occur in the absence of allergy (ie, in nonallergic or vasomotor rhinitis), and is also observed in roughly 40% of allergic rhinitics.[47]

Sinusitis

Few studies have examined the endpoint of sinusitis and occupational exposures. Surveys of furriers, spice workers, vegetable picklers, hemp workers, and grain and flour workers all show increased prevalence rates for self-reported sinusitis.[48–52] Pathophysiologically, the causal sequence for an occupationally induced (or exacerbated) sinusitis may include initial allergic or irritant rhinitis; ciliastasis (with impaired clearance of pathogenic organisms); mucous membrane swelling (with occlusion of sinus ostia and impaired sinus drainage); and infection and mucosal remodeling.

Olfactory Dysfunction

Temporary and long-lasting alterations in olfactory function have been reported among workers exposed to a variety of industrial chemicals. Chemically induced olfactory dysfunction may include quantitative defects, including hyposmia (reduced odor acuity) and anosmia (absent odor perception); or qualitative defects, including olfactory agnosia (decreased ability to identify odors) and various dysosmias (distorted odor perception).

Occupational groups and exposures with which olfactory dysfunction has been associated include alkaline battery workers and braziers (cadmium or nickel exposure); tank cleaners (hydrocarbon exposure); paint formulators (solvent or acrylic acid exposure); and chemical plant workers (ammonia and sulfuric acid exposures).[53–55] In terms of specific olfactory toxicology, hydrogen sulfide produces acute and reversible olfactory paralysis with exposures in excess of roughly 50 parts per million.[56]

Of importance in the differential diagnosis of olfactory dysfunction, competing causes of olfactory impairment include head trauma; chronic nasal obstruction and inflammation caused by rhinitis; postinfectious inflammation; neurodegenerative and endocrine disorders; hepatic and renal disease; neoplasms; various drugs; ionizing radiation; congenital defects (eg, Kallmann syndrome); and selected psychiatric conditions.[57]

Sinonasal Cancer

A variety of occupations and imputed exposures have been linked with the development of malignant neoplasms of the paranasal sinuses. The strongest (and most consistent) associations include cigarette smoking (squamous cell carcinoma) and leather- and wood-dust-exposed workers (adenocarcinoma).[58,59] Workers engaged in nickel refining, chrome refining and plating, and selected aspects of textile and food processing have also been found to be at risk in some studies.[60–62] In addition, the potential of formaldehyde to produce nasopharyngeal cancer in humans is now widely recognized.[63–65]

Vocal Cord Dysfunction

VCD, also referred to as "paradoxic vocal fold motion," is a condition that is frequently confused with asthma. Overlapping symptoms includes episodic dyspnea, cough, and chest tightness. In contrast to asthma, VCD is characterized by inspiratory wheezing (stridor); hoarseness; and a pressure sensation in the throat (globus). VCD involves paradoxic adduction of the vocal cords (folds) during inspiration, as visualized on rhinolaryngoscopy. Alternatively, the condition can be diagnosed on the flow-volume loop with the finding of variable extrathoracic obstruction. Diagnosis is frequently hampered by a lack of reliable provocation maneuvers, although occasional patients with VCD react to inhaled methacholine. A subset of patients with VCD gives a history of initial onset of symptoms in relationship to a one-time, high-level irritant exposure. This diagnostic subgroup has been labeled "irritant-associated VCD."[66]

DIAGNOSIS

Occupational upper airway disorders are diagnosed based on history of exposure at work, physical examination, and for some conditions specialized diagnostic tests. Depending on their availability and degree of standardization, diagnostic techniques are classified here as research versus clinical methods (**Table 3**).[7,67–73]

Occupational and Exposure History

As with any occupational disorder, a careful medical, work, and exposure history is key to recognition and diagnosis. A history of allergies and asthma before the job in question should be clarified. The timing of the onset of symptoms

Table 3
Diagnostic tools for upper airway disorders

General	Specific	Research	Clinical Practice
Medical and exposure history	Occupational and environmental exposure history, temporal relationships between exposures and symptoms	X	X
Questionnaires	Symptom questionnaires	X	X
	Quality-of-life questionnaires	X	X
Direct visualization	Rhinolaryngoscopy	X	X
Allergy testing	In vitro (radioallergosorbent test or enzyme-linked immunosorbent assay)	X	X
	In vivo (skin prick testing)	X	X
Diagnostic radiology	Computerized axial tomography	X	X
Sensory testing	Odor identification (qualitative)	X	X
	Odor detection (quantitative)	X	
Nasal patency	Nasal peak flow	X	X
	Rhinomanometry	X	
	Acoustic rhinometry	X	
	Rhinostereometry	X	
Cytometry	Nasal cytology (curetting)	X	X
	Nasal lavage (cell counts)	X	
Biochemistry	Nasal lavage	X	
Mucociliary clearance	Saccharine transit test	X	

and association with exposures at work, such as improvement away from work, are important to inquire about, as are symptoms among co-workers. As rhinitis becomes more chronic, similar to asthma, patients tend to respond more nonspecifically to a wider array of exposures. Thus, one should inquire about work exposures when rhinitis symptoms first started or became exacerbated.

Questionnaires and Rating Scales

Specialized questionnaires have been developed to document the degree of interference with quality-of-life posed by upper airway allergies. These include the Rhinoconjunctivitis Quality of Life Questionnaire and the Sinonasal Outcome Test.[74,75] These tools can be used to assess symptoms and quality-of-life impairment longitudinally, including documenting the response to therapeutic and environmental interventions.

Physical Examination

Basic physical examination of the upper airway includes anterior rhinoscopy and percussion of the maxillary and frontal sinuses for "tap tenderness." Beyond this basic examination, rhinolaryngoscopy is an easily acquired skill and enables the practiced clinician to visualize the sinus ostia and to more completely evaluate patients for nasal polyposis. Flexible rhinolaryngoscopy also allows for superior visualization of the vocal cords for suspected cases of VCD.

Allergy Testing

The diagnosis of allergic rhinitis is supported by documenting reactivity to the suspect allergen (or mixture). Common practice in North America and in Europe involves either in vivo testing (epicutaneous skin prick) or in vitro serum immunoassays (radioallergosorbent test or enzyme-linked immunosorbent assay) for allergen-specific IgE. Local (nasal) allergen challenge is more commonly performed in Europe than in North America, and has incidentally resulted in the identification of a subset of individuals with positive local challenge but negative evidence for systemic sensitization. This diagnostic subset has given rise to the term "local allergic rhinitis." The implications of local mucosal allergy for occupational rhinitis remain largely unexplored at this time.[76]

Because irritant-associated symptoms, such as nasal congestion and rhinorrhea, may mimic an allergic response, the treating healthcare professional may be faced with a diagnostic challenge in determining responsible etiologic agents and pathophysiologic processes. In contrast to allergy, which typically occurs sporadically among coworkers, a high prevalence rate of symptoms among coworkers favors a diagnosis of irritant rhinitis. In irritant rhinitis the laboratory work-up is characterized by a lack of systemic eosinophilia, the predominance of neutrophils on nasal smear, and when applicable a lack of in vivo or in vitro reactivity to identified workplace allergens. Air monitoring for airborne irritants may be of assistance in industrial settings, but is more often a source of frustration in the investigation of so-called problem buildings.

Diagnostic Radiology

In diagnostic radiology of the upper respiratory tract, computed tomography scanning has largely supplanted the use of plain radiographs. For clinically based research involving sinus computed tomography scans, it is common to use a standardized radiographic scoring system (ie, the Lund-Mackay Score).[77]

Miscellaneous Tests

Of the several tests documenting nasal patency, only nasal peak flow measurement is sufficiently standardized to recommend for routine clinical practice. Nasal peak flow measurements can also be obtained on an ambulatory basis to document the response to allergens (or irritants) encountered on the job. Nasal cytometry, although somewhat laborious, is also sufficiently straightforward to permit incorporation into the clinical work-up. In terms of chemosensory function, the University of Pennsylvania Smell Identification Test is portable and straightforward to administer.

MANAGEMENT
Primary Prevention

Occupational rhinitis and asthma are preventable conditions. In general, primary prevention should follow the so-called hierarchy of industrial hygiene controls: substitution of less hazardous materials; enclosure and ventilation; administrative controls (limited exposure time); and personal protective equipment (eg,. gloves, respirator). This hierarchical approach can, in some instances, prevent incident cases of occupational rhinitis and asthma.[78]

Secondary Prevention

Secondary prevention involves the early detection of disease and interruption of disease progression. Early detection can be achieved by monitoring symptoms (ie, through the use of periodic questionnaires); by documenting physiologic alterations (eg, exaggerated decrements of pulmonary function); or by identifying biomarkers (eg, antigen-specific IgE). The value of surveillance is illustrated by longitudinal studies, which document a higher risk for developing occupational respiratory disorders in the first few years after entering a profession.[79–81] Medical surveillance programs (beginning with preplacement examination, following of workers through apprenticeship, and continuing thereafter) offer the potential for early detection and prevention of disease progression among susceptible individuals.

Tertiary Prevention

For established occupational irritant rhinitis, treatment consists of exposure reduction; nonspecific supportive measures (eg, saline nasal lavage); and occasionally topical steroids. Patients troubled by prominent reflex symptoms (eg, congestion and rhinorrhea) may benefit from the topical cholinergic blocker, ipratropium bromide. In atopic patients with irritant rhinitis, control of intercurrent allergic rhinitis (even if unrelated to the workplace) may also decrease reactivity to chemical irritants.

In occupational allergic rhinitis, timely removal from exposure is the most effective means of preventing disease progression. Effective pharmacotherapy includes topical steroids; selected topical antihistamines (with anti-inflammatory properties); and topical ipratropium bromide for symptomatic treatment of hypersecretion. Oral antihistamines, if used, should be limited to nonsedating varieties. Oral leukotriene receptor antagonists are an option that has been little studied in occupational settings. Nasal irrigation with saline remains a benign intervention that has been reported by some to be of benefit.

SUMMARY

Occupational upper airway disorders are common, and the development of rhinitis likely plays a role in the pathogenesis of lower airway disease. Primary prevention involves exposure controls for irritants and allergens. Secondary prevention (workplace surveillance and selective reassignment) can also help reduce the burden of disease. Tertiary prevention (treatment and disability management) may come into play if a strong sensitizer is involved, or if diagnosis has been delayed and disease progression has occurred.

REFERENCES

1. Laitman JT, Reidenberg JS. Specializations of the human upper respiratory and upper digestive systems as seen through comparative and developmental anatomy. Dysphagia 1993;8:318–25.

2. Baroody FM. Functional anatomy of the upper airway in humans. In: Morris JB, Shusterman DJ, editors. Toxicology of the nose and upper airways. New York: Informa Healthcare; 2010. p. 18–44.

3. Keck T, Leiacker R, Heinrich A, et al. Humidity and temperature profile in the nasal cavity. Rhinology 2000;38:167–71.

4. Snipes MB. Biokinetics of inhaled radionuclides. In: Raabe OG, editor. Internal radiation dosimetry. Madison (WI): Medical Physics Publishing; 1994. p. 181.

5. Cole AM, Dewan P, Ganz T. Innate antimicrobial activity of nasal secretions. Infect Immun 1999;67:3267–75.

6. USPHS. The health consequences of involuntary smoking: a report of the surgeon general. Washington: U.S. Dept. of Health and Human Services, Public Health Service, Centers for Disease Control, Center for Health, Promotion and Education, Office on Smoking and Health; 1986.

7. Solomon WR. Nasal provocative testing. In: Spector SL, editor. Provocation testing in clinical practice. New York: Marcel Dekker; 1995. p. 647–92.

8. Raphael GD, Baraniuk JN, Kaliner MA. How and why the nose runs. J Allergy Clin Immunol 1991; 87:457–67.

9. Baraniuk JN, Merck SJ. Neuroregulation of human nasal mucosa. Ann N Y Acad Sci 2009;1170:604–9.

10. Shusterman D, Hummel T. Nasal trigeminal function: qualitative, quantitative and temporal effects. Ann N Y Acad Sci 2009;1170:181–3.

11. Silver WL, Finger TE. The anatomical and electrophysiological basis of peripheral nasal trigeminal chemoreception. Ann N Y Acad Sci 2009;1170:202–5.

12. Tai CF, Baraniuk JN. Upper airway neurogenic mechanisms. Curr Opin Allergy Clin Immunol 2002; 2:11–9.

13. Braun T, Mack B, Kramer MF. Solitary chemosensory cells in the respiratory and vomeronasal epithelium of the human nose: a pilot study. Rhinology 2011; 49:507–12.

14. Widdicombe J. Nasal and pharyngeal reflexes: protective and respiratory functions. In: Mathew OP, Sant'Ambrogio G, editors. Respiratory function of the upper airway. New York: Marcel Dekker; 1988. p. 233–58.

15. Green BG, Lawless HT. The psychophysics of somatosensory chemoreception in the nose and mouth. In: Getchell T, Doty RL, Bartoshuk LM, et al, editors. Smell and taste in health and disease. New York: Raven Press; 1991. p. 235–53.

16. Cometto-Muniz JE, Cain WS. Sensory irritation: relation to indoor air pollution. Ann N Y Acad Sci 1992; 641:137–51.

17. Hodgson M. Field studies on the sick building syndrome. Ann N Y Acad Sci 1992;641:21–36.

18. Siracusa A, Desrosiers M, Marabini A. Epidemiology of occupational rhinitis: prevalence, aetiology and determinants. Clin Exp Allergy 2000;30:1519–34.

19. Malo JL, Lemiere C, Desjardins A, et al. Prevalence and intensity of rhinoconjunctivitis in subjects with occupational asthma. Eur Respir J 1997;10:1513–5.

20. Slavin RG. The upper and lower airways: the epidemiological and pathophysiological connection. Allergy Asthma Proc 2008;29:553–6.

21. Castano R, Gautrin D, Thériault G, et al. Occupational rhinitis in workers investigated for occupational asthma. Thorax 2009;64:50–4.

22. Fasano MB. Combined airways: impact of upper airway on lower airway. Curr Opin Otolaryngol Head Neck Surg 2010;18:15–20.

23. Redlich CA, Herrick CA. Lung/skin connections in occupational lung disease. Curr Opin Allergy Clin Immunol 2008;8:115–9.

24. Bascom R, Naclerio RM, Fitzgerald TK, et al. Effect of ozone inhalation on the response to nasal challenge with antigen of allergic subjects. Am Rev Respir Dis 1990;142:594–601.

25. Peden DB, Setzer RW Jr, Devlin RB. Ozone exposure has both a priming effect on allergen-induced responses and an intrinsic inflammatory action in the nasal airways of perennially allergic asthmatics. Am J Respir Crit Care Med 1995;151: 1336–45.

26. Fujieda S, Diaz-Sanchez D, Saxon A. Combined nasal challenge with diesel exhaust particles and allergen induces in vivo IgE isotype switching. Am J Respir Cell Mol Biol 1998;19:507–12.

27. Diaz-Sanchez D, Garcia MP, Wang M, et al. Nasal challenge with diesel exhaust particles can induce sensitization to a neoallergen in the human mucosa. J Allergy Clin Immunol 1999;104:1183–8.

28. Diaz-Sanchez D, Rumold R, Gong H Jr. Challenge with environmental tobacco smoke exacerbates allergic airway disease in human beings. J Allergy Clin Immunol 2006;118:441–6.

29. Shusterman D, Murphy MA, Balmes J. Differences in nasal irritant sensitivity by age, gender, and allergic rhinitis status. Int Arch Occup Environ Health 2003; 76:577–83.

30. Shusterman D, Murpy MA, Balmes J. Influence of age, gender and allergy status on nasal reactivity to inhaled chlorine. Inhal Toxicol 2003;15:1179–89.

31. Moscato G, Vandenplas O, Van Wijk RG, et al, European Academy of Allergology and Clinical Immunolgy. EAACI position paper on occupational rhinitis. Respir Res 2009;10:16.

32. Ahman M, Holmstrom M, Cynkier I, et al. Work related impairment of nasal function in Swedish woodwork teachers. Occup Environ Med 1996;53:112–7.

33. Chan OY, Lee CS, Tan KT, et al. Health problems among spice grinders. J Soc Occup Med 1990;40:111–5.

34. Hauser R, Elreedy S, Hoppin JA, et al. Upper airway response in workers exposed to fuel oil ash: nasal lavage analysis. Occup Environ Med 1995;52: 353–8.

35. Torjussen W. Rhinoscopical findings in nickel workers, with special emphasis on the influence of nickel exposure and smoking habits. Acta Otolaryngol 1979;88:279–88.

36. Petruson B, Jarvholm B. Formation of new blood vessels in the nose after exposure to dicumylperoxide at a chemical plant. Acta Otolaryngol 1983;95:333–9.

37. Wiggins P, McCurdy SA, Zeidenberg W. Epistaxis due to glutaraldehyde exposure. J Occup Med 1989;31:854–6.

38. Skoner DP, Hodgson MJ, Doyle WJ. Laser-printer rhinitis [letter]. N Engl J Med 1990;322:1323.

39. Morgan MS, Camp JE. Upper respiratory irritation from controlled exposure to vapor from carbonless copy forms. J Occup Med 1986;28:415–9.

40. Calderon-Garcidueñas L, Osorno-Velazquez A, Bravo-Alvarez H, et al. Histopathologic changes of the nasal mucosa in southwest metropolitan Mexico City inhabitants. Am J Pathol 1992;140:225–32.

41. Calderon-Garcidueñas L, Rodriguez-Alcaraz A, Garcia R, et al. Human nasal mucosal changes after exposure to urban pollution. Environ Health Perspect 1994;102:1074–80.

42. Brooks SM, Weiss MA, Bernstein IL. Reactive airways dysfunction syndrome (RADS): persistent asthma syndrome after high level irritant exposures. Chest 1985;88:376–84.

43. Meggs WJ. RADS and RUDS: the toxic induction of asthma and rhinitis. J Toxicol Clin Toxicol 1994;32:487–501.

44. Meggs WJ, Elsheik T, Metzger WJ, et al. Nasal pathology and ultrastructure in patients with chronic airway inflammation (RADS and RUDS) following an irritant exposure. J Toxicol Clin Toxicol 1996;34:383–96.

45. Krishna G, Mathur JS, Gupta RK. Health hazard amongst chrome industry workers with special reference to nasal septum perforation. Indian J Med Res 1976;64:866–72.

46. Lin SC, Tai CC, Chan CC, et al. Nasal septum lesions caused by chromium exposure among chromium electroplating workers. Am J Ind Med 1994;26:221–8.

47. Shusterman D, Murphy MA. Nasal hyperreactivity in allergic and nonallergic rhinitis: a potential risk factor for nonspecific building-related illness. Indoor Air 2007;17:328–33.

48. Awad el Karim MA, Gad el Rab MO, Omer AA, et al. Respiratory and allergic disorders in workers exposed to grain and flour dusts. Arch Environ Health 1986;41:297–301.

49. Zuskin E, Skuric Z, Kanceljak B, et al. Respiratory findings in spice factory workers. Arch Environ Health 1988;43:335–9.

50. Zuskin E, Skuric Z, Kanceljak B, et al. Respiratory symptoms and lung function in furriers. Am J Ind Med 1988;14:187–96.

51. Zuskin E, Kanceljak B, Pokrajac D, et al. Respiratory symptoms and lung function in hemp workers. Br J Ind Med 1990;47:627–32.

52. Zuskin E, Mustajbegovic J, Schachter EN, et al. Respiratory symptoms and ventilatory capacity in workers in a vegetable pickling and mustard production facility. Int Arch Occup Environ Health 1993;64:457–61.

53. Amoore JA. Effects of chemical exposure on olfaction in humans. In: Barrow CS, editor. Toxicology of the nasal passages. New York: Hemisphere Publishing; 1986. p. 154–90.

54. Cometto-Muniz JE, Cain W. Influence of airborne contaminants on olfaction and the common chemical sense. In: Getchell T, Doty RL, Bartoshuk LM, et al, editors. Smell and taste in health and disease. New York: Raven Press; 1991. p. 765–85.

55. Dalton P. Olfactory toxicity in humans and experimental animals. In: Morris JB, Shusterman DJ, editors. Toxicology of the nose and upper airways. New York: Informa Healthcare; 2010. p. 215–41.

56. Reiffenstein RJ, Hulbert WC, Roth SH. Toxicology of hydrogen sulfide. Annu Rev Pharmacol Toxicol 1992;32:109–34.

57. Snow JB, Doty RL, Bartoshuk LM, et al. Categorization of chemosensory disorders. In: Getchell T, Doty RL, Bartoshuk LM, editors. Smell and taste in health and disease. New York: Raven Press; 1991. p. 445–7.

58. Fukuda K, Shibata A. Exposure-response relationships between woodworking, smoking or passive smoking, and squamous cell neoplasms of the maxillary sinus. Cancer Causes Control 1990;1:165–8.

59. Gordon I, Boffetta P, Demers PA. A case study comparing a meta-analysis and a pooled analysis of studies of sinonasal cancer among wood workers. Epidemiology 1998;9:518–24.

60. Mannetje A, Kogevinas M, Luce D, et al. Sinonasal cancer, occupation, and tobacco smoking in European women and men. Am J Ind Med 1999;36:101–7.

61. Olsen JH. Occupational risks of sinonasal cancer in Denmark. Br J Ind Med 1988;45:329–35.

62. Leclerc A, Luce D, Demers PA, et al. Sinonasal cancer and occupation. Results from the reanalysis of twelve case-control studies. Am J Ind Med 1997;31:153–65.

63. Olsen JH, Jensen SP, Hink M, et al. Occupational formaldehyde exposure and increased nasal cancer risk in man. Int J Cancer 1984;34:639–44.

64. Luce D, Gerin M, Leclerc A, et al. Sinonasal cancer and occupational exposure to formaldehyde and other substances. Int J Cancer 1993;53:224–31.

65. World Health Organization, International Association for Research in Cancer. IARC monographs on the evaluation of carcinogenic risks to humans. Formaldehyde,

2-Butoxyethanol, and 1-tert-Butoxypropan-2-ol, Vol. 88. Geneva (Switzerland): IARC Press; 2006.

66. Perkner JJ, Fennelly KP, Balkissoon R, et al. Irritant-associated vocal cord dysfunction. J Occup Environ Med 1998;40:136–43.

67. Dias MA, Shusterman D, Kesavanthan J, et al. Upper airway diagnostic methods. In: Harber P, Schenker M, Balmes J, editors. Occupational and environmental respiratory disease. St Louis: Mosby-Yearbook; 1996. p. 67–89.

68. Hilberg O, Pederson OF. Acoustic rhinometry: recommendations for technical specifications and standard operating procedures. Rhinol Suppl 2000;16:3–17.

69. Ahman M. Nasal peak flow rate records in work related nasal blockage. Acta Otolaryngol 1992; 112:839–44.

70. Bryan MP, Bryan WT. Cytologic and cytochemical aspects of ciliated epithelium in the differentiation of nasal inflammatory disease. Acta Cytol 1969;13:515.

71. Koster EP. Human psychophysics in olfaction. In: Moulton DG, Turk A, Johnston JW, editors. Methods in olfactory research. New York: Academic Press; 1975. p. 345–74.

72. Corbo GM, Foresi A, Bonfitto P, et al. Measurement of nasal mucociliary clearance. Arch Dis Child 1989;64:546–50.

73. Koren HS, Hatch GE, Graham DE. Nasal lavage as a tool in assessing acute inflammation in response to inhaled pollutants. Toxicology 1990;60:15–25.

74. Juniper EF, Guyatt GH. Development and testing of a new measure of health status for clinical trials in rhinoconjunctivitis. Clin Exp Allergy 1991;21:77–83.

75. Piccirillo JF, Merritt MG Jr, Richards ML. Psychometric and clinimetric validity of the 20-Item sino-nasal outcome test (SNOT-20). Otolaryngol Head Neck Surg 2002;126:41–7.

76. Rondón C, Campo P, Togias A, et al. Local allergic rhinitis: concept, pathophysiology, and management. J Allergy Clin Immunol 2012;129(6):1460–7.

77. Lund VJ, Mackay IS. Staging in rhinosinusitis. Rhinology 1993;31:183–4.

78. Kelly KJ, Wang ML, Klancnik M, et al. Prevention of IgE sensitization to latex in health care workers after reduction of antigen exposures. J Occup Environ Med 2011;53:934–40.

79. Archambault S, Malo JL, Infante-Rivard C, et al. Incidence of sensitization, symptoms, and probable occupational rhinoconjunctivitis and asthma in apprentices starting exposure to latex. J Allergy Clin Immunol 2001;107:921–3.

80. Gautrin D, Ghezzo H, Infante-Rivard C, et al. Long-term outcomes in a prospective cohort of apprentices exposed to high-molecular-weight agents. Am J Respir Crit Care Med 2008;177:871–9.

81. Moscato G, Pala G, Boillat MA, et al. EAACI position paper: prevention of work-related respiratory allergies among pre-apprentices or apprentices and young workers. Allergy 2011;66:1164–73.

Indoor Fuel Exposure and the Lung in Both Developing and Developed Countries: An Update

Akshay Sood, MD, MPH

KEYWORDS

- Biomass • Solid fuel • Chronic obstructive pulmonary disease • Asthma • Lung cancer
- Respiratory tract infection

KEY POINTS

- Around 3 billion people cook and heat their homes with biomass or coal.
- Nearly 2 million people die prematurely from illness attributable to indoor air pollution from household solid fuel use.
- Indoor air pollution from solid fuel use is strongly associated with chronic obstructive pulmonary disease or COPD (both emphysema and chronic bronchitis), acute respiratory tract infections, and lung cancer, and weakly associated with asthma, tuberculosis, and interstitial lung disease.
- Nearly 50% of pneumonia deaths among children less than 5 years of age are due to particulate matter inhaled from indoor air pollution from solid fuel use.
- Worldwide, indoor air pollution from solid fuel use is the number one cause of COPD. Both women and men exposed to indoor smoke are 2 to 3 times more likely to develop COPD than those not similarly exposed.
- Tobacco use potentiates the development of respiratory disease among subjects exposed to solid fuel smoke.
- Additional research to treat diseases caused or exacerbated by pollutants from indoor fuel smoke, including interventional studies, are urgently needed.

INTRODUCTION

There are 4 principal categories of indoor air pollution: combustion products, chemicals, radon, and biologic products. This article focuses on the respiratory health effects of pollutants from combustion of various types of indoor fuels, which is currently a major public health problem in the world.

TYPES OF INDOOR FUELS

Indoor fuels include solid, liquid, and gas fuels (**Box 1**). Solid fuels include biomass and coal.

Biomass fuel refers to any living or recently living plant and/or animal-based material that is deliberately burned by people for fuel such as wood, twigs, dried animal dung (eg, cow dung), charcoal (a product of incomplete burning of wood), grass, or agricultural crop residues (eg, corn husk, straw, and bagasse–biomass remaining after processing sugar cane). Coal, as distinct from charcoal, is a naturally occurring fossil fuel formed from preserved compressed and partially metamorphosed organic material. Coal includes smoky coal (bituminous coal) and smokeless coal (anthracite coal). Liquid fuel includes kerosene and liquefied

Disclosure Statement: The author has no relationship with a commercial company that has a direct financial interest in the subject matter or materials discussed in the article or with a company making a competing product.
Department of Medicine, School of Medicine, Health Sciences Center, University of New Mexico, 1 University of New Mexico, MSC 10 5550, Albuquerque, NM 87131, USA
E-mail address: asood@salud.unm.edu

Clin Chest Med 33 (2012) 649–665
http://dx.doi.org/10.1016/j.ccm.2012.08.003

Box 1
List of indoor fuels

Solid Fuels

    Agricultural crop residues

    Animal dung

    Wood

    Charcoal

    Coal

Liquid Fuels

    Kerosene

    Ethanol and methanol

    LPG

Gas Fuels

    Natural gas

    Methane gas

Electricity

petroleum gas (LPG). Gas fuels include methane and natural gas. LPG and natural gas, in addition to electricity, are widely viewed as clean fuels. The most important determinant of the choice of fuel in a given region of the world is its cost, giving rise to the energy ladder depicted in **Fig. 1**. Worldwide, wood is the most common solid fuel used,

although coal is predominantly used in China and dried cow dung is commonly used in rural South Asia.[1] The primary focus of this review is indoor solid fuels.

BURDEN OF SOLID FUEL-RELATED ADVERSE EFFECTS

In 2007, worldwide, approximately 42% of all households and 76% of all rural households used solid fuels (**Fig. 2**).[2] Most solid fuel users are poor and live in developing countries. Smoke that emanates from the household combustion of solid fuels is thus the most widespread traditional source of indoor air pollution on a global scale. It should, however, be pointed out that solid fuel, primarily wood, is also used in developed countries; 28% of a cohort based in New Mexico, United States, reported wood smoke exposure in a 2010 report.[3] Poorly maintained stoves are an important contributor to indoor air pollution in developed countries as well. Thus, solid fuel use is prevalent in all inhabited continents of the world. Because almost 3 billion people worldwide are exposed to solid fuel smoke, the population at risk worldwide for adverse respiratory effects is very large.

USE OF INDOOR SOLID FUEL

In developing countries, various solid fuels are used primarily for cooking purpose in unvented,

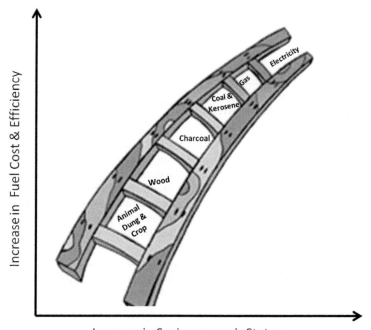

Increase in Fuel Cost & Efficiency

Increase in Socioeconomic Status

Fig. 1. The energy ladder. Fuels lower in the energy ladder are less efficient and produce more pollution, but are less expensive. Conversely, fuels higher in the energy ladder are more efficient and produce less pollution, but are more expensive.

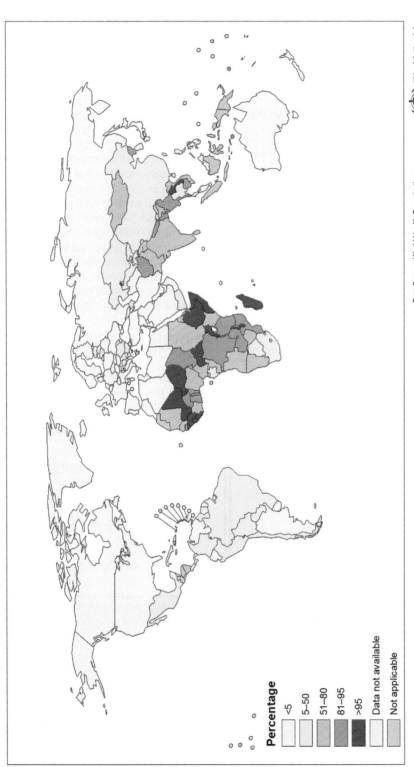

Population using solid fuels (%), 2010
Total

Percentage
- <5
- 5–50
- 51–80
- 81–95
- >95
- Data not available
- Not applicable

The boundaries and names shown and the designations used on this map do not imply the expression of any opinion whatsoever on the part of the World Health Organization concerning the legal status of any country, territory, city or area or of its authorities, or concerning the delimitation of its frontiers or boundaries. Dotted and dashed lines on maps represent approximate border lines for which there may not yet be full agreement.

Data Source: World Health Organization
Map Production: Public Health Information and Geographic Information Systems (GIS) World Health Organization

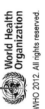 World Health Organization

© WHO 2012. All rights reserved.

Fig. 2. Global use of indoor solid fuels in 2010, as reported in percent, by the World Health Organization (WHO). *(Reproduced from World Health Organization. Global Health observatory map gallery. Map on world populations using solid fuels (%), 2010: total. 2012. Available at: http://gamapserver.who.int/mapLibrary/Files/Maps/Global_iap_2010_total.png; with permission.)*

inefficient, and leaky but inexpensive stoves.[4,5] These stoves typically consist of simple arrangements such as a few stones or a U-shaped hole or a rounded pit and operate under poorly ventilated conditions.[5–7] In developed countries (as well as in developing countries with cold climates), primarily wood is used in home fireplaces and stoves for heating indoors (**Fig. 3**).[8,9]

CONTENTS OF INDOOR SOLID FUEL SMOKE

Indoor solid fuel smoke contains a complex mixture of a large number of pollutants,[10,11] including respirable particulate matter (PM), carbon monoxide, oxides of nitrogen and sulfur, benzene, formaldehyde, 1,3-butadiene, polycyclic aromatic hydrocarbons such as benzo(α)pyrene, free radicals, aldehydes, volatile organic compounds, chlorinated dioxins, oxygenated and chlorinated organic matter, and endotoxin (the latter is raised particularly in smoke from burning maize crop residue and cow dung[1]).

PM Content in Indoor Solid Fuel Smoke

PM_{10} are particles with mass median aerodynamic diameter of less than 10 μm. These particles are easily inhaled and reach the deeper portions of the lung, causing a spectrum of adverse cardiovascular and pulmonary health effects. More recently $PM_{2.5}$ (aerodynamic diameter <2.5 μm)

has been used as a PM metric, reflecting the likelihood that greater toxicity may be attributable to smaller particulates. PM_{10} values ranging from 10,000 to 20,000 μg/m^3 have been reported in households in developing countries[12] that are well above the US Environmental Protection Agency (EPA) national 24-h standard for PM_{10} of 150 μg/m^3.[13] In households with limited ventilation (as is common in many developing countries), exposures experienced by household members may be 100 times higher than World Health Organization (WHO) and EPA guidelines.

Further, smoke from the various solid fuels is not alike. Ellegard reported that wood-burning stoves were associated with a significantly higher release of respirable particles (1260 μg/m^3) compared with either charcoal (540 μg/m^3) or liquefied petroleum gas stoves (200–380 μg/m^3) during cooking time.[14] Some biomass smokes, such as agricultural crop residue smoke, primarily contain particles that are less than 10 μm in diameter and thus may have disproportionately greater respiratory effects than smoke from other biomass fuels.[15]

COMPARISON OF SOLID FUEL SMOKE WITH OTHER COMMON COMBUSTION EMISSIONS

Compared with cleaner indoor fuels (such as kerosene and gas fuels), biomass fuel use is associated with higher concentrations of respirable

Developed Countries	Developing Countries
Primarily residential heating	Primarily cooking activities
Low concentration exposure	High concentration exposure
Both sexes exposed	Women & children highly exposed
Primarily wood	Fuels low on the energy ladder
Single type of exposure	Mixed exposures common

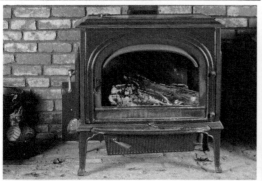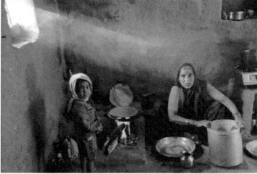

Fig. 3. Key differences in solid fuel exposure between developing and developed countries. (*Adapted from* Salvi SS, Barnes PJ. Chronic obstructive pulmonary disease in nonsmokers. Lancet 2009;374:733–43; with permission.)

particulate matter.[16] Biomass smoke is also associated with greater levels of inflammation and oxidative stress in sputum as well as greater DNA damage in buccal epithelium, as compared with the cleaner fuel LPG.[17] Further, the combustion of biomass is qualitatively similar to the burning of tobacco in terms of emissions of particulate matter and gases, although without the nicotine. Additionally, particles from wood smoke are similar to those from traffic emission in their pro-inflammatory potential, although mediated by different particle characteristics. For example, the organic fraction is the most important particle component in the response to wood smoke, whereas this fraction plays a lesser role in the response to traffic-derived particles.[18] Wood smoke particulate matter also generates greater DNA damage than traffic-generated particulate matter per unit mass in human cell lines, possibly due to the higher level of polycyclic aromatic hydrocarbons in the former.[19]

POPULATIONS MOST AFFECTED BY SOLID FUEL SMOKE

In developing countries, women and young children have the greatest exposure, since they spend the most time near the domestic hearth. Exposure for infants and toddlers is further increased if they are carried on their mother's back while she cooks, a common cultural practice in some regions.[20] The greatest burden among adults in these countries is borne by nonsmoking women,[21] but the process by which solid fuel smoke leads to respiratory disease may begin in early childhood, or even in utero.

In cold climates and highland areas, people spend more time indoors, where they are exposed to fires that burn over extended periods in homes that may have tight construction for space heating.[22] Thus, both pollution levels and exposure times increase, affecting both sexes and children. It is further possible that elderly subjects who spend a majority of their time indoors may also be more vulnerable to the health effects of solid fuel smoke.

MECHANISMS BY WHICH SOLID FUEL SMOKE AFFECTS RESPIRATORY OUTCOMES

There are limited data on the mechanisms by which solid fuel smoke affects the lung (**Box 2**). Macrophage dysfunction, increased proteolytic activity of matrix metalloproteinases (MMPs), greater gene expression of MMP, pulmonary surfactant deactivation, reduced bacterial clearance, and reduced mucociliary clearance have all been reported.[23–29] Chronic obstructive pulmonary

---

Box 2
Mechanisms by which solid fuel smoke may affect respiratory outcomes

Neutrophilic inflammation

Macrophage phagocytic dysfunction and surface adherence

Increased MMP activity (pro-MMP-2; pro-MMP-9, and MMP-9)

Greater MMP gene expression (MMP-2 and MMP-12)

Pulmonary surfactant deactivation

Reduced bacterial clearance

Reduced mucociliary clearance

Up-regulated arginase activity

Greater oxidative stress

Increased apoptosis

DNA damage

Break in integrity of the pulmonary air–blood barrier.

---

disease (COPD) subjects exposed to wood smoke demonstrate an upregulation of arginase activity in their platelets and erythrocytes, which is linked with greater oxidative stress.[30] The high levels of oxidative stress related to wood smoke exposure further mediate increased apoptosis in human cells such as pulmonary artery endothelial cells.[31] In addition, solid fuel smoke produces DNA damage and inflammatory and oxidative stress response gene expression in cultured human cells.[32] Exposure to wood smoke by healthy human volunteers is followed by a rise in serum and urine concentrations of Clara cell protein 16 (CC16), a marker of the integrity of the pulmonary air–blood barrier.[33,34]

LUNG HISTOPATHOLOGICAL EFFECTS OF SOLID FUEL SMOKE EXPOSURE

Rats exposed to chronic wood smoke develop mild bronchiolitis, epithelial cell hyperplasia and hypertrophy, alveolar septal thickening, and emphysema.[35] Similarly, rabbits exposed to dried animal dung smoke show respiratory epithelial cell proliferation, alveolar destruction, and emphysema.[36] Bronchoalveolar lavage obtained from healthy human volunteers acutely exposed to wood smoke reveals a neutrophilic influx.[37]

USEFUL INTERVENTIONS

Intervention studies to modify adverse respiratory outcomes from solid fuel smoke exposure are limited. The most effective way of eliminating exposure to smoke from solid fuels is to switch to cleaner fuels such as electricity, but this option is not always feasible. Other useful interventions reported in the literature for developing countries include the following

- Outdoor relocation of cooking with solid fuels. Women cooking with biomass fuel outdoors are exposed to lower levels of particulate matter as compared with those cooking indoors.[38,39]
- Partitioning of kitchen from living space. The presence of partition to the kitchen does not reduce the exposure of the cook, but reduces exposure to other members in the household.[38]
- Window in kitchen. The presence of an additional window in the kitchen may be associated with lower adverse respiratory effects.[40]
- Improved cook stoves. Improved cook stoves are characterized by a higher efficiency in thermal conversion, a higher heat transfer ratio, and a more complete combustion (and therefore a lower emission of smoke), compared with the traditional counterparts. Improved cook stoves may be accompanied by better removal of smoke by the addition of a chimney. In a parallel randomized wood stove intervention trial in highland Guatemala, the intervention group received an improved stove with chimney, the plancha, whereas the control group continued using open indoor fires.[6] A 50% mean reduction in 48-hour average personal carbon monoxide exposure levels among children 0 to 18 months of age was associated with the improved stove intervention.[6]

Outcomes from interventions, such as better stove design and maintenance, have not been adequately studied in developed countries.

RESPIRATORY OUTCOMES RELATED TO SOLID FUEL SMOKE EXPOSURE

Indoor air pollution from solid fuel use is strongly associated with premature mortality as well as COPD (both emphysema and chronic bronchitis), acute respiratory tract infections, and lung cancer, and weakly associated with asthma, tuberculosis, and interstitial lung disease (**Box 3**).

Overall Mortality

The WHO in its annual report estimated that in 2004 indoor air pollution from solid fuel use was

---

> **Box 3**
> **Diseases associated with smoke from solid fuel use**
>
> Strongly Associated Respiratory Outcomes
>   COPD—emphysema/chronic bronchitis
>   Acute respiratory tract infections/pneumonia
>   Lung cancer (coal smoke)
> Weakly Associated Respiratory Outcomes
>   Asthma
>   Tuberculosis
>   Interstitial lung disease
> Associated non-pulmonary outcomes
>   Cataract
>   Pregnancy-related complications
>   Nasopharyngeal cancer
>   Ischemic heart disease
>   Cor pulmonale

---

responsible for 2.7% of the total annual global burden of disease (over 41 million disability-adjusted life years), and 3.3% of annual premature deaths (almost 2 million), primarily in developing countries.[41] In that report, indoor air pollution ranked tenth on the examined list of risk factor causes of death globally and first among environmental risk factors (ahead of unsafe water/sanitation/hygiene).[41] Further, indoor smoke from solid fuel caused about 21% of lower respiratory tract infections worldwide, 35% of chronic obstructive pulmonary deaths, and about 3% of lung cancer deaths.[41] Unfortunately, the greatest burden of indoor air pollution-related premature deaths is among children from pneumonia.[21]

COPD Outcomes

While cigarette smoking is the leading preventable cause of COPD in the developed world, indoor solid fuel smoke exposure may be the leading preventable cause in lesser developed countries, particularly among women.[42] COPD outcomes studied in relation to solid fuel smoke exposure include emphysema, chronic bronchitis, and poor lung growth. Longitudinal change in lung function attributable to indoor solid fuel smoke exposure has not been studied.

Emphysema
The odds for developing COPD with biomass fuel exposure is about twofold to threefold higher, disproportionately affecting women and young

adults. In one cohort of Colombian women, the population attributable risk for wood smoke causing COPD was 50%.[43]

Cross-sectional studies Multiple cross-sectional studies in developing countries have established an association between biomass fuel use and chronic airflow obstruction.[44–49] A prevalence study of COPD (as defined by postbronchodilator ratio of forced expiratory volume in 1 second to forced vital capacity or FEV_1/FVC <0.70) in 5 cities of Colombia found that biomass stove use for at least 10 years was associated with COPD (odds ratio [OR] 1.50; 95% confidence interval [CI], 1.22–1.86).[48] Further, a study from rural Mexico found that biomass stove use was associated with a 2.8% adjusted decrease in FEV_1/FVC ratio.[49] Additionally, a cross-sectional study of smokers in New Mexico in the United States showed wood smoke exposure to be associated with low postbronchodilator percent predicted FEV_1 and prevalence of COPD with remarkably similar odds ratios (OR 1.96; 95% CI 1.52–2.52) as described in the literature originating from developing countries.[3]

Case–control studies Multiple case–control studies have consistently found an association between cooking with biomass fuel and airflow obstruction.[43,50,51] These studies are from developing countries, with the exception of a study from Barcelona, Spain.[9] The study from Spain (as well as the cross-sectional study from the southwestern United States) suggests that exposed people in developed countries may not be spared from the ill effects of wood smoke.[3,9]

Longitudinal studies Longitudinal studies of the impact of biomass smoke exposure on the development of COPD are few in number, but one study did follow 520 COPD patients over 7 years in Mexico City to assess their mortality risk.[52] Multivariable survival analysis showed that biomass smoke-exposed COPD subjects experienced a similar mortality rate as tobacco smoke-exposed COPD subjects, after adjusting for severity of disease.[52]

Meta-analyses Three meta-analyses show consistent results between biomass smoke exposure and lung function-diagnosed COPD. Kurmi and colleagues[53] examined 13 COPD studies and showed a threefold increased risk (OR 2.96; 95% CI 2.01, 4.37). Hu and colleagues[54] examined 15 studies and showed a 2.4-fold increased risk (OR 2.44; 95% CI 1.9–3.33). Po and colleagues[55] showed a similar risk in women, using 6 studies (OR 2.40; 95% CI 1.47–3.93, **Table 1**). The pooled effect estimates for lung function-diagnosed COPD are generally comparable to those published for chronic bronchitis and higher than those published for doctor-diagnosed COPD.[53]

Interventional studies A Chinese retrospective cohort study found significant reduction in incidence of doctor-diagnosed COPD (relative risk of 0.58 in men, 0.75 in women) in homes where coal was used in improved cooking stoves with chimneys, the effect increasing with time since adoption.[56] There is a need for additional prospective studies and clinical trials to examine changes in incidence and severity of COPD following interventions to decrease solid fuel smoke exposure.

Dose–response relationship Exposure–response analyses show a positive trend, with correlation between developing COPD and increasing level or duration of exposure to biomass smoke.[9,43,48,51,57,58]

Table 1
Overall pooled odds ratios for associations between respiratory outcomes and biomass fuel exposure, compared with other fuel type exposures among children and women

Respiratory Outcome	Number of Studies Included in Meta-analysis	Strength of Association
Acute respiratory tract infection in children[a]	8[b]	3.53 (1.93, 6.43)
Asthma in children	4	0.50 (0.12, 1.98)
Asthma in women	5	1.34 (0.93, 1.93)
Chronic bronchitis in women	6	2.52 (1.88, 3.38)
COPD in women	6	2.40 (1.47, 3.93)

[a] Acute respiratory tract infection in this meta-analysis included both upper and lower respiratory tract infections.
[b] All studies included in the meta-analysis are from developing countries except one study from the United States that examined acute respiratory infections in American Indian children.[73]
Data from Po JY, FitzGerald JM, Carlsten C. Respiratory disease associated with solid biomass fuel exposure in rural women and children: systematic review and meta-analysis. Thorax 2011;66:232–9.

INTERACTION BETWEEN HOST CHARACTERISTICS AND SOLID FUEL SMOKE ON COPD: SEX

While solid fuel-exposed women apparently are at higher risk for developing COPD in developing countries, exposed men may be at higher risk in developed countries.[3] There is possibly no sex predilection toward these outcomes. The higher burden of disease in a certain gender in a region likely reflects the sex-related differences in activities that lead to greater exposure.

Hispanic Ethnicity

In New Mexico in the United States, Hispanic ethnicity may be protective against low lung function and COPD related to wood smoke exposure.[3] Interestingly, Hispanics of New Mexico, characterized by high Native American genetic ancestry, are also similarly protected from COPD due to cigarette smoke exposure.[59]

Cigarette Smoking

Tobacco use may potentiate the development of COPD among subjects exposed to solid fuel smoke.[55] Epidemiologic studies from developing countries demonstrate a greater prevalence of respiratory symptoms and greater degree of airway obstruction in tobacco smokers concomitantly exposed to biomass smoke than either nonbiomass-exposed smokers or nonsmokers exposed to biomass emissions.[54,60,61] A similar additive interaction between wood smoke and cigarette smoke exposures on COPD is described in a study from the United States.[3]

DIFFERENCES BETWEEN SMOKING-RELATED COPD AND BIOMASS-RELATED COPD

Biomass smoke-related COPD is similar to tobacco-smoke related COPD with respect to its clinical, physiologic, and radiological presentation (dyspnea, airway obstruction, air trapping, increased airway resistance, chronic bronchitis, centrilobular emphysema, and pulmonary hypertension); impact on quality of life; mortality rate; histopathological findings (of anthracosis and bronchial squamous metaplasia); and levels of inflammatory cells (neutrophils, eosinophils) and mediators (interleukin [IL]-8, MMP-9 and 8-isoprostanes) in induced sputum.[52,62,63] In contrast, Rivera and colleagues[64] reported that biomass-related COPD was associated with a lesser extent of emphysema and goblet cell metaplasia but greater fibrosis and pigment deposition in the lung parenchyma and thicker pulmonary arterial intima, as compared with cigarette smoke-exposed COPD.

EPIGENETIC SUSCEPTIBILITY

Wood smoke exposure may be more strongly associated with COPD outcomes in the presence of methylated p16 or GATA4 genes in sputum.[3] The study did not find that promoter methylation caused or explained away the wood smoke association with COPD. However, promoter methylation enhanced the susceptibility toward COPD among wood smoke exposed subjects.

COPD-CHRONIC BRONCHITIS

The most common manifestations of domestically acquired particulate lung disease in adults in developing countries are cough-related complaints, specifically chronic bronchitis.

Prevalence

The prevalence rates for chronic bronchitis in communities exposed to indoor biomass smoke are high.[39,46,57,58,60,65] Some of the highest prevalence rates have been reported in rural parts of Nepal (19.8% in nonsmoking women who spent more than 4 hours per day near the fireplace) and Bolivia (22% for all nonsmokers in a village that cooked indoors with cow dung).[39,65]

Strength of Association

Users of biomass fuel had approximately twofold greater rates of chronic bronchitis than those using cleaner fuels such as kerosene or LPG.[60,66] Additionally, a cross-sectional study of smokers in New Mexico showed wood smoke exposure to be associated with chronic bronchitis, with somewhat similar odds ratios (OR 1.64; 95% CI 1.31–2.06), as described in the literature originating from developing countries.[3]

Dose–Response Relationship

In a case–control study of rural nonsmoking Mexican women, the odds for chronic bronchitis were directly related to total cumulative exposure to biomass smoke.[58] Thus, a cumulative exposure of 100 hour–years was associated with an adjusted odds ratio of 9.3, while 200 hour–years of exposure was associated with a higher odds ratio of 15.0 for chronic bronchitis.[58] However, since lower exposures may be associated with higher socioeconomic status and more efficient stove design, these studies are limited by their inability to control for these potential confounders. An interesting occurrence in rural Bolivia has provided an unusual opportunity to control for these factors.[39] Two rural Bolivian villages with no reported tobacco use, identical in every way except for the location of their cooking stoves, were studied.[39] One village had its kitchens indoors (consistent with traditional Bolivian custom), while the other moved their stoves outdoors 50 years earlier due to the perceived ill effects of smoke inhalation on health. The study recorded a twofold higher prevalence of chronic bronchitis in the indoor group compared with the outdoor group (22% vs 13%).[39] By controlling for all confounders including socioeconomic status, floor type, and fuel type, this study provides excellent evidence for the pathogenic role for biomass combustion in the development of chronic bronchitis.

Interventional Studies

In a parallel randomized wood stove intervention trial of Mayan women in highland Guatemala, the intervention group received an improved stove with chimney, the plancha, whereas the control group continued using open indoor fires.[6,67] The intervention group reported a significant reduction in the prevalence of chronic respiratory symptoms, especially wheeze (relative risk for wheeze of 0.42, 95% CI 0.25, 0.70).[67]

POOR LUNG GROWTH AND DEVELOPMENT

Exposure to biomass smoke from an early age may retard lung growth. Various indices of lung function were lower among adolescent and young adult men and women in Nepal (16–25 years old) who were biomass smoke exposed, compared with those who were not.[47] Similarly, lower lung function was observed in school children aged 10 to 13 years living in homes with coal stoves in Chengde and Shanghai cities of China[68] and in 7- to 12-year-old school children exposed to indoor wood stoves in Kuala Lumpur, Malaysia.[69] A retrospective cohort study of 1036 9-year old Polish children living in households heated with gas or coal in the first 6 months of their life, showed that a higher indoor pollution score during the first 6 months of life was strongly associated with lower lung function at age 9 years.[70] These findings suggest an adverse effect of solid fuel smoke exposure on early lung growth. On the other hand, longitudinal decline in lung function has not yet been studied in relation to solid fuel smoke exposure.

ACUTE RESPIRATORY TRACT INFECTIONS

Acute respiratory tract infections (ARIs) can be divided into 2 types—upper respiratory tract

infections (AURIs) and lower respiratory tract infections (ALRIs)—of which ALRIs are associated with a greater risk for death. Infants and children living in homes using solid fuels are at increased risk for developing both AURIs and ALRIs and dying from ALRIs.[23]

Burden Statement

ALRI is a leading contributor to the global burden of disease, accounting for 6.2% of the total disability-adjusted life–years for all ages in the year 2004.[71] ALRI is the primary cause of death in children under 5 years old globally (accounting for 1.4 million deaths in 2010 in this age group).[2] Almost half of deaths in this age group from ALRI are attributable to indoor air pollution from household solid fuel use.[72]

Strength of Association

The odds for ALRIs for children exposed to household biomass smoke have been quantified in a number of studies, the majority from developing countries, but also from the United States and Italy.[50,73,74] Most of these studies have used a case–control design, although several cohort studies have also been done.[75] The overall estimate of the risk of ALRI from 13 studies selected for the meta-analysis conducted by Smith and colleagues[76] for the WHO comparative risk assessment was 2.3 (95% CI 1.9–2.7). The risk was higher among children younger than 2 years (OR 2.5). The highest odds ratio was found for children carried on their mothers' backs while cooking (OR 3.1). An update of this meta-analysis was recently published with a total of 24 studies selected.[77] The overall pooled OR for ALRI in this updated meta-analysis was 1.8 (95% CI, 1.5–2.2). On the other hand, combining acute upper and lower respiratory tract infections in another meta-analysis, higher odds ratio of 3.5 (1.9, 6.4) was described by Po and colleagues.[55]

Dose–Response Relationship

The relationship of the rate of increase in ALRIs on average daily exposure level to PM_{10} is a nonlinear or concave function, with the rate of increase declining for exposures above approximately 1000 to 2000 $\mu g/m^3$.[75]

Mechanism

Impaired respiratory tract defense mechanisms may explain the association between biomass smoke exposure and ARI risk in children.[25,50] Acute exposure to particulate matter reduces mucociliary clearance, resulting in increased residence time of inhaled particles, including microorganisms.[23,24] Animal studies demonstrate impairment in macrophage phagocytic function and surface adherence and reduction in bacterial clearance[25,26] in response to wood smoke (see **Box 2**).

Interventional Trials

In a parallel randomized wood stove intervention trial in highland Guatemala, the intervention group received an improved stove with chimney, the plancha, whereas the control group continued using open indoor fires (**Fig. 4**).[6] The intervention group experienced significant and robust reductions for 3 secondary outcomes: fieldworker-assessed severe pneumonia, physician-diagnosed severe pneumonia, and respiratory syncytial virus-negative severe pneumonia.[6]

LUNG CANCER

Although smoking is the major risk factor for lung cancer worldwide, approximately 1.5% of annual lung cancer deaths are attributed to exposure to carcinogens from indoor solid fuel use.[76] The International Agency for Research on Cancer (IARC) has classified combustion products from coal and biomass fuels as group 1 and group 2A carcinogens, respectively (ie, known and probable carcinogens respectively).[78] Consistent with the IARC classification, the data suggest a stronger association for coal smoke with lung cancer, as compared with exposure to other biomass fuel smoke, in both animals and people.[1,79]

Cross-sectional, case–control, and retrospective longitudinal studies have examined the association between solid fuel smoke and lung cancer. Most, published studies in this field originate from China where smoky (bituminous) coal is widely used for cooking. After adjustment for smoking and chronic airway disease, the 2004 meta-analysis by Smith and colleagues[76] indicated a twofold increase in risk among women from indoor coal smoke exposure (OR 1.94; 95% CI 1.09–3.47), with a lower risk among men (OR 1.51; 95% CI 0.97–2.46). There are fewer studies that examine the risk for lung cancer associated with biomass fuel use. One such study by Behera and Balamugesh[80] reported an adjusted OR of 3.59 (95% CI 1.07–11.97) in an Indian population. Results from a pooled analysis among 4181 cases and 5125 controls from Europe and North America who reported predominant use of wood fuels in their house also showed that wood smoke exposure was associated with increased risk for lung cancer (OR 1.21, 95% CI: 1.06–1.38).[81]

Mechanism

Smoke from solid fuel, particularly bituminous coal, contains high concentrations of carcinogens such as polycyclic aromatic hydrocarbons and benzo[α]pyrene and produces high levels of free radicals and DNA damage in cultured human cells.[32] Further, comparison of various biomass

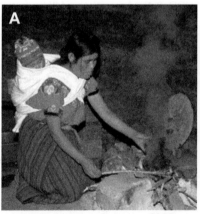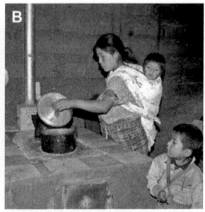

Fig. 4. Traditional open fire used for cooking (*panel A*) and the locally developed and constructed chimney woodstove, the plancha (*panel B*) in Guatemala. The chimney woodstove has a thick metal heating surface for cooking tortillas and holes with removable concentric rings for pots, a firebrick combustion chamber with baffling, a concrete and brick body, tile surfaces around the cooking area, dirt and pumice stone insulation, a metal fuel door, and a metal chimney with damper. Infants and toddlers are highly exposed to combustion smoke as they are carried on their mother's back while she cooks, a common cultural practice in Guatemala and other regions. (*Reprinted from* Smith KR, McCracken JP, Weber MW, et al. Effect of reduction in household air pollution on childhood pneumonia in Guatemala (RESPIRE): a randomised controlled trial. Lancet 2011;378:1719; with permission.)

fuels showed that the DNA damage was most significant with animal dung cake.[17] The direct genotoxicity of solid fuel smoke may thus contribute to the development of lung cancer.

Although it is unclear if the solid fuel smoke affects the histologic distribution of lung cancer among those exposed, a mutation spectrum comprising of TP53 and codon 12 K-ras gene mutations is noted in lung cancers from nonsmokers exposed to smoky coal.[82,83] This mutation spectrum is consistent with an exposure to polycyclic aromatic hydrocarbons, which are the primary component of the smoky coal emissions. In addition, overexpression of the p53 protein is described in coal smoke-related lung cancer tissue.[84,85]

Host Susceptibility Factors

Cigarette smokers may be more susceptible than nonsmokers to developing lung cancer related to exposure to indoor air pollutants.[81,86] This interaction is plausible, given that both tobacco smoke and solid fuel smoke share similar carcinogenic constituents and together may increase the risk for lung cancer to a greater extent than either exposure alone. Further, there may be genetic and epigenetic susceptibility factors. Thus, gene polymorphisms in the glutathione-S-transferase family such as GSTM1 null genotype may increase the susceptibility to lung cancer related to both wood smoke and coal smoke exposures.[84,87] Additionally, promoter methylation of genes (such as p16 gene) in sputum may be associated with greater odds for lung cancer among individuals exposed to smoky coal emissions.[88]

Interventional Study

A retrospective cohort study performed on a cohort of over 20,000 farmers from the Xuan Wei county of China, where smoky coal is used for cooking indoors, lung cancer incidence was noted to be almost halved (hazard ratios of 0.59 among men and 0.54 among women) among residents who had changed from unvented fire pits to stoves with chimneys.[89]

TUBERCULOSIS

There is inconsistent evidence that exposure to biomass smoke increases the risk of either acquiring tuberculosis or progression of tuberculosis to clinical disease.

Mechanism

Exposure to wood smoke results in impaired macrophage phagocytic function and surface adherence, reduced mucociliary clearance,[23] and reduced bacterial clearance.[25,26] These mechanisms may predispose exposed subjects to tuberculosis.[90,91]

Strength of Association

A meta-analysis of 10 studies revealed a pooled effect estimate (OR) of 1.55 (95% CI 1.11, 2.18) for tuberculosis disease.[1] Earlier meta-analyses had yielded similar results.[92]

ASTHMA
Prevalence

Published effect sizes for asthma prevalence in relation to biomass exposure vary considerably. All these studies adopted different techniques to determine asthma prevalence, and none measured actual biomass exposure levels. A meta-analysis of 4 studies showed that exposure to indoor air pollution approximately doubles the risk of developing asthma in children (OR, 1.96; 95% CI 1.29, 2.99).[1] On the other hand, another meta-analysis failed to show a significant association either in children or in women (see **Table 1**).[55]

Severity

Exposure to solid fuel smoke may enhance disease severity among asthmatics. In a small cohort study of children in a boarding house of a metropolitan school in New Zealand, peak levels of air pollution from wood burning were associated with small but statistically significant effects on FEV_1 diurnal variability, morning values of FEV_1, and night time peak expiratory flow rate values in the (doctor-diagnosed) asthmatic students.[93]

Mechanisms

Several mechanisms are hypothesized for the development of asthma due to exposure to solid fuel smoke. High indoor air levels of nitrogen dioxide and sulfur dioxide have been associated with asthma.[94] In the presence of air pollutants, pollen grains become agglomerated with airborne particles.[95] These agglomerated pollens then release higher levels of eicosanoid-like substances that increase serum immunoglobulin (Ig)E, eosinophils, and neutrophils.[96] Samuelsen and colleagues[97] found that particles generated from wood burning had about the same capacity to enhance allergic sensitization as road traffic particles in laboratory animals. Apart from this, biomass smoke contains high levels of endotoxin (especially animal dung smoke) and volatile organic compounds that are risk factors for asthma.[98] Once inhaled, endotoxin stimulates an amplifying series of endotoxin–protein and protein–protein interactions, leading to lung inflammation and oxidative stress, which may contribute to the development of asthma.

INTERSTITIAL LUNG DISEASE (HUT LUNG)

Hut lung, an interstitial lung disease characterized by carbon deposition, dust macules, and mixed dust fibrosis, has been reported in case series primarily of women with chronic high-level exposure to indoor biomass smoke in developing countries.[99–103] This disease has, however, also been described from North Carolina in the United States, where it was attributed to a malfunctioning indoor wood-burning heater.[104]

Although there are currently no longitudinal studies describing the natural history of hut lung, this disease is best described in a case series by Sandoval and colleagues[100] of 30 rural Mexican nonsmoking women in their 60s. These women had a mean exposure to biomass emissions of 400 hour–years. Their main symptoms and signs included dyspnea (100%), cough (93%), cyanosis (63%), and inspiratory crackles on auscultation (70%). Arterial blood gas demonstrated hypoxia with a mean PaO_2 of 45 mm Hg and $PaCO_2$ of 36 mm Hg. Pulmonary function testing usually showed obstruction or mixed obstruction–restriction pattern (although other case series have also described normal lung function[99] or a restrictive pattern[103]). Abnormal chest radiographs were found in 90% of subjects, with 2 to 3 mm reticulonodular opacities the most common findings, followed by cardiomegaly. The opacities closely resembled radiographic categories 2p, 2q, 3p, and 3q for rounded opacities and 2s, 2t, 3s, and 3t for irregular opacities seen in pneumoconiosis.[105] The vast majority had evidence of cor pulmonale with electrocardiographic evidence of right ventricular hypertrophy in 77% of subjects, and a mean pulmonary artery pressure of 46 mm Hg by right heart catheterization. Bronchoscopy revealed grossly visible anthracotic plaques, usually seen at the bifurcations of lobar bronchi. Histopathologic examination of transbronchial biopsy specimens showed thickened basement membranes with diffuse deposition of fine anthracotic particles. Open lung biopsy specimens confirmed the presence of diffuse anthracosis and areas of interstitial fibrosis. Other case series have described the fibrosis as bronchiolocentric in distribution.[103] Although the treatment of this disease is not known, improvement with systemic corticosteroids followed by inhaled corticosteroids has been reported.[103]

HEALTH EFFECTS OF INDOOR COMBUSTION OF CLEANER FUELS
Kerosene

Kerosene is a common cooking fuel in many parts of the world. The emissions and exposures for kerosene combustion are intermediate between those for solid and for gaseous fuels (Smith 1987). However, health effects from kerosene smoke are not adequately studied. In 1 such study, indoor kerosene stoves were associated with low lung function in a cross-sectional evaluation of 7- to 12-year-old Malaysian children.[69] In another cross-sectional study of Indian women, kerosene users had fewer symptoms than biomass fuel users (13% vs 23%) but more than LPG users (8%).[44] A similar trend was noted for lung function in that study.[44]

Gas and Electricity

Studies on the respiratory health effects of exposure to emissions from the 2 major sources of energy used for cooking in developed countries, gas and electricity, have yielded inconsistent results with small effect sizes.[106] Thus, fuels that are highest on the energy ladder do not have the same magnitude of health effects as smoke from solid fuels.

LIMITATIONS OF THE EXISTING LITERATURE

There is a need to address the following critical knowledge gaps:

Lack of actual exposure measurements in most studies adds to misclassification bias. Exposure assessment in most studies is by self-report, and direct measurement of solid fuel smoke exposure is performed in few studies only. Therefore, exposure–response information is also inadequately established in the literature.

Few longitudinal studies have been reported. As a result, the precise effect of solid fuel smoke exposures on longitudinal outcomes (such as decline in lung function or lung growth) or on incidence of chronic diseases is not well understood.

Few interventional studies have been conducted. As a result, the quantification of the effect of improved stoves on longitudinal outcomes or incidence of chronic diseases cannot be accurately assessed.

Small sample size. Studies of small sample size often have insufficient statistical power to reveal possible cause-and-effect relationships.

Inadequate outcome assessment adds to misclassification bias. An example is the use of nonstandard definitions of emphysema or chronic bronchitis. Similarly, the diagnosis of asthma is troublesome, since objective measures of bronchial hyperreactivity have not been used. Therefore, it is not possible to determine whether solid fuel smoke is associated with a pattern of asthma-like symptoms or true asthma. The lack of a uniformly accepted definition of acute respiratory tract infections may similarly cause misclassification bias that may contribute to the heterogeneity in reporting across different studies.

Lack of adjustment for key covariates. Socioeconomic status is an important confounder in these studies, since both solid fuel use and diseases such as tuberculosis and COPD are more prevalent in poorer populations. Cigarette smoking is another important confounder, but no objective measurement of smoking was performed in most studies.

Inadequate understanding of the mechanistic bases for these associations and of the role of genetics and epigenetics in affecting individual susceptibility are additional limitations of this field.

Solid fuel smoke as a risk factor for COPD and lung cancer is not well-characterized in developed countries. This is due to insufficient research on the adverse respiratory effects of relatively lower levels of exposure that are often considered harmless, the overwhelming interest in cigarette smoking as the major risk factor; the mistaken perception among people in these countries that wood (being natural) is benign, and the inadequate awareness that wood smoke may have major respiratory effects when combined with cigarette smoking.

SUMMARY

Smoke from indoor solid fuel combustion for cooking or heating purposes is associated with multiple acute and chronic respiratory conditions. Although indoor solid fuel smoke is likely a greater problem in developing countries, wood-burning populations in developed countries may also be at risk for these conditions, especially when these exposures are combined with cigarette smoking. Studies suggest that lower solid fuel smoke exposure may be associated with lower risk for select respiratory outcomes. It is currently unclear if prevention of chronic disease can be achieved by reducing solid fuel exposure and how much reduction in exposure is required to achieve a useful benefit. It is important to increase awareness about the health effects of solid fuel smoke inhalation among physicians and patients and promote preventive initiatives through education, research, and policy change.

REFERENCES

1. Kurmi OP, Lam KB, Ayres JG. Indoor air pollution and the lung in low and medium income countries. Eur Respir J 2012;40(1):239–54.
2. World Health Organization. World health statistics, 2010. Geneva (Switzerland): World Health Organization; 2010.
3. Sood A, Petersen H, Blanchette CM, et al. Wood smoke exposure and gene promoter methylation are associated with increased risk for COPD in smokers. Am J Respir Crit Care Med 2010;182: 1098–104.
4. Legros G, Havet I, Briuce N, et al. The energy access situation in developing countries: a review focusing on the least developed countries and sub-Saharan Africa. New York: United Nations Development Program; 2009.
5. Miah MD, Rashid HA, Shin MY. Wood fuel use in the traditional cooking stoves in the rural floodplain areas of Bangladesh: a socio-environmental perspective. Biomass Bioenergy 2009;33:70–8.
6. Smith KR, McCracken JP, Weber MW, et al. Effect of reduction in household air pollution on childhood pneumonia in Guatemala (RESPIRE): a randomised controlled trial. Lancet 2011;378:1717–26.
7. Balmes JR. When smoke gets in your lungs. Proc Am Thorac Soc 2010;7:98–101.
8. Semple S, Garden C, Coggins M, et al. Contribution of solid fuel, gas combustion, or tobacco smoke to indoor air pollutant concentrations in Irish and Scottish homes. Indoor Air 2012;22:212–23.
9. Orozco-Levi M, Garcia-Aymerich J, Villar J, et al. Wood smoke exposure and risk of chronic obstructive pulmonary disease. Eur Respir J 2006; 27:542–6.
10. Sallsten G, Gustafson P, Johansson L, et al. Experimental wood smoke exposure in humans. Inhal Toxicol 2006;18:855–64.
11. Zhang J, Smith KR. Indoor air pollution: a global health concern. Br Med Bull 2003;68:209–25.
12. Ezzati M, Kammen DM. The health impacts of exposure to indoor air pollution from solid fuels in developing countries: knowledge, gaps, and data needs. Environ Health Perspect 2002;110: 1057–68.
13. Environmental Protection Agency. National ambient air quality standards for particulate matter; final

rule: 40 CFR part 50. Washington, DC: Federal Register, Government Printing Office; 2006. p. 61144–233.

14. Ellegard A. Cooking fuel smoke and respiratory symptoms among women in low-income areas in Maputo. Environ Health Perspect 1996; 104:980–5.

15. Awasthi A, Singh N, Mittal S, et al. Effects of agriculture crop residue burning on children and young on PFTs in North West India. Sci Total Environ 2010;408:4440–5.

16. Mukkanawar U, Sambhudas S, Juvekar S, et al. Indoor PM2.5 levels in homes using different types of cooking fuels in a rural Indian population and its association with COPD. 183s: Abstract No: P1033. European Respiratory Society Annual Congress. Amsterdam, September 25, 2011.

17. Mondal NK, Bhattacharya P, Ray MR. Assessment of DNA damage by comet assay and fast halo assay in buccal epithelial cells of Indian women chronically exposed to biomass smoke. Int J Hyg Environ Health 2011;214:311–8.

18. Kocbach A, Namork E, Schwarze PE. Proinflammatory potential of wood smoke and traffic-derived particles in a monocytic cell line. Toxicology 2008;247:123–32.

19. Danielsen PH, Loft S, Kocbach A, et al. Oxidative damage to DNA and repair induced by Norwegian wood smoke particles in human A549 and THP-1 cell lines. Mutat Res 2009;674:116–22.

20. Armstrong JR, Campbell H. Indoor air pollution exposure and lower respiratory infections in young Gambian children. Int J Epidemiol 1991; 20:424–9.

21. Ezzati M, Lopez AD, Rodgers A, et al. Selected major risk factors and global and regional burden of disease. Lancet 2002;360:1347–60.

22. Davidson CI, Lin SF, Osborn JF, et al. Indoor and outdoor air pollution in the Himalayas. Environ Sci Technol 1986;20:561–7.

23. Rinne ST, Rodas EJ, Rinne ML, et al. Use of biomass fuel is associated with infant mortality and child health in trend analysis. Am J Trop Med Hyg 2007;76:585–91.

24. Loke J, Paul E, Virgulto JA, et al. Rabbit lung after acute smoke inhalation. Cellular responses and scanning electron microscopy. Arch Surg 1984;119:956–9.

25. Zelikoff JT, Chen LC, Cohen MD, et al. The toxicology of inhaled woodsmoke. J Toxicol Environ Health B Crit Rev 2002;5:269–82.

26. Fick RB Jr, Paul ES, Merrill WW, et al. Alterations in the antibacterial properties of rabbit pulmonary macrophages exposed to wood smoke. Am Rev Respir Dis 1984;129:76–81.

27. Feldbaum DM, Wormuth D, Nieman GF, et al. Exosurf treatment following wood smoke inhalation. Burns 1993;19:396–400.

28. Nieman GF, Clark WR Jr, Wax SD, et al. The effect of smoke inhalation on pulmonary surfactant. Ann Surg 1980;191:171–81.

29. Montano M, Beccerril C, Ruiz V, et al. Matrix metalloproteinases activity in COPD associated with wood smoke. Chest 2004;125:466–72.

30. Guzman-Grenfell A, Nieto-Velazquez N, Torres-Ramos Y, et al. Increased platelet and erythrocyte arginase activity in chronic obstructive pulmonary disease associated with tobacco or wood smoke exposure. J Investig Med 2011;59:587–92.

31. Liu PL, Chen YL, Chen YH, et al. Wood smoke extract induces oxidative stress-mediated caspase-independent apoptosis in human lung endothelial cells: role of AIF and EndoG. Am J Physiol Lung Cell Mol Physiol 2005;289:L739–49.

32. Danielsen PH, Moller P, Jensen KA, et al. Oxidative stress, DNA damage, and inflammation induced by ambient air and wood smoke particulate matter in human A549 and THP-1 cell lines. Chem Res Toxicol 2011;24:168–84.

33. Stockfelt L, Sallsten G, Olin AC, et al. Effects on airways of short-term exposure to two kinds of wood smoke in a chamber study of healthy humans. Inhal Toxicol 2012;24:47–59.

34. Barregard L, Sallsten G, Andersson L, et al. Experimental exposure to wood smoke: effects on airway inflammation and oxidative stress. Occup Environ Med 2008;65:319–24.

35. Lal K, Dutta KK, Vachhrajani KD, et al. Histomorphological changes in lung of rats following exposure to wood smoke. Indian J Exp Biol 1993;31: 761–4.

36. Fidan F, Unlu M, Sezer M, et al. Acute effects of environmental tobacco smoke and dried dung smoke on lung histopathology in rabbits. Pathology 2006;38:53–7.

37. Ghio AJ, Soukup JM, Case M, et al. Exposure to wood smoke particles produces inflammation in healthy volunteers. Occup Environ Med 2012;69: 170–5.

38. Balakrishnan K, Sankar S, Parikh J, et al. Daily average exposures to respirable particulate matter from combustion of biomass fuels in rural households of southern India. Environ Health Perspect 2002;110:1069–75.

39. Albalak R, Frisancho AR, Keeler GJ. Domestic biomass fuel combustion and chronic bronchitis in two rural Bolivian villages. Thorax 1999;54: 1004–8.

40. Kodgule R, Salvi S. Exposure to biomass smoke as a cause for airway disease in women and children. Curr Opin Allergy Clin Immunol 2012;12:82–90.

41. World Health Organization. Global health risks mortality and burden of disease attributable to selected major risks. Geneva (Switzerland): World Health Organization; 2009.

42. Salvi S, Barnes PJ. Is exposure to biomass smoke the biggest risk factor for COPD globally? Chest 2010;138:3–6.

43. Dennis RJ, Maldonado D, Norman S, et al. Woodsmoke exposure and risk for obstructive airways disease among women. Chest 1996;109: 115–9.

44. Dutt D, Srinivasa DK, Rotti SB, et al. Effect of indoor air pollution on the respiratory system of women using different fuels for cooking in an urban slum of Pondicherry. Natl Med J India 1996;9:113–7.

45. Fullerton DG, Suseno A, Semple S, et al. Wood smoke exposure, poverty and impaired lung function in Malawian adults. Int J Tuberc Lung Dis 2011;15:391–8.

46. Golshan M, Faghihi M, Marandi MM. Indoor women jobs and pulmonary risks in rural areas of Isfahan, Iran, 2000. Respir Med 2002;96:382–8.

47. Kurmi OP, Devereux GS, Smith WC, et al. Reduced lung function due to biomass smoke exposure in young adults in rural Nepal. Eur Respir J 2012. [Epub ahead of print].

48. Caballero A, Torres-Duque CA, Jaramillo C, et al. Prevalence of COPD in five Colombian cities situated at low, medium, and high altitude (PREPOCOL study). Chest 2008;133:343–9.

49. Regalado J, Perez-Padilla R, Sansores R, et al. The effect of biomass burning on respiratory symptoms and lung function in rural Mexican women. Am J Respir Crit Care Med 2006;174:901–5.

50. Torres-Duque C, Maldonado D, Perez-Padilla R, et al. Biomass fuels and respiratory diseases: a review of the evidence. Proc Am Thorac Soc 2008;5:577–90.

51. Dossing M, Khan J, al-Rabiah F. Risk factors for chronic obstructive lung disease in Saudi Arabia. Respir Med 1994;88:519–22.

52. Ramirez-Venegas A, Sansores RH, Perez-Padilla R, et al. Survival of patients with chronic obstructive pulmonary disease due to biomass smoke and tobacco. Am J Respir Crit Care Med 2006;173: 393–7.

53. Kurmi OP, Semple S, Simkhada P, et al. COPD and chronic bronchitis risk of indoor air pollution from solid fuel: a systematic review and meta-analysis. Thorax 2010;65:221–8.

54. Hu G, Zhou Y, Tian J, et al. Risk of COPD from exposure to biomass smoke: a meta-analysis. Chest 2010;138:20–31.

55. Po JY, FitzGerald JM, Carlsten C. Respiratory disease associated with solid biomass fuel exposure in rural women and children: systematic review and meta-analysis. Thorax 2011;66:232–9.

56. Chapman RS, He X, Blair AE, et al. Improvement in household stoves and risk of chronic obstructive pulmonary disease in Xuanwei, China: retrospective cohort study. BMJ 2005;331:1050.

57. Pandey MR. Domestic smoke pollution and chronic bronchitis in a rural community of the Hill Region of Nepal. Thorax 1984;39:337–9.

58. Perez-Padilla R, Regalado J, Vedal S, et al. Exposure to biomass smoke and chronic airway disease in Mexican women. A case–control study. Am J Respir Crit Care Med 1996;154:701–6.

59. Bruse S, Sood A, Petersen H, et al. New Mexican Hispanic smokers have lower odds of chronic obstructive pulmonary disease and less decline in lung function than non-Hispanic whites. Am J Respir Crit Care Med 2011;184:1254–60.

60. Behera D, Jindal SK. Respiratory symptoms in Indian women using domestic cooking fuels. Chest 1991;100:385–8.

61. Anderson HR. Chronic lung disease in the Papua New Guinea Highlands. Thorax 1979;34: 647–53.

62. Brashier B, Vanjare N, Londhe J, et al. Comparison of airway cellular and mediator profiles between tobacco smoke-induced COPD and biomass fuel exposure-induced COPD in an Indian population. 2011 European Respiratory Society Annual Congress. Amsterdam, September 25, 2011.

63. Moran-Mendoza O, Perez-Padilla JR, Salazar-Flores M, et al. Wood smoke-associated lung disease: a clinical, functional, radiological and pathological description. Int J Tuberc Lung Dis 2008;12:1092–8.

64. Rivera RM, Cosio MG, Ghezzo H, et al. Comparison of lung morphology in COPD secondary to cigarette and biomass smoke. Int J Tuberc Lung Dis 2008;12:972–7.

65. Pandey MR, Regmi HN, Neupane RP, et al. Domestic smoke pollution and respiratory function in rural Nepal. Tokai J Exp Clin Med 1985;10: 471–81.

66. Malik SK. Exposure to domestic cooking fuels and chronic bronchitis. Indian J Chest Dis Allied Sci 1985;27:171–4.

67. Smith-Sivertsen T, Diaz E, Pope D, et al. Effect of reducing indoor air pollution on women's respiratory symptoms and lung function: the RESPIRE Randomized Trial, Guatemala. Am J Epidemiol 2009;170:211–20.

68. Shen S, Qin Y, Cao Z, et al. Indoor air pollution and pulmonary function in children. Biomed Environ Sci 1992;5:136–41.

69. Azizi BH, Henry RL. Effects of indoor air pollution on lung function of primary school children in Kuala Lumpur. Pediatr Pulmonol 1990;9: 24–9.

70. Jedrychowski W, Maugeri U, Jedrychowska-Bianchi I, et al. Effect of indoor air quality in the postnatal period on lung function in pre-adolescent children: a retrospective cohort study in Poland. Public Health 2005;119:535–41.

71. World Health Organization. The global burden of disease: 2004 update. Geneva (Switzerland): World Health Organization; 2008.

72. World Health Organization. The world health report 2002: reducing risks, promoting healthy life. Available at: http://www.who.int/heli/risks/indoorair/indoorair/en/.

73. Morris K, Morgenlander M, Coulehan JL, et al. Wood-burning stoves and lower respiratory tract infection in American Indian children. Am J Dis Child 1990;144:105–8.

74. Simoni M, Scognamiglio A, Carrozzi L, et al. Indoor exposures and acute respiratory effects in two general population samples from a rural and an urban area in Italy. J Expo Anal Environ Epidemiol 2004;14(Suppl 1):S144–52.

75. Ezzati M, Kammen D. Indoor air pollution from biomass combustion and acute respiratory infections in Kenya: an exposure–response study. Lancet 2001;358:619–24.

76. Smith KR, Mehta S, Maeusezahl-Feuz M. Indoor air pollution from household use of solid fuels: comparative quantification of health risks. In: Ezzati ML, Rodgers A, Murray CJ, editors. Global and regional burden of disease attributable to selected major risk factors. Geneva (Switzerland): World Health Organization; 2004. p. 1435–93.

77. Dherani M, Pope D, Mascarenhas M, et al. Indoor air pollution from unprocessed solid fuel use and pneumonia risk in children aged under five years: a systematic review and meta-analysis. Bull World Health Organ 2008;86:390C–8C.

78. IARC. Household use of solid fuels and high-temperature frying. IARC Monogr Eval Carcinog Risks Hum 2010;95:1–430.

79. Liang CK, Quan NY, Cao SR, et al. Natural inhalation exposure to coal smoke and wood smoke induces lung cancer in mice and rats. Biomed Environ Sci 1988;1:42–50.

80. Behera D, Balamugesh T. Indoor air pollution as a risk factor for lung cancer in women. J Assoc Physicians India 2005;53:190–2.

81. Hosgood HD 3rd, Boffetta P, Greenland S, et al. In-home coal and wood use and lung cancer risk: a pooled analysis of the International Lung Cancer Consortium. Environ Health Perspect 2010;118: 1743–7.

82. DeMarini DM, Landi S, Tian D, et al. Lung tumor KRAS and TP53 mutations in nonsmokers reflect exposure to PAH-rich coal combustion emissions. Cancer Res 2001;61:6679–81.

83. Keohavong P, Lan Q, Gao WM, et al. K-ras mutations in lung carcinomas from nonsmoking women exposed to unvented coal smoke in China. Lung Cancer 2003;41:21–7.

84. Lee KM, Chapman RS, Shen M, et al. Differential effects of smoking on lung cancer mortality before and after household stove improvement in Xuanwei, China. Br J Cancer 2010;103:727–9.

85. Mumford JL, Tian D, Younes M, et al. Detection of p53 protein accumulation in sputum and lung adenocarcinoma associated with indoor exposure to unvented coal smoke in China. Anticancer Res 1999;19:951–8.

86. Tang L, Lim WY, Eng P, et al. Lung cancer in Chinese women: evidence for an interaction between tobacco smoking and exposure to inhalants in the indoor environment. Environ Health Perspect 2010;118:1257–60.

87. Malats N, Camus-Radon AM, Nyberg F, et al. Lung cancer risk in nonsmokers and GSTM1 and GSTT1 genetic polymorphism. Cancer Epidemiol Biomarkers Prev 2000;9:827–33.

88. Liu Y, Lan Q, Shen M, et al. Aberrant gene promoter methylation in sputum from individuals exposed to smoky coal emissions. Anticancer Res 2008;28:2061–6.

89. Lan Q, Chapman RS, Schreinemachers DM, et al. Household stove improvement and risk of lung cancer in Xuanwei, China. J Natl Cancer Inst 2002;94:826–35.

90. Mishra VK, Retherford RD, Smith KR. Cooking with biomass fuels increases the risk of tuberculosis. Natl Fam Health Surv Bull 1999;13:1–4.

91. Mishra VK, Retherford RD, Smith KR. Biomass cooking fuels and prevalence of tuberculosis in India. Int J Infect Dis 1999;3:119–29.

92. Slama K, Chiang CY, Hinderaker SG, et al. Indoor solid fuel combustion and tuberculosis: is there an association? Int J Tuberc Lung Dis 2010; 14:6–14.

93. Epton MJ, Dawson RD, Brooks WM, et al. The effect of ambient air pollution on respiratory health of school children: a panel study. Environ Health 2008;7:16.

94. Tunnicliffe WS, Burge PS, Ayres JG. Effect of domestic concentrations of nitrogen dioxide on airway responses to inhaled allergen in asthmatic patients. Lancet 1994;344:1733–6.

95. Chehregani A, Majde A, Moin M, et al. Increasing allergy potency of zinnia pollen grains in polluted areas. Ecotoxicol Environ Saf 2004;58:267–72.

96. Behrendt H, Kasche A, Ebner von Eschenbach C, et al. Secretion of proinflammatory eicosanoid-like substances precedes allergen release from pollen grains in the initiation of allergic sensitization. Int Arch Allergy Immunol 2001;124:121–5.

97. Samuelsen M, Nygaard UC, Lovik M. Allergy adjuvant effect of particles from wood smoke and road traffic. Toxicology 2008;246:124–31.

98. Semple S, Devakumar D, Fullerton DG, et al. Airborne endotoxin concentrations in homes burning biomass fuel. Environ Health Perspect 2010; 118:988–91.

99. Gold JA, Jagirdar J, Hay JG, et al. Hut lung. A domestically acquired particulate lung disease. Medicine 2000;79:310–7.

100. Sandoval J, Salas J, Martinez-Guerra ML, et al. Pulmonary arterial hypertension and cor pulmonale associated with chronic domestic wood smoke inhalation. Chest 1993;103:12–20.

101. Grobbelaar JP, Bateman ED. Hut lung: a domestically acquired pneumoconiosis of mixed aetiology in rural women. Thorax 1991;46:334–40.

102. Ozbay B, Uzun K, Arslan H, et al. Functional and radiological impairment in women highly exposed to indoor biomass fuels. Respirology 2001;6:255–8.

103. Churg A, Myers J, Suarez T, et al. Airway-centered interstitial fibrosis: a distinct form of aggressive diffuse lung disease. Am J Surg Pathol 2004;28:62–8.

104. Ramage JE Jr, Roggli VL, Bell DY, et al. Interstitial lung disease and domestic wood burning. Am Rev Respir Dis 1988;137:1229–32.

105. Merchant JA, Schwartz DA. Chest radiography for the assessment of the pneumoconioses. In: Rom WN, editor. Environmental and occupational medicine. 3rd edition. Philadelphia: Lippincott-Raven; 1998. p. 293–304.

106. Basu RS. A review of the epidemiological evidence on health effects of nitrogen dioxide exposure from gas stoves. J Environ Med 1999;1:173–87.

Newly Recognized Occupational and Environmental Causes of Chronic Terminal Airways and Parenchymal Lung Disease

Maor Sauler, MD[a], Mridu Gulati, MD, MPH[a,b,*]

KEYWORDS

- Occupational lung disease • Diffuse parenchymal lung disease • Indium lung
- Nylon flock worker's lung • Flavorings-related lung disease • "Popcorn worker's lung"
- World Trade Center lung • Nanoparticles

KEY POINTS

- Occupational health investigators continue to uncover associations between novel exposures and chronic forms of diffuse parenchymal lung disease and terminal airways disease.
- This article details several newly recognized chronic parenchymal and terminal airways diseases related to exposure to indium, nylon flock, diacetyl used in the flavorings industry, nanoparticles, and the World Trade Center disaster are reviewed.
- Additionally, this article reviews methods in worker surveillance and the potential use of biomarkers in the evaluation of exposure–disease relationships.

INTRODUCTION

Chronic parenchymal lung disease comprises a heterogeneous group of disorders that have overlapping clinical, physiologic, and radiologic features. Exposure-related chronic parenchymal lung diseases were thought to be limited to the pneumoconioses and hypersensitivity pneumonitis. However, recent studies have linked new causative occupational and environmental agents with terminal airways disease and parenchymal lung disease. This research has also elucidated the contribution of these exposures to the burden of the so-called idiopathic interstitial pneumonias.[1]

Exploring causality in patients who develop an acute parenchymal process immediately after a high-intensity exposure is usually straightforward; however, inferring causality when chronic lower-level exposures occur over many months to years is challenging. Inferring such associations requires a high index of suspicion, a careful exposure history in individual patients, and a meticulous evaluation of respiratory surveillance data for larger worker cohorts.

Over the years, such agencies as the National Institute for Occupational Safety and Health (NIOSH) have worked with industry to conduct

Disclosures: None.
[a] Section of Pulmonary and Critical Care Medicine, Yale School of Medicine, 15 York Street, New Haven, CT 06510, USA; [b] Yale Occupational and Environmental Medicine Program, Yale School of Medicine, 135 College Street, 3rd Floor, New Haven, CT 06510, USA
* Corresponding author. Section of Pulmonary and Critical Care Medicine, Yale School of Medicine, 135 College Street, 3rd Floor, New Haven, CT 06510.
E-mail address: mridu.gulati@yale.edu

Clin Chest Med 33 (2012) 667–680
http://dx.doi.org/10.1016/j.ccm.2012.09.002
0272-5231/12/$ – see front matter © 2012 Elsevier Inc. All rights reserved.

exposure assessments, review historical and current medical surveillance data, and implement prospective medical surveillance strategies.

This article reviews selected newly identified occupational and environmental causes of chronic terminal airways disease and diffuse parenchymal lung disease during the past 20 years, including indium lung, nylon worker's lung, diacetyl-induced bronchiolitis obliterans, and respiratory disorders related to exposure to toxicants at the site of the attack on the World Trade Center (WTC). The potential toxicity of emerging technologies, such as nanoparticles, is also discussed. Newly recognized causes of acute lung injury, hypersensitivity pneumonitis, pneumoconiosis, and disease related to military service are reviewed elsewhere in this issue. Although the term "diffuse parenchymal lung disease" is preferable for these disorders, given that many affect anatomic structures other than the interstitium, the commonly used term interstitial lung disease (ILD) is also used.

EMERGING DISEASES
Indium Lung

The recent story of indium lung illustrates that new occupational diseases can emerge with the novel use of existing materials. Although the US Bureau of Mines listed indium as a commodity in 1936,[2] the industrial use of this malleable and fusible posttransition metal was limited to production of bearing and dental alloys, nuclear reactor control rods, and semiconductor research until the 1990s. The use of indium–tin oxide for the production of transparent conductive coatings for liquid crystal display and plasma display televisions stimulated an increase in worldwide demand for indium from 371 tons in 1999 to 1340 tons in 2007.[3]

In 2003, Homma and colleagues[4] published the first case report of indium lung in a 27-year-old previously healthy Japanese man who worked on wet-surface polishing of indium–tin oxide targets used for the transparent coatings. The patient developed interstitial pneumonitis three years after he began employment and died four years after clinical presentation. This dramatic case prompted Japanese investigators to conduct epidemiologic investigations to better characterize the burden of disease among workers. Cases have not been limited to Japan. For example, NIOSH concluded that lung disease occurred as a consequence of hazardous levels of indium–tin oxide in a Rhode Island factory prompting the development of formal recommendations to improve the safety of the workers.[5]

Subsequently, investigators have evaluated the prevalence of respiratory symptoms along with physiologic and radiographic abnormalities among indium workers. For example, Chonan and colleagues[6] reported radiographic interstitial changes in 21% of indium workers (23 of 108). In another evaluation conducted in a liquid manufacturing display facility, 53% of workers (8 of 15) in the same job as an employee with documented indium lung left employment before receiving a diagnosis.[6–9]

A multidisciplinary panel consisting of a chest radiologist, a pulmonologist, epidemiologists, and industrial hygienists reviewed the 10 cases of indium lung disease known as of May 2010 (seven in Japan, two in the United States, and one in China). These patients were employed in production, use and reclamation jobs.[4] The two primary findings were pulmonary alveolar proteinosis (PAP) and pulmonary fibrosis. The patients were all men; had a median age at diagnosis of 35 years; presented with the insidious onset of cough, dyspnea, and sputum production. One patient had hemoptysis. The latency period from initial employment to diagnosis was 6 years. Auto-antibodies to granulocyte-macrophage colony–stimulating factor, which have been implicated in the pathogenesis of PAP, were also detected in one patient. Although indium is not known to be carcinogenic, lung cancer has been reported.[10]

The disease process stabilized or improved in only 2 of the 10 patients, one treated with whole-lung lavage and the second without treatment. Two of the eight patients whose condition deteriorated died. Only one of seven patients treated with inhaled or oral corticosteroids had objective improvement, although it was not sustained. Only one of the three patients receiving whole-lung lavage, a treatment used for PAP, had sustained improvement.[7]

Radiographic features of patients with indium lung include PAP patterns and interstitial fibrosis patterns. Chest computed tomography (CT) scan of patients with PAP showed the classic "crazy paving pattern" consisting of ground-glass opacities superimposed on interlobular septal thickening (**Fig. 1**). CT scan of patients with interstitial fibrosis showed traction bronchiectasis, bronchiolectasis, and septal thickening.

Histopathologic evaluation in patients classified as PAP and interstitial fibrosis showed common features. Transbronchial biopsies or surgical biopsies were almost universally obtained. Although only three cases were initially diagnosed histopathologically as PAP, most of the cases deemed to be ILD also had the granular eosinophilic and intra-alveolar exudates characteristic of

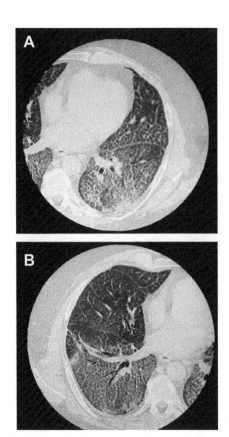

Fig. 1. High-resolution computed tomography scan of indium lung. The left chest (*A*) and right chest (*B*) showing bilateral ground glass opacities, centrilobular nodules, and intralobular and interlobular septal thickening. (*From* Cummings K, Donat W, Ettensohn D. Pulmonary alveolar proteinosis at an indium processing facility. Am J Respir Crit Care Med 2010;181:458–64; with permission.)

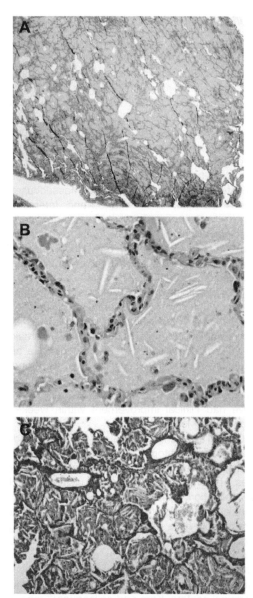

PAP. In addition, fibrosis was noted in all cases, even those initially diagnosed as PAP. Cholesterol clefts with associated granulomas were also noted in all cases (**Fig. 2**). Lung tissue particle analysis confirmed the presence of indium in six patients. Inductively coupled mass spectrometry conducted in one case showed an indium concentration 29.3 μg/g of lung tissue.

A relationship between indium exposure and disease has been suggested based on biomarkers of ILD. For example, KL-6 and surfactant protein D have been shown to be increased in patients exposed to indium in a dose-dependent manner.[10]

Recently, the Japanese Society for Occupational Health has recommended a comparatively much lower serum indium occupational exposure limit of less than 3 μg/L. Routine medical monitoring with symptom surveys and spirometry and baseline chest CT scan was also recommended.[11,12]

Fig. 2. Histopathologic sections of lung biopsy, hematoxylin and eosin stain. (*A*) Low-power overview showing filling of alveolar spaces by eosinophilic material (magnification ×10). (*B*) High-power view showing granular eosinophilic material and cholesterol clefts (magnification ×200). Birefrigent particles were identified with polarizing microscopy, consistent with the presence of crystalline indium–tin oxide. (*C*) Periodic acid–Schiff stain after diastase digestion, showing granular, periodic acid–Schiff positive intraalveolar material, and cholesterol clefts (magnification ×100). (*From* Cummings K, Donat W, Ettensohn D. Pulmonary alveolar proteinosis at an indium processing facility. Am J Respir Crit Care Med 2010;181:458–64; with permission.)

Nylon Flock Worker's Lung

In 1996, NIOSH and Brown University's Program in Occupational Medicine launched an epidemiologic investigation after two young male workers employed in the same Rhode Island nylon flocking plant presented with ILD. The employer requested the assistance of NIOSH through the Health Hazard Evaluation Program to conduct a formal worksite evaluation. Further investigation identified a cluster of eight workers who worked with rotary cut flock. Subsequent study detected affected workers in Rhode Island, Massachusetts, North Carolina, and Ontario, and internationally.[13-16] Even workers who had not sought medical evaluation had evidence of subclinical disease. For example, in one study, 19 of 32 asymptomatic workers had radiographic abnormalities on chest CT scan.[15]

The nylon flock–exposed workers commonly presented with chronic respiratory symptoms over several years, but subacute presentations also occurred. For example, in a Canadian outbreak, 5 of 88 exposed workers developed disease after exposure occurring over several days.[17] A temporal relationship between work and symptoms has not consistently been reported, although many workers have had clinical improvement within weeks to months after leaving work.

Clinical assessment reveals characteristic radiographic and histopathologic patterns (**Figs. 3** and **4**). CT scan shows diffuse micronodular opacities, patchy ground glass opacities, patchy consolidation, and honeycombing. Restrictive ventilatory defects are most common, but obstructive defects have been reported. Histopathologic evaluation commonly shows a nonspecific interstitial pneumonia pattern with characteristic lymphocytic bronchiolitis with peribronchovascular interstitial lymphoid infiltrates with or without germinal centers. Kern and colleagues[14] reported one case of desquamative interstitial pneumonia and another case of bilateral synchronous adenocarcinoma in patients exposed to nylon flock.

NIOSH investigators conducted qualitative and quantitative exposure assessments and medical surveillance that implicated respirable nylon fibers as the causative agent. Toxicologic study showed that rats exposed to intratracheal instillation of nylon flock developed bronchiolocentric inflammation.[16]

Pulmonary disease has been reported only in workers exposed to rotary cut flock as opposed to guillotines, which are most frequently used in this industry. When cutters are not appropriately sharpened and become dull, melting and tailing of the nylon flock ends occur and they tend to break off during milling. High levels of these small

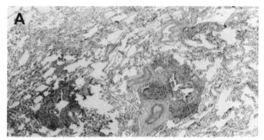

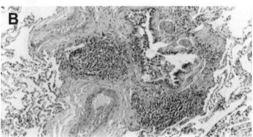

Fig. 3. Nylon flock worker's lung histopathology. Photomicrographs of thoracoscopic lung biopsy specimen from nylon flock plant worker. Histology reveals lymphocyte-predominant infiltrate surrounding bronchiole in center of lobule. Original magnification of photomicrographs (*A*) ×3100 and (*B*) ×3250. (*Data from* Eschenbacher W, Kreiss K, Lougheed D, et al. Nylon flock-associated interstitial lung disease. Am J Respir Crit Care Med 1999;159:2003–8).

respirable particles were found in the flocking room.[18]

The story of flock worker's lung demonstrates the effect of a comprehensive industrial hygiene assessment and control strategy. NIOSH investigations helped lead to the implementation of exposure control measures that have reduced the incidence of the disease over recent years. After initial reports, the American Flock Association established an Occupational Health Committee for the approximately 3000 US employees. Industry efforts to reduce exposure including exhausting of process cyclones to outside, reduction in the use of compressed air for cleaning, improved cutter maintenance, and implementation of medical surveillance programs have reduced the number of reported cases.

WTC-Related Lung Disease

The destruction of the WTC towers on September 11, 2001, resulted in unprecedented respiratory exposure for thousands of rescue workers and residents. For those exposed, irritant-induced asthma or asthmatic bronchitis has received the greatest attention; however, terminal airways disease and ILD, including sarcoidosis and acute eosinophilic pneumonia, have been reported.

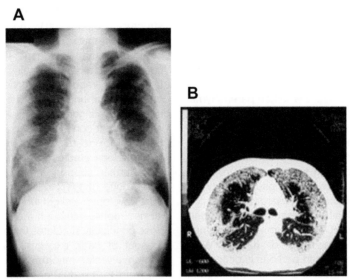

Fig. 4. (*A*) Chest radiograph and (*B*) CT scan results for one of the cases of interstitial lung disease associated with nylon flock processing. The diffuse interstitial involvement is predominantly in a peripheral pattern. (*Data from* Eschenbacher W, Kreiss K, Lougheed D, et al. Nylon flock-associated interstitial lung disease. Am J Respir Crit Care Med 1999;159:2003–8.)

Prezant and colleagues[19–21] reported the phenomenon of "WTC cough" in 332 firefighters and demonstrated a dose-dependent response: 8% of firefighters with peak high exposure (those present at the time of the collapse of the towers), versus 3% with moderate exposure (those present within the first 2 days) and 1% with low exposure (those present within 3–7 days) developed the cough. A prospective cohort of 20,834 responders enrolled in the WTC Medical Monitoring and Treatment Program had an increased lifetime prevalence of asthma from 3% in 2000 to 19% in 2007. An increased prevalence of respiratory symptoms has also been reported in persons living near the towers.

Bronchiolitis has also been reported in persons exposed to WTC dust. Mann and colleagues[22] reported a pathologically confirmed case of chronic bronchiolitis with focal obliterative bronchiolitis that stabilized and improved after azithromycin therapy. In 2010, Wu and colleagues[23] reported the histopathologic presence of small airways disease among seven previously healthy first responders who developed respiratory impairment or radiologic abnormalities.

Like asthma, bronchiolitis may present with dyspnea and cough. Also as in asthma, diagnostic assessment may reveal physiologic airway obstruction and normal chest radiographs. Radiography may show air trapping, a feature commonly overlooked if high-resolution chest CT scans with inspiratory and expiratory images are not performed. Other possible findings include bronchial wall thickening, bronchiectasis, ground-glass opacities, and centrilobular nodules with tree-in-bud appearance. Investigational impulse oscillometry in persons exposed to WTC dust has shown increased airway resistance, reflecting the distal airway abnormalities that occur in terminal airways disease.[24]

Other ILDs reported in patients exposed to the dust include two cases of eosinophilic pneumonitis, including a sentinel case of acute eosinophilic pneumonia in a New York City firefighter whose disorder responded to systemic corticosteroid therapy. Bronchoalveolar lavage revealed 70% eosinophils, and CT scan showed patchy ground-glass density, thickened bronchial walls, and bilateral pleural effusion. Minerologic analysis revealed commercial asbestosis fibers, fly ash, and degraded fiberglass.[25]

Imaging and histopathologic studies have suggested the presence of interstitial fibrosis after exposure to WTC dust. Caplan-Shaw and colleagues[26] reported diverse pathologic findings of patchy interstitial fibrosis and small airway findings with scant lymphoid aggregates. Wu and colleagues[23] reported four cases of diffuse interstitial fibrosis.

Among the terminal airways and interstitial diseases reported in association with WTC dust exposure, sarcoidosis has received the greatest attention. Izbicki and colleagues[27,28] reported 26 cases of sarcoidosis among New York Fire Department rescue workers within 5 years of September 11, 2001, half of whom presented within the first year. The WTC Registry and the WTC Medical Monitoring and Treatment Program have also reported sarcoidosis, including such extrapulmonary findings as uveitis, dermatologic involvement, arthralgias, seizures, and cardiac arrhythmias. All sarcoidosis stages have been reported, including patients with stage I disease with intrathoracic lymphadenopathy and patients with stage II and III disease who had parenchymal disease. In Izbicki's series four of eight patients improved or resolved with corticosteroid therapy.

Establishing causal links between exposure to WTC dust and disease is complicated by several considerations, including limited exposure data, the latency period between exposure and onset of disease, and concerns regarding detection and surveillance bias. General prevalence and incidence data for ILDs are limited, and thus comparing prevalence rates of ILD in WTC exposed versus unexposed persons is difficult.

Additionally, WTC dust is a complex amalgam, and it is difficult to identify the specific toxic components. There exists a complexity of different exposures at different time points because the fires burned during the ensuing months and rescue efforts resuspended settled dust. Because the event was unanticipated and unprecedented, air samples representing the peak exposure at the time of collapse are unavailable. Existing environmental air monitoring stations set up to provide air pollution monitoring surveillance did not capture all pollutants of interest.

Analysis of the coarse medium-sized and large respirable particles of alkaline pH has revealed a mixture of fiberglass, asbestos, aluminum, calcium silicates, and polycyclic hydrocarbons. Asbestos was used only in the early part of the construction of WTC Tower 1 and not at all in Tower 2. In addition to asbestos, the dust contained other materials with fibrogenic potential, such as silica and man-made vitreous fibers. The dust analysis has not demonstrated metals, such as beryllium, zirconium, and tungsten, which have been associated with granulomatous or fibrotic lung disease.[28–31]

Lung tissue analyses support causal relationships between exposure to WTC dust exposure and disease. Mineralogic analysis of the bronchoalveolar lavage fluid from the sentinel case of eosinophilic pneumonia revealed asbestos fibers, degraded fiberglass, and fly ash particles.[25] Induced sputum from New York City firefighters demonstrated particles with minerals, including titanium.[32] In another study, tissue mineralogic analyses from seven responders revealed aluminum, magnesium silicates, asbestos, phosphate, and calcium sulfate and shards of glass containing silica and magnesium. Nanomaterials, such as carbon nanotubes, were detected in three patients. Carbon nanotubes were unlikely present in the building structure before 2001; however, investigators postulated that high temperatures from fuel combustion may have generated large number of carbon nanotubes.[23] Finally, Caplan-Shaw and colleagues[26] reported a study of 12 patients undergoing surgical lung biopsy who demonstrated opaque and birefingent particles within macrophages, particles that containing silica, aluminum silicates, titanium dioxide, talc, and metals.

Toxicology studies in animals and in cultured cells further support the biologic plausibility of the toxicity of WTC dust. Mice exposed to the dust developed a slight increase in bronchoalveolar neutrophils, although the study dust exposure dose principally simulates the high exposure levels present at peak exposure. Studies of cultured human alveolar macrophages and type II cells exposed to the dust showed a dose-dependent increase in proinflammatory cytokines, such as tumor necrosis factor (TNF)-α, interleukin (IL)-6 and -8, and γ-glutamyl transpeptidase.[30,31]

Flavoring-Related Lung Disease (Popcorn Worker's Lung)

In 2000, the Missouri Department of Health received a report of bronchiolitis obliterans in eight workers formerly employed in a microwave popcorn production facility.[33] The Missouri Department of Health in collaboration with industry subsequently enlisted the assistance of NIOSH to develop a protocol to protect the safety of current workers, measure the disease burden among other workers, and investigate and identify the respiratory intoxicant. Mixers and microwave packaging workers were found to be at highest risk. Industrial hygiene sampling demonstrated more than 100 volatile compounds. The greatest risk of airflow obstruction was in workers exposed to high levels of diacetyl, a water-soluble volatile diketone that readily vaporizes and that is used in popcorn production and other food flavoring industries.[34]

Monitoring programs of food flavoring workers expanded, and the California Department of Public Health and the California Division of Occupational Safety and Health (Cal/OSHA) implemented a major public health surveillance program for workers from 20 different flavoring manufacturing companies. Of the 677 workers evaluated, 23% had abnormal spirometry, 4.9% had airways obstruction, and approximately 9.6% had excessive FEV_1 decline with rates of decline greater in companies using more than 800 lb of diacetyl per year. One patient lost 1 L of FEV_1 after approximately 4 months of exposure, a finding that suggests that annual spirometry may not be sufficiently frequent to detect disease.[35] There have been additional case reports from other food plants using flood flavorings that contain diacetyl, such as a British worker at a potato chip factory.[36] Lung disease has also been reported in workers employed at a chemical plant in the Netherlands that produced diacetyl but not other food flavorings, supporting the conclusion that diacetyl is the most likely causative agent.[37]

Studies in animals experimentally exposed to diacetyl have shown evidence of airway tissue injury and necrosis. Continuous exposure to high and subchronic diacetyl concentrations and high brief intense bursts have been associated with injury.[38,39]

Preliminary NIOSH studies suggest that of diacetyl substitutes, such as 2,3-hexanedione, 2,3-heptanedione, and diacetyl trimer, may also have respiratory toxicity. Preliminary NIOSH studies have demonstrated potential toxicity.[40]

Workers with diacetyl lung disease commonly present with cough and exertional dyspnea. Irritation of the eye, nose, and throat and skin involvement may also occur in exposed workers. Both the insidious and rapid onset of disease has been reported. Diagnostic work-up includes pulmonary function testing that shows evidence of obstruction without bronchodilator response. Recent evidence suggests using a cutoff of a 15% decline in FEV_1 per year may not be adequately sensitive to screen for disease. Alternative methods, such as calculating the longitudinal limit of decline, which incorporates data precision, may allow for earlier detection of excessive lung function loss.[41]

Chest radiography is unremarkable, whereas high-resolution CT scan shows subtle findings of bronchial wall thickening and air trapping detectable only on inspiratory and expiratory images (**Fig. 5**). Histopathologic evaluation shows constrictive bronchiolitis obliterans characterized by inflamed and scarred small airways (**Fig. 6**). Induced sputum from workers with high levels of diacetyl exposure show inflammatory responses as evidenced by higher neutrophil counts and levels of IL-8 and eosinophilic cationic protein.[42] Nonsmokers may be at higher risk than smokers.

OSHA issued a Hazard Communication regarding diacetyl that did not establish an occupational exposure limit but did require that manufacturers supply workers with updated toxicologic information and health effects information. With respect to control measures, OSHA suggested effective respiratory protection for workers with higher exposure, including air purifying respirators, and suggested that manufacturers consider industrial hygiene

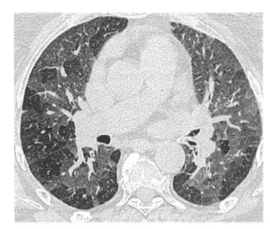

Fig. 5. Bronchiolitis obliterans. High-resolution computed tomography chest scan. Expiratory imaging showing patchy air trapping. (*Courtesy of* Ami Rubinowitz, MD, Yale School of Medicine, New Haven, CT.)

sampling and medical surveillance. In 2011, NIOSH issued a draft criteria document for diacetyl exposure, proposing a recommended exposure limit of 5 parts per billion as an 8-hour time-weight average and a short-term exposure limit of 25 parts per billion. Recommendations for 2,3-pentanedione were also proposed.[43]

Nanoparticles

The implementation of nanoscale materials has the potential to revolutionize multiple industries. Investigators are currently studying the toxicity of nanoparticles as a potential source of occupational lung disease. Nanoparticles have at least one dimension smaller than 100 nm and are further characterized by such physicochemical properties as size, surface area, structure, agglomerativity,

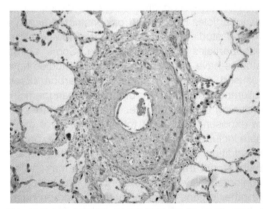

Fig. 6. Constrictive bronchiolitis. Marked submucosal fibrosis causing severe narrowing of the airway lumen. (*Courtesy of* Robert Homer, MD, PhD, Yale School of Medicine, New Haven, CT.)

and solubility. The various categories of nanoparticles include carbon-based (nanotubes); metal-based (eg, titanium dioxide); and biologic (eg, viruses designed for drug delivery). These nanoparticles may lead to more efficient water purification, stronger and lighter building materials, increased computing power, and new nanomedical devices. However, the small size of nanoparticles may result in a range of toxicity.

The interest in nanoparticle toxicity has evolved. In the past, the term ultrafine particles has been used to refer to unintentionally generated nanoparticles, such as those found in air pollution, and nanoparticles that have been intentionally manufactured. Ambient air pollution studies have suggested an association between exposure to the unintentionally generated ultrafine particles and increased cardiopulmonary toxicity.[44] This has contributed to an interest in the potential toxicity of the manufactured nanoparticles. Oberdorster and coworkers[45] published a highly cited paper on the emerging discipline of nanotoxicology and the journal Nanotoxicology began publication in 2007. NIOSH and various international agencies have funded hazard and risk assessments of nanomaterials. The Project on Emerging Technologies at the Woodrow Wilson International Center for Scholars (www.wilsoncenter.org/nano) maintains an updated list of such particles.[46–48]

Although nanoparticles may be ingested or penetrate the skin, nanoparticles easily penetrate the alveoli and can enter the blood circulation reaching the liver, heart, and nervous system within hours. Nanoparticles may be ineffectively cleared by alveolar macrophages if the nanoparticles are agglomerated. The adherence of metals or other organic compounds to nanoparticles may also contribute to toxicity. There are few human studies of the effects of nanoparticles. Computer models have suggested increased deposition of nanoparticles in diseased or constricted airways. Animal studies have demonstrated low levels of nanoparticles distal to the lung. Some animal studies have shown lung toxicity.[49] Studies have focused on carbon nanotubes, carbon black, fullerenes, silica, and metal-based nanoparticles including titanium dioxide. The method and route of exposure can affect toxicity. Routes of exposure include dermal and gastrointestinal exposure in addition to inhalational exposure through the respiratory tract. These factors may affect agglomerativity and the potential for translocation to other organs distal to the lung. Carbon nanotubes have been shown to induce fibrotic and inflammatory responses.[45–48]

There are several pathophysiologic mechanisms through which nanoparticles can cause toxicity. After being ingested, nanoparticles may activate macrophages that then release such proinflammatory mediators as IL-1, IL-6, TNF-α, macrophage inhibitory protein, and monocyte chemotactic protein. Nanoparticles can also lead to the generation of reactive oxygen species and oxidative stress. The proinflammatory and oxidative stress induced by nanoparticles contribute to a milieu that may promote the development of diffuse ILD.

Recently, a case of bronchiolitis obliterans with organizing pneumonia was reported in a 58-year-old man after a 3-month exposure at a polyester powder plant. Transmission electron microscopy of the lung tissue demonstrated the presence of titanium dioxide. With the explosion of nanomaterials in manufacturing, medical surveillance in the workplace is recommended.[50]

Idiopathic Interstitial Pneumonias

The contribution of occupational and environmental exposures to "idiopathic" diseases is likely underappreciated. However, epidemiologic studies have been hampered by the relatively low prevalence and heterogeneity of ILD, limited exposure data, and variability in individual susceptibility to exposure.[51]

Exposure to some agents can cause patterns similar to those seen in specific "idiopathic" interstitial pneumonias. For example, asbestos can cause radiographic changes indistinguishable from idiopathic pulmonary fibrosis, the most common form of idiopathic interstitial pneumonia. A careful occupational history and an evaluation for markers of asbestos exposure, such as pleural plaques on chest CT scans or asbestos bodies on histopathologic examination, can differentiate asbestosis from idiopathic pulmonary fibrosis.[52] Nonspecific interstitial pneumonia may represent the pathologic manifestation of hypersensitivity pneumonitis from exposure to organic antigens, such as avian proteins in bird fancier's lung.[53]

The epidemiologic and pathologic evidence supporting the link between chronic occupational and environmental exposures and the broader group of "idiopathic" interstitial pneumonias has evolved over the years. In the 1980s, several case reports demonstrated a relationship between ILD and exposures in aluminum welders, dairy workers, domestic wood burning, dental technicians, and diamond polishing.[54,55] Lung mineral analyses have also supported the relationship between exposures to mineral dusts and parenchymal lung disease.[56–58]

In 2006, Taskar and Coultas[59] reviewed epidemiologic evidence supporting the causal link between occupational exposures and "idiopathic" interstitial pneumonia. The literature, predominantly based on case-control studies in the United States, Japan, and the United Kingdom, showed an increased risk of ILD was associated with agricultural exposures, livestock, wood dust, metal dust, stone/sand/silica, and smoking. Inconsistent associations between exposure and disease have been noted with textile dust, mold, and wood fires. Dose-dependent associations have been shown for cigarette smoke, metal, and wood exposure.[59-63] A recent study that includes patients in a Swedish oxygen registry suggested associations of ILD in patients with exposure to birch and hardwood dust,[64] and a 2011 Mexican study showed that patients with idiopathic pulmonary fibrosis were more likely than unaffected persons to be former smokers and more likely to have been exposed to "dusts, smokes, gases and chemicals."[65]

Chronic silica exposure has traditionally been linked to the development of simple silicosis or progressive massive fibrosis, but two recent Japanese studies have linked chronic silica exposure to the development of clinicoradiographic patterns characteristic of the idiopathic interstitial pneumonias. Arakawa and coworkers[66] reported that 12% of patients with mixed dust pneumoconioses or silicosis had radiographic evidence of chronic interstitial pneumonia, including idiopathic pulmonary fibrosis. Kitamura and coworkers[67] reported the presence of inorganic dust particles, including silica, in the hilar lymph nodes of patients with idiopathic pulmonary fibrosis. Finally, a recent autopsy study of California farm workers detected increased small airways disease and pneumoconiosis and findings of interstitial fibrosis. Crystalline silica and aluminum silicate particles as demonstrated by scanning electron microscopy and x-ray spectrometry were more prevalent in farm workers than in nonfarm workers.[56]

FUTURE DIRECTIONS IN OCCUPATIONAL AND ENVIRONMENTAL TERMINAL AIRWAYS AND DIFFUSE PARENCHYMAL LUNG DISEASE
Evaluating Causality

Recent discoveries of new causes for interstitial and small airway disease highlight some of the difficulties in recognizing the role of occupational and environmental exposures, including clinician awareness and recognition, misdiagnosis, and limited information on work and environmental exposures, and the presentation of variable clinical phenotypes in response to a single exposure.

The contribution of occupational and environmental exposures should be considered in all patients with diffuse pulmonary diseases (Table 1).

Individual workers with small airways disease and ILD disease are often misdiagnosed with chronic obstructive pulmonary disease or idiopathic pulmonary fibrosis.

Most important, a high index of suspicion and a thorough occupational and environmental history is essential. For more chronic diseases and those with a long latency between exposure and the development of disease, such as asbestosis, it is important to ask about past jobs, which is subject to recall bias. A unique or unusual presentation of disease, such as the presentation of ILD in a younger patient, should prompt a careful exposure history. Investigators should inquire about respiratory symptoms among coworkers or other individuals sharing similar exposures. Clinicians can solicit crude yet effective exposure information from patients by asking simple questions, such as whether visible dust, gases, or fumes are present in the work environment and whether personal protective equipment, such as respirators, is used.

Routine evaluation tools, such as plain chest radiography or office spirometry, may be insufficient to detect terminal airways disease or interstitial disease. For example, air trapping in patients with popcorn worker's lung or subtle reticular markings or ground glass in patients with other forms of interstitial disease, easily missed on chest radiograph, can be detected on high-resolution CT scan. Restrictive ventilatory defects and diffusion impairments require full pulmonary function testing and are missed by routine office spirometry.

When an index case of possible work-related lung disease is identified, the possibility that coworkers may also be affected should always be considered. Ideally, regulatory agencies, industrial hygienists specializing in exposure assessments, and pulmonary medicine and occupational health providers collaborate to investigate the possibility of work-related disease among coworkers or other cohorts with similar exposures. For example, recent reports of indium lung and flavoring-related lung disease in individual patients prompted further investigation by NIOSH, and implementation of medical surveillance, that revealed a greater burden of clinical and subclinical disease among larger cohorts of workers.

When one suspects a correlation between exposure and disease has occurred in one individual patient, it can be difficult to determine if there is a more widespread effect of any particular exposure. Exposures rarely occur without other confounding exposures and can be difficult to measure. The goal of epidemiologic studies is to estimate the relevant exposure and try to find association with disease. Case-control studies

Table 1
Methods for exploring suspected exposure-disease relationships

Methods	Benefits	Limitations
Full Environmental and Occupational History		
• Past and Present exposures • Specific Job tasks • Coworkers or acquaintances with similar disease • Presence of visible dusts, gases, or fumes • Use of a respirator	• Inexpensive • Often available in large datasets (spirometry surveillance)	• Recall Bias • Latency Period • Measure of exposure not specific
Imaging		
• Plain chest radiograph	• Inexpensive • Routinely done in surveillance programs	• May be insensitive to detect subtle abnormalities in terminal airway or Interstitial lung disease
• High Resolution Chest CT (with inspiratory and expiratory imaging)	• Detects more subtle disease such as reticular markings, ground glass and air trapping	• Expensive • Not routinely done in industry surveillance programs • Requires experienced radiologist
Pulmonary Function Testing		
• Spirometry	• Widely available/portable • Longitudinal data records exist • Routine in many surveillance programs	• Often insufficient to detect terminal airway disease or interstitial disease • May misdiagnose terminal airway disease as asthma • Longitudinal surveillance required as accelerated lung function loss may be earliest manifestation
• Lung Volumes and DLCO	• Required for the diagnosis of interstitial and terminal airway disease	• Increased cost • Decreased availability
Exposure Assessment		
• Qualitative exposure: Job type	• Readily available	• Qualitative assessments imprecise
• Quantitative exposure	• Required or performed by industry routinely • Can test suspected agent found in an investigation • Historical data often available • Precise measurements allow for assessment of dose dependence	• Low level exposures or short term peak exposure data may be missing • Often unavailable or insufficient sampling
Animal Toxicology and In-vitro studies	• Provides biologic evidence of toxicity for a suspected agent • Allows investigation into disease mechanisms	• Costly • Requires knowledge of the offending agent • Limitations in extrapolating understanding human disease from animals or in-vitro data
Biomarkers	• Demonstrates biologic effect • Surrogate endpoint for lung injury	• Field still in its infancy • Lack of validation data with disease and disease severity

often use measures of exposure, such as self-report or job exposure or tasks from administrative datasets, but these may be crude or inaccurate. Quantitative exposure assessments that establish dose relationships are preferable but such measurements are often lacking and not mandated or performed in industry. For example, quantitative exposure assessments of respiratory intoxicants at the time of collapse of the WTCs were not available; however, a qualitative measure of exposure (the physical presence of a patient at the actual time of the collapse) has been shown to be an effective means to classify individuals with the highest level of exposure. When new causes of occupational diseases are identified, the causative agent is not always evident. For example, the specific component of WTC dust responsible for disease is still not clear given the number of different exposures that occurred. Industries are required to conduct routine industrial hygiene sampling only for certain specific exposures. Therefore, historical databases of exposures are often unavailable. Finally, even when a novel occupational disease is suspected to correlate with one specific exposure, recommended or required exposure limits for a respiratory toxicant may be completely lacking or far above what has actually caused toxicity in susceptible workers.

Animal studies can support the biologic plausibility of a given exposure causing disease and better understand dose-response relationships and possible mechanisms. Such studies have been performed, for example, in the case of indium lung, nylon flock worker's lung, and diacetyl-induced lung disease.

Detection of foreign material in lung tissue using such methods as polarizable light microscopy or scanning electron microscopy and energy dispersive x-ray spectroscopy, can help evaluate inhalational exposures. For example, scanning electron microscopy and energy dispersive x-ray spectroscopy revealed opaque and birefringent particles with macrophages that contained silica, aluminum silicates, titanium oxide, talc, and metals in a series of patients with ILD exposed to WTC dust.[26] However, the significance of these findings is unclear, given lack of controls and the small sample size. In the case of indium lung, biopsy specimens have confirmed presence of indium in lung tissue. Such methods may also advance the understanding of "idiopathic" lung diseases.

Respiratory Surveillance Programs

Workplace medical surveillance programs can help detect early lung disease and lead to improved preventive strategies. Such programs are based on serial periodic spirometry and symptom surveys and can help detect disease in an individual patient or identify risk factors for disease in an at-risk cohort of workers, such as certain tasks or processes. When lung disease presents in a single or few workers, medical surveillance can help estimate the burden of disease among other workers with similar exposures.

Detecting disease in a working population can be particularly challenging because many workers have "supranormal" lung function or above average levels of spirometric function. This is caused by the healthy worker phenomenon that arises because individuals entering the working force are in general healthier than the general population. The evaluation of longitudinal changes in lung function can help identify workers with excessive declines in lung function, despite apparently normal-appearing lung function. Given the significant variability between individuals, longitudinal changes in individual workers effectively compares an individual to himself or herself. Ideally longitudinal spirometry also includes baseline spirometric testing before the onset of exposure. The case of diacetyl induced lung disease as described previously, for example, clearly demonstrated excessive declines in lung function.[35]

The performance and evaluation of spirometry in workers over time is challenging, including issues related to the quality of the spirometry testing and analysis and interpretation of the results, recently reviewed by Hnizdo and coworkers.[68] Defining excessive declines of lung function over time has been challenging and depend on the quality of the spirometry obtained. Recommendations have varied from greater than 15% yearly FEV_1 loss, or absolute loss of 60 mL/year, or 90 mL/year. Recently, NIOSH has developed a program called Spirometry Longitudinal Data Analysis that can help determine excessive longitudinal lung function loss. This program takes into account the quality and precision of the spirometry testing and calculates a longitudinal limit of normal for lung function decline.

One difficulty with spirometry is the lack of sensitivity or specificity for restrictive disease, which is common in ILD. A reduced forced vital capacity may suggest restrictive disease; however, a formal measurement of total lung capacity is required to make a formal diagnosis. It should be remembered that spirometry and questionnaires performed in the work setting are designed to identify those with possible early lung disease who may need further evaluation, such as full pulmonary function tests and diffusing capacity, and chest imaging. A normal spirometry does not rule out lung disease, and should be interpreted in the context of symptom questionnaire and other relevant information.

Plain chest radiography is insensitive for detecting subtle changes, such as air trapping, groundglass, or reticular markings common in patients with terminal airways disease and interstitial disease. High-resolution chest CT scan can be helpful and detect subtle reticular markings or ground glass opacities. Inspiratory and expiratory imaging can reveal mosaic or air trapping in individuals with terminal airways disease.

Biomarkers

The use of biomarkers of disease in conjunction with epidemiologic data may improve diagnostic capabilities and understanding of occupational disease. Such markers can measure exposure, susceptibility, and effect. Biomarkers of exposure (eg, serum indium concentrations) confirm the presence of a biologic dose and decrease the possibility of exposure misclassification.

Many biomarkers have been evaluated in fibrotic lung disease. KL-6 is a mucin-like protein that is chemotactic for fibroblasts and has been used as a biomarker for ILD. Surfactant proteins and matrix metalloproteases have also been shown to be elevated in ILD. Other implicated proteins include certain chemokines, such as CCL2, YKL-40, and osteopontin. Recent investigations of newly diagnosed terminal airways disease and ILD have used these biomarkers as evidence of lung injury in exposed workers with and without clinically apparent disease. Investigators seeking to characterize the toxicity of indium, for example, use KL-6 and surfactant proteins as biomarkers of effect. Multiple biomarkers have been suggested for silica and coal workers pneumoconioses, including such markers of inflammation as TNF-α, IL-1B, and IL-8 and markers of oxidant injury, such as 8-isoprostanes and glutathione peroxidase activity.[69] Nonetheless, the field is still in its infancy. The validity of using such biomarkers to indicate of disease or disease severity must still be established.

SUMMARY

During the past 20 years several important new causes of occupational and environmental terminal airways disease and diffuse parenchymal lung disease have been recognized, including indium lung, flock-worker's lung, diacetyl lung, the spectrum of WTC lung diseases, WTC lung, and nanoparticle-related lung disease. Despite the increased recognition of occupation hazards in the workplace, these examples highlight the difficulty in evaluating causality despite

advances in the understanding of diffuse parenchymal lung disease. Given that new potential hazards, such as engineered nanoparticles, and unanticipated exposures, such as after the collapse of the WTC, continue to occur, the individual clinician must carefully consider the potential role of occupational exposures in the diagnosis of chronic parenchymal lung and terminal airways disease.

REFERENCES

1. Blanc P. Emerging occupational and environmental respiratory diseases. PCCSU 2009;23.
2. Tyler PM. Minor metals, in minerals. US Bureau of Mines; 1937. p. 759–86.
3. Minami H. Trend of demand, supply and price of indium and gallium. Kinzoku-Shigen Report 2010;81–93.
4. Homma T, Ueno T, Sekizawa K, et al. Interstitial pneumonia developed in a worker dealing with particles containing indium-tin oxide. J Occup Health 2003;45(3):137–9.
5. Cummings KJ, Donat WE, Ettensohn DB, et al. Pulmonary alveolar proteinosis in workers at an indium processing facility. Am J Respir Crit Care Med 2010;181(5):458–64.
6. Chonan T, Taguchi O, Omae K. Interstitial pulmonary disorders in indium-processing workers. Eur Respir J 2007;29(2):317–24.
7. Cummings KJ, Nakano M, Omae K, et al. Indium lung disease. Chest 2012;141(6):1512–21.
8. Nakano M, Omae K, Tanaka A, et al. Causal relationship between indium compound inhalation and effects on the lungs. J Occup Health 2009;51(6):513–21.
9. Nogami H, Shimoda T, Shoji S, et al. Pulmonary disorders in indium-processing workers. Nihon Kokyuki Gakkai Zasshi 2008;46(1):60–4 [in Japanese].
10. Omae K, Nakano M, Tanaka A, et al. Indium lung: case reports and epidemiology. Int Arch Occup Environ Health 2011;84(5):471–7.
11. Ministry of Health, Labor, and Welfare. Technical guidelines for preventing health impairment in the indium tin oxide handling process. 2010. Cited 2012 July 28. Available at: http://www.hourei.mhlw.go.jp/cgi-.
12. ACGIH. Documentation of the threshold limit values and biological exposure indices. ACIGI Hygienists, Editor 2001: Cincinnati.
13. Kern DG, Crausman RS, Durand KT, et al. Flock worker's lung: chronic interstitial lung disease in the nylon flocking industry. Ann Intern Med 1998;129(4):261–72.
14. Kern DG, Kuhn C III, Ely EW, et al. Flock worker's lung: broadening the spectrum of clinicopathology,

narrowing the spectrum of suspected etiologies. Chest 2000;117(1):251–9.

15. Weiland DA, Lynch DA, Jensen SP, et al. Thin-section CT findings in flock worker's lung, a work-related interstitial lung disease. Radiology 2003; 227(1):222–31.

16. Porter DW, Castranova V, Robinson VA, et al. Acute inflammatory reaction in rats after intratracheal instillation of material collected from a nylon flocking plant. J Toxicol Environ Health A 1999; 57(1):25–45.

17. Lougheed MD, Roos JO, Waddell WR, et al. Desquamative interstitial pneumonitis and diffuse alveolar damage in textile workers. Potential role of mycotoxins. Chest 1995;108(5):1196–200.

18. Eschenbacher WL, Kreiss K, Lougheed MD, et al. Nylon flock-associated interstitial lung disease. Am J Respir Crit Care Med 1999;159(6):2003–8.

19. Prezant DJ, Weiden M, Banauch GI, et al. Cough and bronchial responsiveness in firefighters at the World Trade Center site. N Engl J Med 2002; 347(11):806–15.

20. Reibman J, Lin S, Hwang SA, et al. The World Trade Center residents' respiratory health study: new-onset respiratory symptoms and pulmonary function. Environ Health Perspect 2005;113(4):406–11.

21. Guidotti TL, Prezant D, de la Hoz R, et al. The evolving spectrum of pulmonary disease in responders to the World Trade Center tragedy. Am J Ind Med 2011;54(9):649–60.

22. Mann JM, Sha KK, Kline G, et al. World Trade Center dyspnea: bronchiolitis obliterans with functional improvement: a case report. Am J Ind Med 2005; 48(3):225–9.

23. Wu M, Gordon RE, Herbert R, et al. Case report: lung disease in World Trade Center responders exposed to dust and smoke: carbon nanotubes found in the lungs of World Trade Center patients and dust samples. Environ Health Perspect 2010; 118(4):499–504.

24. Friedman SM, Maslow CB, Reibman J, et al. Case-control study of lung function in World Trade Center Health Registry area residents and workers. Am J Respir Crit Care Med 2011;184(5):582–9.

25. Rom WN, Weiden M, Garcia R, et al. Acute eosinophilic pneumonia in a New York City firefighter exposed to World trade center dust. Am J Respir Crit Care Med 2002;166(6):797–800.

26. Caplan-Shaw CE, Yee H, Rogers L, et al. Lung pathologic findings in a local residential and working community exposed to World Trade Center dust, gas, and fumes. J Occup Environ Med 2011;53(9): 981–91.

27. Crowley LE, Herbert R, Moline JM, et al. "Sarcoid like" granulomatous pulmonary disease in World Trade Center disaster responders. Am J Ind Med 2011;54(3):175–84.

28. Izbicki G, Chavko R, Banauch GI, et al. World Trade Center "sarcoid-like" granulomatous pulmonary disease in new York City Fire Department rescue workers. Chest 2007;131(5):1414–23.

29. McGee JK, Chen LC, Cohen MD, et al. Chemical analysis of World Trade Center fine particulate matter for use in toxicologic assessment. Environ Health Perspect 2003;111(7):972–80.

30. Gavett SH, Haykal-Coates N, Highfill JW, et al. World Trade Center fine particulate matter causes respiratory tract hyperresponsiveness in mice. Environ Health Perspect 2003;111(7):981–91.

31. Lioy PJ, Georgopoulos P. The anatomy of the exposures that occurred around the World Trade Center site: 9/11 and beyond. Ann N Y Acad Sci 2006; 1076:54–79.

32. Fireman EM, Lerman Y, Ganor E, et al. Induced sputum assessment in New York City firefighters exposed to World Trade Center dust. Environ Health Perspect 2004;112(15):1564–9.

33. Kreiss K, Gomaa A, Kullman G, et al. Clinical bronchiolitis obliterans in workers at a microwave-popcorn plant. N Engl J Med 2002;347(5):330–8.

34. Centers for Disease Control and Prevention. Fixed obstructive lung disease in workers at a microwave popcorn factory–Missouri, 2000-2002. JAMA 2002; 287(22):2939–40.

35. Kreiss K, Fedan KB, Nasrullah M, et al. Longitudinal lung function declines among California flavoring manufacturing workers. Am J Ind Med 2012;55(8): 657–68.

36. Hendrick DJ. "Popcorn worker's lung" in Britain in a man making potato crisp flavouring. Thorax 2008;63(3):267–8.

37. van Rooy FG, Rooyackers JM, Prokop M, et al. Bronchiolitis obliterans syndrome in chemical workers producing diacetyl for food flavorings. Am J Respir Crit Care Med 2007;176(5):498–504.

38. Morgan DL, Flake GP, Kirby PJ, et al. Respiratory toxicity of diacetyl in C57BL/6 mice. Toxicol Sci 2008;103(1):169–80.

39. Hubbs AF, Goldsmith WT, Kashon ML, et al. Respiratory toxicologic pathology of inhaled diacetyl in Sprague-Dawley rats. Toxicol Pathol 2008;36(2):330–44.

40. Flake GP, Kirby PJ, Price HC, et al. Bronchiolitis obliterans-like lesions in rats treated with diacetyl, acetoin, or acetyl propionyl by intratracheal instillation. The Toxicologist–An official Journal of the Society of Toxicology 2010;114.

41. Chaisson NF, Kreiss K, Hnizdo E, et al. Evaluation of methods to determine excessive decline of forced expiratory volume in one second in workers exposed to diacetyl-containing flavorings. J Occup Environ Med 2010;52(11):1119–23.

42. Akpinar-Elci M, Stemple KJ, Enright PL, et al. Induced sputum evaluation in microwave popcorn production workers. Chest 2005;128(2):991–7.

43. document, n.d., 2011.

44. Donaldson K, Stone V, Seaton A, et al. Ambient particle inhalation and the cardiovascular system: potential mechanisms. Environ Health Perspect 2001;109(Suppl 4):523–7.

45. Oberdorster G, Oberdorster E, Oberdorster J. Nanotoxicology: an emerging discipline evolving from studies of ultrafine particles. Environ Health Perspect 2005;113(7):823–39.

46. Bonner JC. Nanoparticles as a potential cause of pleural and interstitial lung disease. Proc Am Thorac Soc 2010;7(2):138–41.

47. Morimoto Y, Kobayashi N, Shinohara N, et al. Hazard assessments of manufactured nanomaterials. J Occup Health 2010;52(6):325–34.

48. Castranova V. Overview of current toxicological knowledge of engineered nanoparticles. J Occup Environ Med 2011;53(Suppl 6):S14–7.

49. Choi HS, Ashitate Y, Lee JH, et al. Rapid translocation of nanoparticles from the lung airspaces to the body. Nat Biotechnol 2010;28(12):1300–3.

50. Cheng TH, Ko FC, Chang JL, et al. Bronchiolitis obliterans organizing pneumonia due to titanium nanoparticles in paint. Ann Thorac Surg 2012;93(2):666–9.

51. Glazer CS, Newman LS. Occupational interstitial lung disease. Clin Chest Med 2004;25(3):467–78, vi.

52. American Thoracic Society. Diagnosis and initial management of nonmalignant diseases related to asbestos. Am J Respir Crit Care Med 2004;170(6):691–715.

53. Vourlekis JS, Schwarz MI, Cool CD, et al. Nonspecific interstitial pneumonitis as the sole histologic expression of hypersensitivity pneumonitis. Am J Med 2002;112(6):490–3.

54. Pujol JL, Barneon G, Bousquet J, et al. Interstitial pulmonary disease induced by occupational exposure to paraffin. Chest 1990;97(1):234–6.

55. Sherson D, Maltbaek N, Heydorn K. A dental technician with pulmonary fibrosis: a case of chromium-cobalt alloy pneumoconiosis? Eur Respir J 1990;3(10):1227–9.

56. Schenker MB, Pinkerton KE, Mitchell D, et al. Pneumoconiosis from agricultural dust exposure among young California farmworkers. Environ Health Perspect 2009;117(6):988–94.

57. Pariente R, Berry JP, Galle P, et al. A study of pulmonary dust deposits using the electron microscope in conjunction with the electron sound analyser. Thorax 1972;27(1):80–2.

58. Monso E, Tura JM, Marsal M, et al. Mineralogical microanalysis of idiopathic pulmonary fibrosis. Arch Environ Health 1990;45(3):185–8.

59. Taskar VS, Coultas DB. Is idiopathic pulmonary fibrosis an environmental disease? Proc Am Thorac Soc 2006;3(4):293–8.

60. Baumgartner KB, Samet JM, Coultas DB, et al. Occupational and environmental risk factors for idiopathic pulmonary fibrosis: a multicenter case-control study. Collaborating Centers. Am J Epidemiol 2000;152(4):307–15.

61. Baumgartner KB, Samet JM, Stidley CA, et al. Cigarette smoking: a risk factor for idiopathic pulmonary fibrosis. Am J Respir Crit Care Med 1997;155(1):242–8.

62. Hubbard R, Cooper M, Antoniak M, et al. Risk of cryptogenic fibrosing alveolitis in metal workers. Lancet 2000;355(9202):466–7.

63. Hubbard R, Lewis S, Richards K, et al. Occupational exposure to metal or wood dust and aetiology of cryptogenic fibrosing alveolitis. Lancet 1996;347(8997):284–9.

64. Gustafson T, Dahlman-Hoglund A, Nilsson K, et al. Occupational exposure and severe pulmonary fibrosis. Respir Med 2007;101(10):2207–12.

65. Garcia-Sancho C, Buendia-Roldan I, Fernandez-Plata MR, et al. Familial pulmonary fibrosis is the strongest risk factor for idiopathic pulmonary fibrosis. Respir Med 2011;105(12):1902–7.

66. Arakawa H, Johkoh T, Honma K, et al. Chronic interstitial pneumonia in silicosis and mix-dust pneumoconiosis: its prevalence and comparison of CT findings with idiopathic pulmonary fibrosis. Chest 2007;131(6):1870–6.

67. Kitamura H, Ichinose S, Hosoya T, et al. Inhalation of inorganic particles as a risk factor for idiopathic pulmonary fibrosis: elemental microanalysis of pulmonary lymph nodes obtained at autopsy cases. Pathol Res Pract 2007;203(8):575–85.

68. Hnizdo E, Glindmeyer HW, Petsonk EL. Workplace spirometry monitoring for respiratory disease prevention: a methods review. Int J Tuberc Lung Dis 2010;14(7):796–805.

69. Gulumian M, Borm PJ, Vallyathan V, et al. Mechanistically identified suitable biomarkers of exposure, effect, and susceptibility for silicosis and coal-worker's pneumoconiosis: a comprehensive review. J Toxicol Environ Health B Crit Rev 2006;9(5):357–95.

Occupational and Environmental Causes of Lung Cancer

R. William Field, PhD, MS[a],*, Brian L. Withers, DO[b]

KEYWORDS

- Lung • Cancer • Environmental • Occupational • Carcinogen • Epidemiology
- International Agency for Research on Cancer

KEY POINTS

- If considered independently from tobacco smoking, environmentally and occupationally related causes of lung cancer are among the top 10 causes of cancer mortality in the United States.
- The goal of this review was to describe the occurrence and recent findings of the 27 agents currently listed by the International Agency for Research on Cancer (IARC) as lung carcinogens, including the categories of ionizing radiation, chemicals and mixtures, occupational exposures, metals, dust and fibers, personal habits, and other exposures.
- Supplementary new information, with a focus on analytic epidemiologic studies that have become available since IARC's most recent evaluation, is also discussed.

BRIEF EPIDEMIOLOGY OF LUNG CANCER

Although lung cancer incidence rates started to slowly decrease for men in the 1980s followed by declining incidence rates for women in the late 1990s,[1] lung and bronchus cancer remain the leading cause of cancer mortality in the United States, with an estimated 87,750 and 72,590 deaths predicted to occur in men and women, respectively, in 2012.[2] Globally, approximately 75% of lung cancer cases are attributable in part to smoking tobacco, with a higher estimate of 85% to 90% for the United States.[3–6] Of note, women are more likely than men to have nonsmoking-related lung cancer.[7,8] In a study of 6 large prospective epidemiologic cohort studies primarily performed in the United States, Wakelee and colleagues[8] found that the age-adjusted lung cancer incidence rates for individuals 40 to 79 years of age who never smoked ranged from 14.4 to 20.8 per 100,000 person-years in women and 4.8 to 13.7 per 100,000 person-years in men.

Because tobacco smoking is a potent carcinogen, secondary causes of lung cancer are often diminished in perceived importance. If considered in its own disease category, however, lung cancer in never smokers would represent the seventh leading cause of cancer mortality globally, surpassing cancers of the cervix, pancreas, and prostate,[5] and among the top 10 causes of death in the United States.[7,9] Because of the significant number of lung cancer deaths occurring among individuals who have never

Funding sources: Dr Field: NIOSH Grant T42 OH008491, NIEHS Grant P30 ES05605. Dr Withers: NIOSH Grant T42 OH008491.
Conflict of interest: No Conflicts.
[a] Department of Occupational and Environmental Health, Department of Epidemiology, College of Public Health, University of Iowa, 105 River Street, Iowa City, IA 52242, USA; [b] Department of Occupational and Environmental Health, Occupational Medicine, Heartland Center for Occupational Health and Safety, College of Public Health, University of Iowa, 105 River Street, Iowa City, IA 52242, USA
* Corresponding author.
E-mail address: bill-field@uiowa.edu

Clin Chest Med 33 (2012) 681–703
http://dx.doi.org/10.1016/j.ccm.2012.07.001

smoked, it is apparent that there are important risk factors for lung cancer other than tobacco smoking that can contribute substantially to the lung cancer mortality in never smokers.[5,7,9–12] In fact, these other lung carcinogens often act in an additive or synergistic manner in individuals who smoke tobacco products.[13,14]

In a frequently cited paper published in 1981, Doll and Peto[15] estimated that occupational exposures are responsible for 15% and 5% of lung cancer in men and women, respectively, in the United States. The 2008 to 2009 President's Cancer Panel Report[16] indicated that the cancer risk estimates suggested by Doll and Peto,[15] as well as risk estimates from similar studies,[17,18] "are woefully out of date, given our current understanding of cancer initiation as a complex multifactorial, multistage process."

To complicate risk assessment further, the Panel[16] pointed out that fewer than 10% of the more than 80,000 chemicals currently in use in the United States have been evaluated for safety. The primary objective of this article is to provide a brief overview of the environmental and occupational lung carcinogens currently listed by the International Agency for Research on Cancer (IARC) as known human lung carcinogens. Supplementary new information, with a focus on analytic epidemiologic studies that have become available since IARC's most recent evaluation, is also discussed.

IARC GROUP 1 LUNG CARCINOGENS AND CARCINOGENIC AGENTS

The IARC prepares, with the assistance of international working groups of experts, evaluations of carcinogenicity for a wide range of human exposures. The IARC classifies agents as follows:

- Carcinogenic to humans (Group 1)
- Probably carcinogenic to humans (Group 2A)
- Possibly carcinogenic to humans (Group 2B)
- Not classifiable as to its carcinogenicity to humans (Group 3)
- Probably not carcinogenic to humans (Group 4)

Agents classified as known Group 1 lung carcinogens are listed in **Table 1** and include the categories of ionizing radiation, chemicals and mixtures, occupational exposures, metals, dust and fibers, personal habits, and other exposures. Starting in 2009, several IARC panels reassessed the carcinogenicity of Group 1 agents in each of the categories listed. The assessments were published in 2012 as Volume 100 C through F of the IARC Monographs, see http://monographs.iarc.fr/ENG/Monographs/PDFs/index.php.

One of the agents, indoor emissions from household combustion (eg, coal), is predominantly an environmental lung carcinogen; 16 agents are primarily occupational lung carcinogens (although environmental exposures occur); and 8 agents are both potential environmental and occupational lung carcinogens. For purposes of this overview on occupational and environmental lung carcinogens, the chemotherapy regimen of mechlorethamine, oncovin, procarbazine, and prednisone (MOPP), which was developed in the 1960s to treat Hodgkin lymphoma,[19] as well as the well-known IARC Group 1 carcinogens (tobacco smoking, indoor emissions from household combustion [eg, coal], and secondhand tobacco smoke, also referred to as environmental tobacco smoke), are not discussed. A detailed discussion on secondhand smoke is presented in an earlier article by Dela Cruz and colleagues[14] in this journal. Discussion concerning the health effects of tobacco smoking[14,20] are limited to describing selected interactions with other lung carcinogens.

IARC Group 1 Lung Carcinogens: Ionizing Radiation

All types of ionizing radiation have been documented to be carcinogenic to humans (ie, Group 1). The types of radiation primarily identified as lung carcinogens are α-particles, γ-rays, and x-rays.[21] **Fig. 1** displays the relative contribution of the various sources of radiation to the US population.[22] Nearly half (48%) of the average individual's radiation exposure in the United States comes from medically related procedures, with most of the remaining radiation exposure coming from exposure to radon-222 decay products.[22]

Ionizing radiation: α-particles

All internalized radionuclides that emit α-particles, including radon-222 decay products and plutonium-239, are classified as Group 1 carcinogens by IARC.[23] Alpha-particles are somewhat unique among occupational and environmental carcinogens, because of their ability to produce a higher relative rate of double-strand DNA breaks compared with other types of ionizing radiation. Cells that have been hit by an α-particle, as well as nearby cells (ie, the so-called "bystander effect"),[24] may undergo genetic changes that lead to cancer.[25] Alpha-particles can also produce reactive oxygen intermediates that can produce oxidative damage to the DNA.[25] A single bronchial epithelial cell that has sustained genetic damage can initiate lung cancer.[25] Because cancer is thought to originate from a single cell (ie, monoclonal) that has completed the process of malignant transformation, it is unlikely a threshold exists for α-particle–induced

Table 1
Group 1 IARC carcinogens with sufficient evidence of causing lung cancer in humans and primary type of exposure

Agent	Primary Exposure Type
Ionizing radiation-all types	
• Alpha-particle emitters	E,O
○ Radon-222 and its decay products	E,O
○ Plutonium-239	O
• X-radiation, gamma-radiation	E,O
Chemicals and mixtures	
• Bis(chloromethyl)ether; chloromethyl methyl ether	O
• Coal-tar pitch	O
• Soot	O
• Sulfur mustard	O
• Diesel exhausts	E,O
Occupations	
• Aluminum production	O
• Coal gasification	O
• Coke production	O
• Hematite mining (underground)	O
• Iron and steel founding	O
• Painting	O
• Rubber production industry	O
Metals	
• Arsenic and inorganic arsenic compounds	E,O
• Beryllium and beryllium compounds	O
• Cadmium and cadmium compounds	O
• Chromium (VI) compounds	O
• Nickel compounds	O
Dust and fibers	
• Asbestos (all forms)	E,O
• Silica dust, crystalline	E,O
Personal habits	
• Coal, indoor emissions from household combustion	E
• Tobacco smoke, secondhand	E,O
Other exposures	
• Tobacco smoking	—
• MOPP (vincristine-prednisone-nitrogen mustard-procarbazine mixture)	—

Abbreviations: E, environmental exposure; IARC, International Agency for Research in Cancer; O, occupational exposure.

lung cancer.[25] For additional information on the lung cancer risk posed by alpha particles, see http://monographs.iarc.fr/ENG/Monographs/vol100D/mono100D.pdf.

Ionizing radiation (α-particles): radon-222 and its decay products Radon-222 (radon) and its decay products are the oldest known occupational carcinogens.[26–29] Radon is a colorless radioactive noble gas with a half-life of 3.8 days that is formed as part of the uranium-238 decay chain.[30] Because several of the radionuclides (ie, uranium-234, thorium-230, and radium-226) between uranium-238 and radon-222 have relatively long half-lives,

there is a constant source of radon production in the ground (eg, soil, rocks, groundwater). Although radon occurs naturally outdoors, radon can accumulate in underground structures, such as mines, as well as built environments, such as homes, offices, and schools.[30] The potential for radon exposure varies by geographic areas (eg, see http://www.epa.gov/radon/pdfs/zonemapcolor.pdf); however, even structures built in areas with low radon potential can exhibit greatly elevated radon concentrations.

As radon undergoes radioactive decay, it produces a series of solid radioactive decay products that can be inhaled. Two of the short-lived

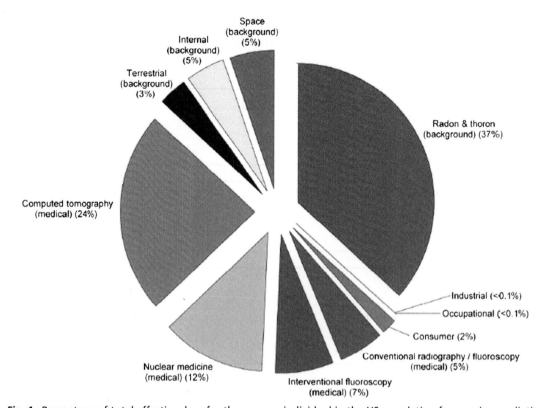

Fig. 1. Percentage of total effective dose for the average individual in the US population from various radiation sources. Percent values rounded to the nearest 1%, except for those <1%. (*Reprinted* with permission of the National Council on Radiation Protection and Measurements, http://NCRPpublications.org.)

radon decay products, polonium-218 and polonium 214, deliver most of the radiation dose, via α-decay, to the bronchial epithelial cells. Deposition of radon decay products in the lung depends on several factors, including particle size, tidal lung volume, respiratory rate, and lung volume.[25,30]

The causative link between protracted radon decay product exposure and lung cancer has been firmly documented in the numerous retrospective mortality studies of uranium and hard rock underground miners performed throughout the world. In the late 1990s, the National Research Council's Biologic Effects of Ionizing Radiation (BEIR) VI Committee pooled the raw data from 11 major retrospective mortality studies of uranium and hard rock underground miners.[25] The study included approximately 68,000 miners with 1.2 M person-years of follow-up and more than 2700 lung cancer deaths. Each of the 11 studies reported significantly increased lung cancer mortality with increasing exposure to radon decay products and a synergistic (albeit sub-multiplicative) interaction between cigarette smoking and radon decay product exposure. The BEIR VI committee also

performed a subset study of miners who had a mean radon exposure of 14.8 Working Level Months (WLMs) (14×10^{-5} per mJ h m^{-3}). The risk estimates for this subgroup that was exposed to radon exposures comparable to protracted exposure at the Environmental Protection Agency's (EPA) action level of 4 pC/L (ie, 14.8 WLMs) were similar to the findings using the overall pooled data set.[25,31] Based on the pooled results, the International Commission on Radiological Protection[32] recently indicated that a lifetime excess absolute risk of 5×10^{-4} per WLM should be used as the nominal probability coefficient for radon progeny-induced lung cancer.

Although **Fig. 1** indicates that occupational exposure to ionizing radiation accounts for less than 0.1% of the average individual's radiation exposure in the United States, 30 years of exposure at the current Mine Safety and Health Administration's and Occupational Safety and Health Administration's (OSHA) permissible exposure limit for cumulative radon decay product exposure of 4 WLMs per year would result in a 6% increase in lifetime risk of lung cancer.[33] Since the publication of the BEIR VI report, additional miner studies have been published that continue to support the original risk estimates from the miner cohort studies.[32–37]

In addition to radon's role as an occupational lung carcinogen, radon exposure occurring outside the workplace also presents an important environmental lung cancer risk. Based on projections from the radon-exposed underground miner studies, the BEIR VI Committee estimated (ie, central risk estimate based on 2 models) that approximately 18,600 lung cancer deaths occur each year in the United States from nonoccupational radon decay product exposure.[25] In 2003, the EPA updated the estimate to 21,100 (13.4%) of the total 157,400 lung cancer deaths that occurred in the United States in 1995.[37] The EPA projected that a lifetime exposure at the EPA's radon action level (ie, 4 pCi/L) yields a 2.3% risk of lung cancer for the US population overall, 4.1% for individuals who smoked at least 100 cigarettes in their lives, and 0.73% for individuals who never smoked.[38]

To directly examine the risk of protracted radon exposure in the residential setting, 22 major case-control residential radon studies were performed in the late 1980s and 1990s.[30,31,39–42] Two of the studies were performed in China,[39] 13 in Europe,[40] and 7 in North America.[41] Of the 22 case-control studies, 19 reported increased risk estimates at 2.7 pCi/L (100 Bq/m^3),[31] which is below the EPA radon action level of 4 pCi/L. The raw data from Chinese, North American, and European studies were pooled to increase study power. The pooled odds ratios (ORs) at 2.7 pCi/L (100 Bq/m^3) for the China, Europe, and North America case control studies were 1.13 (95% confidence interval [CI] 1.01–1.36), 1.08 (95% CI 1.03–1.16), and 1.11 (95% CI 1.00–1.28), respectively. After corrections for random uncertainties in radon assessment, the OR for the European pooling increased to 1.16 (95% CI 1.05–1.31). A similar increase in the OR was also noted for the North American pooled analyses when data were restricted on the basis of completeness of radon measurement data. Although other potential sources of nondifferential radon exposure misclassification could not be ruled out, it would tend to bias the observed association toward the null (eg, the true effect is underestimated).[42]

In summary, after stratification for smoking, the pooled analyses provided direct evidence of an association between protracted residential radon exposure and lung cancer. The studies exhibited a linear dose-response relationship with no evidence of a threshold with risk estimates very comparable to the OR of 1.12 (95% CI 1.02–1.25) extrapolated from the BEIR VI risk models for radon. The findings of the pooled analyses suggest that 8% to 15% of the lung cancer risk in Europe and North America is attributable to radon decay product exposure.[41] Because of the large population at risk and the widespread potential for protracted exposures, residential radon decay products are likely the leading environmental cause of cancer mortality in the United States[30,43] and the seventh leading cause of cancer mortality overall (**Fig. 2**). For additional information on the lung cancer risk posed by radon, see www.breathingeasier.info.

Ionizing radiation (α-particles): plutonium-239 Plutonium-239 (^{239}Pu) is a manmade silvery gray radioactive metal, with a 24,110-year half-life, that undergoes radioactive decay by α-particle emission. Its primary use is in nuclear weapons and nuclear power production (ie, mixed-oxide fuel).[44] In the United States, workers involved with the chemical or mechanical processing of plutonium for nuclear weapons production are at greatest risk of exposure.[44] The primary source of exposure for nuclear workers is inhalation of dust contaminated with ^{239}Pu. After inhalation of ^{239}Pu, it is redistributed primarily to lung, liver, and bone.[44,45] Pulmonary absorption of inhaled plutonium follows a 2-phase model with absorption half-times of months and years.

The IARC's 2001 evaluation of the carcinogenicity of ^{239}Pu relied primarily on the dose-response relationship findings[45] for ^{239}Pu exposure and lung cancer for highly exposed workers at the Mayak Nuclear Processing Plant in the Russian Federation. Although studies[46–48] performed in the United States have only suggested increased lung cancer risk for ^{239}Pu-exposed workers, the causal relationship was strengthened in IARC's 2012 evaluation,[45] which reported on several follow-up studies of ^{239}Pu-exposed Mayak workers that incorporated improved assessment of smoking, dosimetry, and work history data.[46–55] Overall, the follow-up studies reported a statistically significant dose-response relationship between estimated ^{239}Pu lung dose and lung cancer, with no observed departure from linearity or threshold. The most recent follow-up study,[53] published in 2008, estimated excess relative risks for lung cancer per gray (Gy) at attained age 60 years, with adjustment for smoking, was 7.1 (95% CI 4.9–10.0) for males and 15 (95% CI 7.6–29.0) for females. For additional information on ^{239}Pu, see http://monographs.iarc.fr/ENG/Monographs/vol100D/mono100D.pdf.

Ionizing Radiation: X-rays and γ-Rays

A large proportion of the x-ray dose received by the average person in the United States each year is from medically related external exposure from computed tomography (24%), interventional fluoroscopy (7%), or conventional radiography and fluoroscopy procedures (5%) (see **Fig. 1**). The

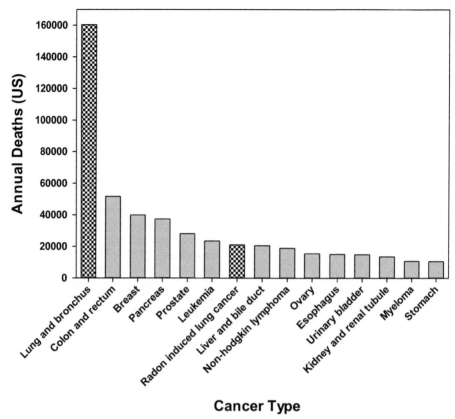

Fig. 2. Estimated number of cancer deaths in the United States for 2012. (*Source*: http://onlinelibrary.wiley.com/doi/10.3322/caac.20138/full#fig1.)

percentage of the total effective dose has increased for these procedures, as well as for nuclear medicine procedures that often use γ-ray emitting radioisotopes (eg, inhalation of technetium-99 m for lung scans). In fact, the collective dose received by the US population in the early 1980s was 7 times lower than in 2006.[22] The low proportion of occupational exposure (ie, <0.1%) observed in **Fig. 1** reflects the low percentage of workers in the United States who are at risk for radiation exposure (eg, nuclear power workers, x-ray technicians), as well as the low percentage who received recordable radiation doses.

The IARC previously classified x-rays and γ-rays as Group 1 lung carcinogens in 2000[23] based primarily on the findings of the Lifespan Study (LSS) of atomic bomb survivors in Hiroshima and Nagasaki, Japan. Lung cancer was the second leading type of cancer, following stomach cancer, in the LSS cohort. The recent 2012 IARC monograph[23] continues to update x-ray and γ-ray cancer risk estimates based primarily on findings from the LSS cohort,[56,57] as well as with supplemental findings from populations exposed to medical procedures.[58]

In a more recent study, not included in the IARC review,[45] that included 105,404 LSS subjects and 1803 primary lung cancer incident cases that were identified for the period 1958 to 1999, Furukawa and colleagues[59] reported that relative to individuals who never smoked, the joint effect between radiation and smoking was supermultiplicative for light or moderate smokers, with a rapid increase in excess risk with smoking intensity up to about 10 cigarettes per day. For smokers who smoked a pack or more per day, however, the investigators reported the joint effect was additive or subadditive. The non–gender-specific average excess relative risk per Gy at attained age 70 was 0.59 (95% CI 0.31–1.00) for nonsmokers, with a female:male ratio of 3.1. The investigators concluded that the "joint effect of smoking and radiation on lung cancer in the LSS is dependent on smoking intensity and is best described by the generalized interaction model rather than a simple additive or multiplicative model." For additional information on the lung cancer risk posed by x-ray and γ-ray exposure, see http://monographs.iarc.fr/ENG/Monographs/vol100D/index.php.

IARC Group 1 Lung Carcinogens: Chemicals and Mixtures

Bis(chloromethyl)ether; technical-grade chloromethyl methyl ether

Bis(chloromethyl)ether (BCME) and technical-grade chloromethyl methyl ether (CMME) were manufactured before 1976 in the United States, but because of their lung carcinogenicity, the use of these chemicals has been reduced substantially in the United States.[60] BCME and CMME were used as alkylating agents and chemical intermediates. Technical-grade CMME contains 1% to 8% BCME.[61] The greatest potential for past occupational exposure to BCME or CMME was for ion-exchange resin makers, chemical plant workers, laboratory workers, and specialty polymer makers.[60]

In a worker survey conducted from 1981 to 1983, the National Institute for Occupational Safety and Health (NIOSH) estimated that a total of 14 laboratory workers were potentially exposed to BCME.[61] There was no estimate of potential exposure to CMME. In the past, a significant potential for environmental exposure to BCME arose from the use of mosquito coils that contain octachlorodipropyl ether, also referred to as "S-2." Although the EPA does not register S-2 for any current use, there have been some concerns about illegal sales of imported mosquito coils containing S-2.[62] BCME can be produced by the burning of mosquito coils from impurities present in the S-2 or by the thermolytic degradation of S-2.[63]

Based on numerous studies of exposed workers, the IARC states that BCME is among the most potent human carcinogens known. The fact that BCME and CMME are both alkylating agents provides support that their mode of action is genotoxic. Six epidemiologic studies performed in 1970 documented statistically significant increases in the relative risks for lung cancer for exposures to BCME. In 4 of the studies, the primary exposure was from technical-grade CMME with 1% to 8% contamination from BCME.[64] The histologic type of lung cancer most often associated with the exposures was small cell carcinoma.[65] For additional information on the lung cancer risk posed by BCME and CMME, see http://monographs.iarc.fr/ENG/Monographs/vol100F/mono100F-25.pdf.

Sulfur mustard

Sulfur mustard, called mustard gas in the military sector, is primarily a chemical warfare agent. Occupational exposures can also occur during its storage and destruction or from inadvertent exposure near dumping areas or areas where contamination may have occurred in the past (eg, military installations, demolition of old buildings). Findings from numerous studies performed between 1950 and 2000 detailing the adverse effects of short-term battlefield exposure and prolonged exposure in chemical factories firmly established the lung carcinogenicity of sulfur mustard.[66] The genotoxicity of sulfur mustard is primarily attributed to its behavior as a bi-functional alkylating agent.[67] For additional information on the lung cancer risk posed by sulfur mustard, see http://monographs.iarc.fr/ENG/Monographs/vol100F/mono100F-30.pdf.

Coal-tar pitch

Coal-tar pitch is the solid residue remaining from the distillation of coal tars. The actual composition of coal-tar pitch depends on the source materials used that resulted in the coal tars and the distillation temperature. Coal tars are composed primarily (90%) of 3-membered to 7-membered polycyclic aromatic hydrocarbons (PAHs), as well as their methylated derivative with lower concentrations of phenolic compounds and nitrogen bases.[68] Potential sources of occupational exposure to volatile PAHs (eg, acridine, anthracene, benzo[a]pyrene, chrysene, pyrene, phenanthrene) from coal tar include foundry and coal gasification processes and the production of coke, aluminum (eg, carbon electrode-manufacturing), pavement tar, roofing tar, coal tar paints, sealants, and refractory bricks.[68]

IARC working groups that met in 2005 and again in 2009 determined that there was sufficient evidence from epidemiologic studies of road pavers and roofers to support the carcinogenicity of coal-tar pitch.[68,69] Even though coal-tar pitch was phased out in the 1960s and 1970s in many of the European countries where the epidemiologic studies were performed, studies focused on the adverse health effects of bitumen exposure continue to observe suggestive evidence of coal tar's lung carcinogenicity.[70,71] For additional information on the lung cancer risk posed by coal tar pitch, see http://monographs.iarc.fr/ENG/Monographs/vol100F/mono100F-17.pdf.

Soot, as found in occupational exposure of chimney sweeps

Soot is a carbonaceous by-product material produced from the incomplete conversion of fossil fuel or other carbon-containing material (eg, paper, plastics) to combustion products (eg, water vapor, CO_2). Soot contains up to 60% carbon, inorganic material, and a soluble fraction consisting primarily of PAHs.[72] Occupations with higher potential for soot exposure include chimney sweeps; firefighters; brick masons and helpers; heating, ventilation, and air conditioning personnel; and others that require work near where organic matter is burned.[72]

Chimney sweeps, in particular, have a high potential for exposure to soot. In 2006, there were more than 1000 members of the National Chimney Sweep Guild, which represents fewer than 50% of the chimney sweeps in the United States.[73]

Two epidemiologic studies of chimney sweeps performed in Sweden and Finland in the 1990s reported elevated lung cancer risks for chimney sweeps from soot exposure. These studies provided the basis for the IARC to classify soot, as found in occupational exposure of chimney sweeps, a human lung carcinogen.[74] Adjustment for smoking was performed at the group level for the Swedish study and by use of social class for the Finnish study. An occupational cohort study by Pukkala and colleagues[75] that accessed 45 years of cancer incidence data by occupational category for individuals aged 30 to 64 years in the 1960, 1970, 1980/1981, and/or 1990 censuses provided further support that soot is a lung carcinogen. In the study published in 2009,[75] a total of 212 incident lung cancers were observed in chimney sweeps from Denmark, Finland, Norway, and Sweden, resulting in a standardized incidence ratio of 1.49 (95% CI 1.3–1.7) for lung cancer for chimney sweeps. For additional information on the lung cancer risk posed by soot, see http://monographs.iarc.fr/ENG/Monographs/vol100F/mono100F-21.pdf.

Diesel engine exhaust

According to McDonald and colleagues,[76] diesel engine exhaust contains a variety of gas and particulate matter constituents, including black carbon, organic carbon, nitrate, carbon monoxide, nonmethane volatile organic compounds, sulfate,

ammonium, alkanes, naphthalenes, phenanthrenes, and various polyaromatic hydrocarbons. In addition, the relative composition of the exhaust is significantly influenced by fuel type, engine type and condition, engine operation, engine load, and pretreatment (eg, particle traps) of exhaust.[76] Certain occupations (eg, underground miners, truck and bus drivers, toll booth attendants, construction workers) are known to have increased risk of exposure to diesel exhaust, with documented higher exposures of elemental carbon associated with enclosed underground mining and construction operations.[77] There is also widespread diesel engine exhaust exposure to the general population.

Diesel engine exhaust had been listed by the IARC since 1998 as possibly carcinogenic to humans (Group 2B).[78] Because of increasing epidemiologic evidence, however, originating from a variety of occupational settings, that exposure to diesel engine exhaust is a human carcinogen, the IARC convened a working group to review the existing evidence.[79] After review of the available information, the IARC work group added diesel engine exhaust as a Group 1 carcinogen on June 12, 2012 (**Fig. 3**).[80] Although the specific findings supporting their decision had not yet been published in monograph form at the time of this writing, the IARC indicated that their decision was based on the mounting evidence,[81] including 2 meta-analyses and a pooled epidemiologic study, that diesel engine exhaust is a known human lung carcinogen. The IARC specifically mentioned the recent results of a nested study performed by Silverman and colleagues[82] within a cohort of workers from 8 nonmetal mining facilities that provided strong

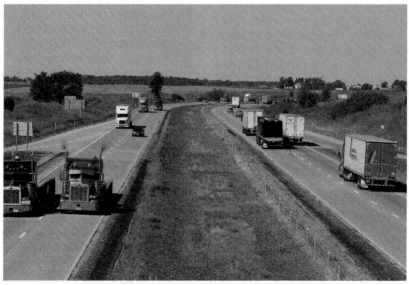

Fig. 3. The International Agency for Research on Cancer added diesel engine exhaust to the list of Group 1 carcinogens in 2012. (*Courtesy of* Centers for Disease Control/The National Institute for Occupational Safety and Health (NIOSH).)

support for the lung carcinogenicity of diesel engine exhausts.

The study by Silverman and colleagues,[82] which included 198 lung cancer deaths, reported a statistically significant positive trend between estimated respirable elemental carbon exposure (used as a marker of the mixed particulate and gaseous components of diesel exhaust), lagged 15 years, and a statistically significant increased lung cancer risk ($P = .001$) after adjustment for smoking and other potential confounders. For workers with heavy exposure to respirable elemental carbon (ie, above the median of the top quartile [respirable elemental carbon ≥ 1005 $\mu g/m^3 - y$]), the reported risk was approximately 3 times greater (OR = 3.20, 95% CI = 1.33–7.69) as compared with workers in the lowest quartile of exposure. The effect of cigarette smoking among study subjects was attenuated among workers with higher past diesel exposure estimated using respirable elemental carbon. Dr Kurt Straif, head of the IARC Monographs Program, stated that although IARC's conclusions regarding the lung carcinogenicity of diesel engine exhaust were based on rigorous epidemiologic studies of highly exposed workers, "we have learned from other carcinogens, such as radon, that initial studies showing a risk in heavily exposed occupational groups were followed by positive findings for the general population. Therefore actions to reduce exposures should encompass workers and the general population."[80] For additional information on the lung cancer risk associated with diesel exposure, see http://www.iarc.fr/en/media-centre/iarcnews/2012/mono105-backgrounderQ_A.php.

IARC GROUP 1 LUNG CARCINOGENS: OCCUPATIONS AND MANUFACTURING PROCESSES

The 2009 IARC work group determined that there was sufficient evidence in humans for the carcinogenicity of occupational exposures occurring during work activities in the following 6 discrete occupational categories[83]:

- Coal gasification
- Coke production
- Iron and steel founding
- Aluminum production
- Painting
- Rubber production industry

Coal Gasification, Coke Production, Iron and Steel Founding, Aluminum Production

The occupational groupings of coal gasification, coke production, iron and steel founding, and aluminum production, all have potential for high exposure to PAHs, as well as to other chemicals, especially in the 1950s to 1990s when many of the occupational cohort epidemiologic studies were performed. The evidence for the positive dose-response relationship noted for many of the cohort studies, which were cited by the IARC[83] to help establish the evidence for the carcinogenicity of that occupational grouping, used benzo(a)pyrene as a surrogate exposure measure of PAHs. It is noteworthy that although IARC has not listed benzo(a)pyrene as a lung carcinogen based on epidemiologic data, it has listed benzo(a)pyrene as a Group 1 carcinogen based on mechanistic and experimental animal studies indicating that it is likely to be a human carcinogen.

In a combined study of cohorts of workers exposed to PAHs published in 2007, Bosetti and colleagues[84] reported a pooled relative risk of 1.51 (95% CI 1.28–1.78) for roofers, 2.58 (95% CI 2.28–2.92) for coal gasification, 1.58 (95% CI 1.47–1.69) for coke production, and 1.40 (95% CI 1.31–1.49) for iron and steel foundries. A non–statistically significant pooled relative risk of 1.03 (95% CI 0.95–1.11) was found for aluminum production workers. For additional information on the lung cancer risk posed by coal gasification, coke production, iron and steel founding, and aluminum production, see http://monographs.iarc.fr/ENG/Monographs/vol100F/index.php.

Painting

The increased use of water-based paints and the intentional reduction of some of the toxic agents in paints, such as benzene, phthalates, lead oxides, and chromates, have reduced the risk of adverse health outcomes related to painting. Nonetheless, painters continue to have the potential for exposure to hundreds of hazardous chemicals (eg, dichloromethane, diisocyanates, amines, esters, chromates, nickel, ketones).[85] For additional details, see http://monographs.iarc.fr/ENG/Monographs/vol100F/mono100F-35.pdf.

More than 50 epidemiologic studies (ie, cohort and case-control) were published between 1951 and 2010 that overall demonstrate a relatively consistent increased risk for painters. A 2010 meta-analysis based on census reports, and case-control and cohort studies published through 2008,[86] reported a summary risk estimate for lung cancer among painters of 1.29 (95% CI 1.10–1.51) for case-control studies and 1.22 (95% CI 1.16–1.29) and 1.36 (95% CI 1.34–1.41) for lung cancer incidence and mortality studies, respectively. A second large meta-analysis published in 2010,[87] which included more than 11,000 incident lung cancer cases or deaths among painters, reported a summary risk estimate for lung cancer of 1.35 (95% CI 1.29–1.41) and 1.35 (95% CI 1.21–1.51) after controlling for smoking. In addition, the exposure-response relationship suggested the risk increased with duration of employment. For additional information on the lung cancer risk associated with painting as a profession, see http://monographs.iarc.fr/ENG/Monographs/vol100F/mono100F-35.pdf.

Rubber Manufacturing Industry

Rubber production workers are exposed to fumes with a complex chemical composition generated during the heating and curing of rubber compounds. The cyclohexane-soluble fraction of fumes often serves as an indicator to assess total particulate fume contamination.[88] In addition, high concentrations of nitrosamines are formed in rubber manufacturing during the vulcanizing process.[89,90] Furthermore, other likely exposures include carbon black, asbestos-contaminated talc, solvents, phthalates, and PAHs.[88,91]

The 2009 IARC work group concluded that there was sufficient evidence in humans for the carcinogenicity of occupational exposures in the rubber-manufacturing industry based in large part on retrospective cohort mortality studies that reported increased lung cancer risks among rubber workers involved with mixing and milling, vulcanization, tire-curing departments, and in cohorts of workers exposed to high concentrations of fumes and/or solvents.[88] Overall, there has been a high degree of heterogeneity of findings for both cohort and case-control studies. A 2006 meta-analysis that included 24 cohort studies of workers in the synthetic rubber-producing industry[92] reported a summary Standardized Mortality Ratio (SMR) of 1.05 (95% CI 0.94–1.18). Several other recent cohort studies of rubber workers performed in Germany, the United Kingdom, and Italy reported similar findings.[93–95] It is unknown to what extent these recent studies were affected by the Healthy Worker Effect. For additional information on the lung cancer risk associated with rubber manufacturing, see http://monographs.iarc.fr/ENG/Monographs/vol100F/mono100F-36.pdf.

IARC GROUP 1 LUNG CARCINOGENS: METALS
Arsenic and Inorganic Arsenic Compounds

Arsenic, a chemical element classified as a metalloid, is both an environmental and occupational lung carcinogen. The most common forms of arsenic in the environment are arsenite and arsenate. Arsenic compounds linked with carbon and hydrogen are considered organic; those combined with oxygen, chlorine, sulfur, and so forth, but without carbon are considered inorganic. Occupational exposures occur primarily among workers who breathe dust from lead, gold, and copper ore mines and smelters. Another potential source of exposure that has diminished in the past 10 years owing to declining use, occurred during the production and application of arsenical insecticides (eg, lead arsenate, calcium arsenate), herbicides, and wood preservatives. Arsenic is also used[96] in the production of the following products or processes:

- Glassware production
- Pigment reduction
- Solders
- Semiconductors
- Ceramics
- Fireworks
- Textiles

Sources of airborne exposures include emissions from smelting of metals (eg, nickel copper smelters), from insecticide/herbicide application, and natural releases from volcanic sources. A significant source of human exposure occurs from consumption of fish and seafood.[96] Over the past 10 years, a major source of environmental exposure of concern with regard to lung cancer is drinking water containing arsenic from groundwater sources.

In addition to studies of historical exposure from pesticidal and pharmaceutical uses, the 2009 IARC work group reviewed a large body of findings from 2 primary routes of arsenic exposure: occupational groups who had exposure to a mixture of inorganic arsenic compounds in contaminated air and nonoccupational studies of individuals who ingested arsenic (ie, arsenite and arsenate) in drinking water over a protracted period. The IARC concluded that the cohort and nested case-control studies provided fairly consistent exposure-response evidence that arsenic exposure via inhalation increases (eg, Standardized Mortality Ratio (SMR) range 2–3) lung cancer risk[97]; however, the quality of the exposure data for inorganic arsenic did not allow a separation of the risk based on a particular arsenic species. In a study of more than 8000 Montana copper smelters employed through 1989, Lubin and colleagues[98] reported a linear exposure-response between cumulative estimated inhaled inorganic arsenic and respiratory cancer mortality. The person-year–weighted mean cumulative arsenic exposure was 3.7 mg/m³-years with a reported SMR for respiratory cancer of 1.56 (95% CI 1.4–1.7). The investigators also noted that "inhalation of higher concentrations of arsenic over shorter durations was more deleterious than inhalation of lower concentrations over longer durations."

The IARC detailed the results of numerous ecologic studies and case-control studies performed in Argentina, Bangladesh, Chile, and Taiwan that examined the associations between higher concentrations (eg, >100 µg/L) of arsenic in drinking water and lung cancer. Overall, the ecologic (eg, studies that use aggregate or summary data to assess both exposure and often adverse health outcomes) studies reported significantly increased risks with increasing estimated levels of arsenic exposure.[97] A case-control study performed by Ferreccio and colleagues[99] reported ORs of 1.0, 1.6 (95% CI 0.5–5.3), 3.9 (95% CI 1.2–12.3), 5.2 (95% CI 2.3–11.7), and 8.9 (95% CI 4.0–19.6) for long-term exposure to ingested waterborne arsenic concentrations of less than 10, 10 to 29, 30 to 49, 50 to 199, and 200 to 400 µg/L, respectively. The investigators also observed a synergistic (ie, greater than additive) effect between waterborne arsenic concentrations and smoking.

Studies examining the association between drinking water with lower concentrations of arsenic and lung cancer are less supportive of an association between ingested arsenic in drinking water and lung cancer. It is not known if the lack of evidence of an association below 100 µg/L is the result of a threshold effect or an attenuation of the observed risk from nondifferential exposure misclassification.[100] Because of the large population at risk from exposure to arsenic in their drinking water, arsenic exposure may represent a substantial public health problem if a risk threshold does not exist. For additional information on the lung cancer risk posed by exposure to arsenic and arsenic compounds, see http://monographs.iarc.fr/ENG/Monographs/vol100C/mono100C-6.pdf.

Beryllium and Beryllium Compounds

Beryllium is a silver-gray metallic divalent element that occurs naturally in the earth's crust.[101,102] Airborne concentrations are generally low and originate primarily form windblown dusts. Higher atmospheric concentrations of beryllium have been detected in the vicinity of coal-generating plants, municipal waste incineration, and beryllium ore processing and production plants,[101,102] and between 1959 and 1970 near the burning of solid rocket fuel.[103] The United States, China, and Kazakhstan are the only countries currently involved in the industrial-scale extraction of beryllium.[104]

A large proportion of the beryllium manufactured is in the form of copper-beryllium alloys. High rigidity, thermal stability, thermal conductivity, low density, and antispark properties make beryllium an important material[101–103] for numerous products, including the following:

- Aircraft
- Missiles
- Space vehicles
- Communication satellites
- Automotive (eg, antilock breaking systems)
- Consumer products (eg, camera shutters)
- Energy and electrical
- Tools
- Sporting goods (eg, golf clubs)
- Electronics, biomedical (eg, dental braces and bridges, x-ray tube windows)
- Jewelry
- Scrap recovery and recycling
- Defense
- Nuclear industries

Kreiss and colleagues[105] estimated that more than 134,000 US workers have been exposed to beryllium. Beryllium that is inhaled may slowly dissolve in the lungs and move into the bloodstream. Some beryllium may be expectorated from the lungs and swallowed, although once engulfed by macrophages the particles have clearance rate half-times of hundreds to thousands of days.[106,107] The IARC has classified beryllium as a Group 1 known human carcinogen since 1981. The IARC based its 1993 review of the lung carcinogenicity of beryllium primarily on studies from US Beryllium Case Registry cases and from the findings of a cohort study of 9225 workers employed at 7 beryllium-processing plants.[108] In the 2009 IARC working group assessment of the lung carcinogenicity of beryllium,[102] the work group references a nested case-control study performed by Schubauer-Berigan and colleagues[109] that included 142 lung cancer cases each matched to 5 controls as supporting the lung carcinogenicity of beryllium. The investigators reported a significant relationship between average, but not cumulative, beryllium exposure and lung cancer risk after adjusting for birth year. Even though the study was criticized for methodological issues related to selection of controls,[110] the IARC working group noted that the criticisms did not undermine their confidence in the findings referencing several publications that supported the methodology used in the analyses.[102]

Two subsequent studies by Schubauer-Berigan and colleagues[111,112] published since the IARC's 2009 review provide further support for the lung carcinogenicity of beryllium. The first study[111] extended the mortality follow-up (1940 through 2005) for 9199 workers from the 7 beryllium-processing plants. The study reported elevated lung cancer rates as compared with the US population (SMR 1.17, 95% CI 1.08–1.28) and intracohort analysis found that workers with maximum beryllium exposure of 10 µg/m³ or higher had higher rates of lung cancer. Positive trends with cumulative beryllium exposure were observed for lung cancer ($P = .01$) when short-term workers were excluded. The second study performed by Schubauer-Berigan and colleagues[112] examined the shape of exposure-response associations between various exposure metrics and lung cancer, while adjusting for potential confounders (ie, race, plant, professional and short-term work status, and exposure to other lung carcinogens). The investigators reported positive associations between lung cancer and mean ($P<.0001$) and maximum ($P<.0001$) beryllium exposure with adjustment for age, birth cohort, and plant, as well as positive associations for cumulative ($P = .0017$) beryllium exposure with adjustment for the previous factors plus short-term work status and exposure to asbestos.

Despite IARC's listing of beryllium as a Group 1 carcinogen, some researchers continue to reject the validity of the science on which the IARC based their decision, as well as the validity of the findings from the recent studies by Schubauer-Berigan and colleagues.[111,112] In a review of epidemiologic data, supported by an unrestricted grant from Materion Brush, Inc, Boffetta and colleagues[113] assert that most epidemiologic studies examining the association between beryllium exposure and lung cancer have likely failed to adequately address confounding by smoking and other occupational and lifestyle factors, claiming, "Overall, the available evidence does not support a conclusion that a causal association has been established between occupational exposure to beryllium and the risk of cancer." For additional information on the lung cancer risk posed by exposure to beryllium and beryllium compounds, see http://monographs.iarc.fr/ENG/Monographs/vol100C/mono100C-7.pdf.

Cadmium and Cadmium Compounds

Cadmium is a soft, bluish-white metal recovered as a by-product of zinc mining and refining. The zinc-to-cadmium ratios in most zinc ores range from 200:1 to 400:1.[114] Cadmium use has decreased over time, except with its use in nickel-cadmium batteries, "silver solder" containing cadmium, and cadmium-telluride solar panels. These declines have come about because of its toxicity, the resulting regulations, and alternate technologies.[115] This decrease in consumption was offset by the increased demand for cadmium in nickel-cadmium batteries, which accounted for 81% of the cadmium used as of 2006 in the United States.[114]

Environmental exposures to cadmium are primarily the result of volcano emissions, fossil fuel and wood combustion, forest fires, phosphate fertilizers, iron and steel production emissions, cement production and use, releases from phosphoric acid processes, smelting of nonferrous metals production, and municipal solid waste incineration.[96] In addition, cigarettes contain varying concentrations of cadmium (in the microgram level) and approximately 10% of the cadmium is inhaled when a cigarette is smoked.[115]

The primary route of cadmium exposure in work areas is via the respiratory tract. The highest potential for occupational exposures occurs during the following work processes[115,116]:

- Welding or remelting cadmium-coated steel
- Smelting zinc and lead ores
- Work involving solders containing cadmium
- Battery production
- Pigment production
- Plastics production
- Processing, producing, and handling cadmium powders

In 2010, Alaska, Idaho, Missouri, and Tennessee produced zinc concentrate containing cadmium; cadmium metal was produced at a primary electrolytic zinc refinery at the Clarksville refinery in Tennessee and at secondary smelters in Ohio and Pennsylvania.[117]

Cohort epidemiologic studies of workers in the nickel alloy, nickel smelting, and nickel-cadmium battery operations that were performed primarily between 1976 and 1998, as well as findings from a prospective population-based study in a cadmium-contaminated area in Belgium, formed the basis for the IARC's decision to classify cadmium and cadmium compounds as Group 1 carcinogens.[118] The 2009 IARC working group noted that interpretation of findings from cohorts exposed are limited by small numbers of workers with high long-term exposures, a scarcity of cadmium exposure data, ability to compare exposure gradients between studies, and difficulty accounting for possible confounding by smoking. Among studies published since the IARC's 2009 review, Beveridge and colleagues[119] reported an increased OR of 4.7 (95% CI 1.5–14.3) only among former or nonsmokers with exposure to cadmium in 2 population-based case control studies in Montreal. Cadmium exposure did not produce an observable increased risk among smokers, however. Park and colleagues[120] recently reported findings from a reanalysis of cadmium smelter workers that incorporated a retrospective exposure assessment for arsenic (As), updated mortality information for 1940 to 2002, a revised cadmium exposure matrix, and improved work history information. The investigators reported an increased lung cancer risk from airborne cadmium exposure independent of arsenic exposure (SMR = 3.2 for 10 mg-year/m^3 cadmium, P = .012). For additional information on the lung cancer risk posed by exposure to cadmium and cadmium compounds, see http://monographs.iarc.fr/ENG/Monographs/vol100C/mono100C-8.pdf.

Chromium (VI) Compounds

Chromium is the 21st most abundant element in the earth's crust, occurring mainly in a trivalent state; however, hexavalent chromium (chromium VI) compounds are classified as Group 1 lung carcinogens and are produced primarily from industrial processes. OSHA classifies chromium (VI) compounds by their water solubility, specifically as follows: water insoluble (solubility <0.01 g/L), slightly soluble (solubility 0.01 g/L–500 g/L), and highly water soluble (solubility ≥500 g/L).[121] Exposure to chromium (VI) trioxide results in damage to the nasal mucosa and possible perforation of the nasal septum, whereas exposure to insoluble chromium (VI) compounds results in damage to the lower respiratory tract.[122]

The Agency for Toxic Substances and Disease Registry reports that about 9000 tons of chromium (VI) are released to the air each year in the United States.[122] The potential for airborne environmental exposure to chromium (VI) compounds is higher for individuals living near anthropogenic sources of chromium production.[122] Although studies based on aggregate measures of exposure and lung cancer outcome (ie, ecologic studies) have been published suggesting an association between environmental exposure to chromium exposure and lung cancer, these types of studies are reserved for hypothesis generating rather than assessing risk.[123]

Based on a 2006 OSHA contractor's report,[124] the following US industries with the highest number of workers exposed to chromium (VI) include:

- Welding
- Painting
- Electroplating
- Steel mills
- Iron and steel foundries
- Paint and coating production
- Plastic colorant production and use
- Chromium catalyst production
- Chromate chemical production
- Plating mixture production
- Printing ink production
- Chromium metal producers
- Chromate pigment production
- Chromated copper arsenate production

The IARC concluded from a review of more than 25 cohort studies published between 1952 and 2006 that there was sufficient evidence in humans for the lung carcinogenicity of chromium (VI) compounds, especially for highly exposed workers in the chromate production, chromate pigment production, and chromium-plating industries.[125] The 2009 IARC working group pointed out that because of the mixed exposures workers received and the increased lung cancer risk observed in diverse industries that exposed workers to varying chromium (VI) compounds, the IARC recommended that the broad category of chromium (VI) be listed a Group 1 carcinogen.

Studies of workers with lower estimated exposures of chromium (VI) that have been published since 2000 have produced mixed results. For example, a recent pooled analysis of 2 case-control studies of Montreal workers exposed to lower estimated concentrations (ie, exposed/unexposed) of chromium (VI) reported ORs of 2.4 (95% CI 1.2–4.8) for nonsmoking, chromium (VI)–exposed workers versus 1.0 (95% CI 0.7–1.3) for chromium (VI)–exposed workers who smoked.[119,125] It should be noted that the results for the nonsmoking workers were based on findings from only 46 controls and 12 cases. For additional information on the lung cancer risk posed by exposure to chromium (VI) compounds, see http://monographs.iarc.fr/ENG/Monographs/vol100C/mono100C-9.pdf.

Nickel Compounds

Nickel is a silvery white metal that occurs naturally, as the 24th most abundant element, in the earth's crust, generally accompanying sulfide and silica-oxides ores. The mining of these ores, which contain less than 3% nickel, occurred in the United States from the late 1950s to 1998.[126–128] New US nickel-mining sites have been developed in Minnesota and Michigan. The potential for low-level atmospheric nickel exposure arises from natural sources (eg, windblown dust, volcanoes, forest, and wildfires) and anthropogenic activities (eg, mining, refining, smelting, manufacture of nickel-containing alloys and stainless steel, fossil fuel combustion, waste incineration).[129] The EPA estimates that in 2007, 1027 facilities released 30.5 million pounds of nickel compounds[127]; however, atmospheric concentrations of nickel compounds in the United States are reported to be 100,000 to 1 million times lower than the concentrations reported to increase cancer rates.[130] Although studies have shown an association between aggregate measures of environmental exposure to nickel compounds and lung cancer, these types of studies (ie, ecologic studies) are generally reserved for hypothesis generating rather than testing.[123]

Occupations that have the potential for exposure to nickel compounds include[126–130] the following:

- Battery makers, storage
- Catalyst workers
- Ceramic makers
- Chemists
- Disinfectant makers
- Dyers
- Electroplaters
- Enamellers
- Ink makers
- Magnet makers
- Nickel-alloy makers
- Mold makers
- Nickel miners
- Nickel refiners
- Nickel smelters
- Nickel workers
- Organic chemical synthesizers
- Paint makers
- Petroleum refinery workers
- Stainless-steel makers
- Textile dyers
- Vacuum tube makers
- Varnish makers
- Welders

The primary evidence demonstrating the human lung carcinogenicity of nickel compounds and nickel metal is based on epidemiologic findings from nickel refinery and nickel smelter workers. The 2009 IARC working group concluded,[129] after a detailed review of pertinent epidemiologic studies, that strong evidence for the carcinogenicity of nickel compounds exists for nickel chloride,[131] nickel sulfate, water-soluble nickel compounds in general,[131,132] insoluble nickel compounds, nickel oxides,[131,133] nickel sulfides,[134] and mostly insoluble nickel compounds.[133]

The investigators[135] of a study funded by Nickel Producers Environmental Research Association contend that, in addition to lack of adequate control for confounding, the epidemiologic studies focusing on soluble nickel compounds cannot differentiate between nickel compounds, and therefore some of the increased risk attributed to soluble nickel compounds may be from other nickel species. However, the IARC[129] cites the studies of Norwegian refinery workers[131,132,136] to support the basis for the human lung carcinogenicity of soluble nickel because of the availability of cigarette smoking data and the adjustments that were performed to reduce

potential confounding. The IARC's[129] 2009 evaluation of nickel as a lung carcinogen concludes that there is "sufficient evidence in humans for the carcinogenicity of mixtures that include nickel compounds and nickel metal. The evidence is strongest for soluble nickel compounds; there is also independent evidence for the carcinogenicity of oxidic and sulfidic nickel compounds."

The IARC's position is further supported by a recent study by Grimsrud and Andersen[137] who assert that the claimed absence of nickel-related respiratory cancer among electrolysis workers resulted from "an arbitrary overemphasis of biased and inconclusive findings" by some researchers.[135] Another recent case-control study performed in Italy[138] that used a lifetime job exposure matrix, estimated an OR of 1.18 (95% CI 0.90–1.53) among workers with relatively low exposures of combined nickel-chromium exposure (eg, metal mechanics). For additional information on the lung cancer risk posed by exposure to nickel compounds, see http://monographs.iarc.fr/ENG/Monographs/vol 100C/mono100C-10.pdf.

IARC GROUP 1 LUNG CARCINOGENS: DUST AND FIBERS
Asbestos (All Forms)

Asbestos is a naturally occurring fibrous silicate mineral that exists in 2 forms: serpentine (ie, chrysotile) and amphibole (ie, actinolite, amosite, anthophyllite, crocidolite, and tremolite). Chrysotile, anthophyllite, amosite, and crocidolite asbestos have been used commercially.[139] Widespread application of asbestos materials in various settings in the United States did not occur until the early 1930s; however, by 1980, the construction industry accounted for more than two-thirds of the total asbestos demand.

A 1989 EPA ban on most asbestos-containing products was overturned in 1991 by a federal court; however, a ban continues on several items (eg, flooring felt, roll board, and certain types of specialty paper), as well as for products that have not historically contained asbestos, otherwise referred to as "new uses" of asbestos.[140] Asbestos is not currently mined in the United States, and the use of asbestos in 2011 was similar to the level (ie, 1000 ton/y) of use in 1909.[141] Most of the asbestos currently used in the United States, which is primarily chrysotile asbestos, is imported from Canada.[141]

Because of the past widespread use of asbestos-containing products, the potential for exposure is widespread, but nonetheless has decreased each year since the partial ban. The primary sources of exposure for members of the general public include releases of asbestos (eg, friable asbestos-containing building materials and insulation) from older buildings, brake linings, demolition of older buildings, living near asbestos-containing waste sites or asbestos-related industries, asbestos-contaminated vermiculite, exposure to poorly contained asbestos removal operations, and exposure to talc containing asbestiform fibers.[142,143] "Bystander exposure" to asbestos fibers can also take place by contact with asbestos workers or their clothes.

Occupational exposures in the past were much more prevalent and included[142–144] the following:

- Asbestos mining and processing operations
- Talc mining and processing (talc containing asbestiform fibers)
- Asbestos insulation
- Textile work
- The manufacture of asbestos-containing products
- Ship building
- Construction
- Numerous other industries

Occupational exposures still occur among workers who work with asbestos-containing end products,[142–144] including the following occupations:

- Asbestos insulation workers
- Automotive repair and maintenance workers
- Building maintenance workers
- Building demolition workers and abatement workers (eg, materials: roof shingles, drywall, flooring, cement, fireproofing, insulation)

The 3 lung-specific adverse health outcomes associated with exposure to asbestos are asbestosis, lung cancer, and mesothelioma (which can be of the pleura as well as the peritoneum, but is not further considered in this review of lung cancer). A long-standing controversy not addressed in a substantive manner by the IARC[137] is whether the risk of lung cancer is associated with asbestos exposure alone and/or asbestosis.[14,143] The 2009 IARC working group concluded that all forms of asbestos cause lung cancer,[144] however, while acknowledging that controversies remain regarding the potency differences for fibers of different types (eg, low potency of chrysotile versus high potency of amphiboles)[145–147] and dimensions (eg, lower potency of shorter and wider fibers versus higher potency of thinner and longer fibers).[148,149]

The 2009 IARC working group indicated that some of the heterogeneity in findings between studies may not be related to differences in potency for different fiber types, but rather differences in rigor of exposure assessment. The investigators of a meta-analysis published in 2011 reported[150] that studies with higher-quality asbestos exposure data produced higher meta-estimates of the lung cancer risk per unit of exposure and that discerning potency differences between chrysotile versus amphibole asbestos–exposed cohorts was more challenging when the meta-analyses are limited to a smaller number of studies with questionable exposure assessment methods.

Nonetheless, several studies[151,152] reported an increased risk for lung cancer associated with chrysotile asbestos exposure. In a retrospective cohort study of 5770 textile workers in North Carolina, Loomis and colleagues[153] reported an SMR of 1.96 (95% CI 1.7–2.2) for lung cancer. In addition, a 2008 retrospective cohort study of 3072 workers at a South Carolina textile plant reported that lung cancer was most strongly associated with exposure to thin (<0.25 μm) and longer (>10 μm) fibers. A recent pooled analysis[154] of 3717 men and 2419 women employed at any of the 4 textile mills in North or South Carolina before 1973 reported a pooled relative rate for lung cancer of 1.11 (95% CI 1.06–1.16) when comparing exposures at 100 f-y/mL to 0 f-y/mL. A subsequent analysis[155] found that whereas lung cancer mortality was associated with particles of any size, exposure to longer (ie, >5–10 μm) and thinner (<0.25 μm) fibers presented a greater risk. For additional information on the lung cancer risk posed by exposure to asbestos, see http://monographs.iarc.fr/ENG/Monographs/vol100C/mono100C-11.pdf.

Silica Dust, Crystalline, in the Form of Quartz or Cristobalite

Silicon is the second most common element in the Earth's crust. Two allotropes of silicon, amorphous and crystalline, exist at room temperature. The compound silica, also known as silicon dioxide (SiO_2), makes up more than 25% of the Earth's crust. Amorphous silica usually occurs as a brown powder as compared with the metallic luster and a grayish color of crystalline silica.[156] Crystalline silica exists as quartz, cristobalite, tridymite, and 4 other very rare forms (ie, keatite, coesite, stishovite, and moganite).[157] Quartz is the most common form of crystalline silica and the primary component of sand and of dust in the air.[156]

Environmental exposures to silica can arise from natural (eg, forest fires, volcanic eruptions, wind erosion) and anthropogenic activities (eg, construction, gravel roads, demolition, quarrying, mining, and farming activities—tilling). The potential for occupational exposure to silica is widespread. Potential occupational exposures to silica include a wide variety of occupations and industries,[157–159] including the following:

- Oil and gas extraction
- Bituminous coal and lignite mining
- Mining and quarrying of nonmetallic minerals (except most fuels) including silica sand mining
- Hydraulic fracturing for natural gas development (**Fig. 4**)
- Metal mining
- Masonry, stonework, tile setting, and plastering
- Services to dwellings and other buildings
- Concrete, gypsum, and plaster products
- Roofing and sheet metal work
- Construction (eg, bridge, tunnel, and elevated highway)
- Agricultural activities
- Wrecking and demolition activities
- Medical and dental laboratories work
- Foundry work (ferrous and nonferrous)
- Vitreous enameling
- Glass manufacturing
- Manufacturing of soaps and detergents
- Shipyard work

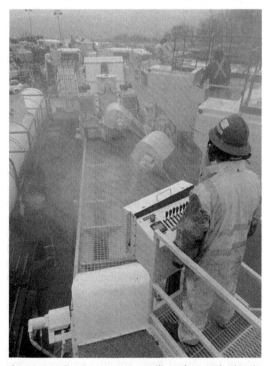

Fig. 4. Worker exposure to silica during hydraulic fracturing. Silica dust created by worker conducting sand transfer operations. Photo shows sand mover and transfer system. (*Courtesy of* Centers for Disease Control/The National Institute for Occupational Safety and Health (NIOSH).)

- Railroads
- Automotive repair shops
- Production of pottery and related items

The 2009 IARC working group's reaffirmation of the lung carcinogenicity of silica focused on the epidemiologic findings from 5 primary occupational settings: ceramics, diatomaceous earth, ore mining, quarries, and sand and gravel.[159] Among these industries, the IARC assumed sand and gravel operations, quarries, and diatomaceous earth facilities had the least potential for confounding and reported that studies with quantitative exposures generally report increased lung cancer rates with increasing exposure to crystalline silica. However, the IARC indicates the strongest evidence supporting the lung carcinogenicity of crystalline silica was from the pooled epidemiologic studies[160,161] that revealed a clear exposure-response relationship and an overall increased lung cancer risk for the meta-analyses from a diverse number of industries.[162,163] Debate continues that the inflammation caused by crystalline silica exposure, and perhaps the resulting silicosis, is the driving force for the development of cancer.[162,164–166] For additional information on the lung cancer risk posed by exposure to silica dust, crystalline, in the form of quartz or cristobalite, see http://monographs.iarc.fr/ENG/Monographs/PDFs/index.php.

IARC GROUP 2 LUNG CARCINOGENS

Group 2–listed human lung carcinogens include the following:

- Acid mists, strong inorganic
- Art glass, glass containers, and pressed ware (manufacture of)
- Biomass fuel (primarily wood) indoor emissions from household combustion of
- Bitumens, oxidized, and their emissions during roofing
- Bitumens, hard, and their emissions during mastic asphalt work
- Carbon electrode manufacture
- alpha-Chlorinated toluenes (benzal chloride, benzotrichloride, benzyl chloride) and benzoyl chloride (combined exposures)
- 2,3,7,8-tetrachlorodibenzo-para-dioxin
- Cobalt metal with tungsten carbide
- Creosotes
- Frying, emissions from high temperature
- Insecticides, nonarsenical (occupational exposures in spraying and application)
- Printing processes (occupational exposures in)
- Welding fumes

Scientific evidence is also mounting that other Group 2 human lung carcinogens[167] should receive greater consideration as Group 1 carcinogens. Fortunately, several potential lung carcinogens (eg, welding; motor vehicle emissions; carbon-based nanoparticles; crystalline fibers other than asbestos; outdoor air pollution, including sulfur oxides, nitrogen oxides, ozone, and dusts; ultrafine particles) are listed as priority agents for future review.[168]

SUMMARY

The IARC's updated assessments, published in 2012 as Volume 100 C through F of the IARC Monographs, provide a long overdue resource for consensus opinions on the carcinogenic potential of various agents. Unfortunately, many of the studies reviewed by IARC, which attempted to identify whether or not a causal association existed between various exposures and lung cancer, were often impeded by confounding from smoking and poor retrospective exposure assessment. As pointed out in the President's Cancer Panel's 2010 report,[16] research on environmental and occupational causes of cancer have been limited by low priority and inadequate funding. This is especially true for lung cancer research. The large percentage of lung cancer deaths caused by smoking often obscures the fact that nonsmoking-related lung cancer is 1 of the top 10 causes of cancer mortality and, in some cases (eg, medically related radiation exposures, radon), the attributable risk of the agent is increasing. The foregoing data also underscore that in the clinical assessment of lung cancer risk, ascertaining past occupational exposures as well clarifying selected environmental risks should hold an equal place to quantifying cumulative cigarette smoking in pack years.

REFERENCES

1. Howlader N, Noone AM, Krapcho M, et al, editors. SEER cancer statistics review, 1975-2008. Bethesda (MD): National Cancer Institute; 2011. Available at: http://dccps.nci.nih.gov/ocs/prevalence/prevalence.html.
2. Siegel R, Naishadham D, Jemal A. Cancer statistics 2012. CA Cancer J Clin 2011;62(1):10–29.
3. U.S. Center for Disease Control. Annual smoking-attributable mortality, years of potential life lost, and productivity losses—United States, 1997–2001. MMWR Morb Mortal Wkly Rep 2005;54:625–8.
4. Thun MJ, Henley SJ, Burns D, et al. Lung cancer death rates in lifelong nonsmokers. J Natl Cancer Inst 2006;98:691–9.
5. Sun S, Schiller JH, Gazdar AF. Lung cancer in never smokers—a different disease. Nat Rev Cancer 2007;7:778–90.
6. Ferlay J, Shin H-R, Bray F, et al. Estimates of worldwide burden of cancer in 2008: GLOBOCAN 2008. Int J Cancer 2010;127(12):2893–917.
7. Couraud S, Zalcman G, Milleron B, et al. Lung cancer in never smokers—a review. Eur J Cancer 2012. Available at: http://dx.doi.org/10.1016/j.ejca.2012.03.007. Accessed June 1, 2012.
8. Wakelee HA, Chang ET, Gomez SL, et al. Lung cancer incidence in never smokers. J Clin Oncol 2007;25(5):472–8.
9. Blair A, Freeman LB. Lung cancer among nonsmokers. Epidemiology 2006;17(6):601–13.
10. Subramanian J, Govindan R. Lung cancer in never smokers: a review. J Clin Oncol 2007;25(5):561–70.
11. Samet JM, Avila-Tang E, Boffetta P, et al. Lung cancer in never smokers: clinical epidemiology and environmental risk factors. Clin Cancer Res 2009;15(18):5626–45.
12. Neuberger J, Field RW. Occupation and lung cancer in nonsmokers. Rev Environ Health 2003;18(4):251–67.
13. Spitz MR, Wu X, Wilkinson A, et al. Cancer of the lung. In: Schottenfeld D, Fraumei J, editors. Cancer epidemiology and prevention (third edition). New York, NY: Oxford University Press; 2006. p. 638–58.
14. Dela Cruz CS, Tanoue LT, Matthay RA. Lung cancer: epidemiology, etiology, and prevention. Clin Chest Med 2011;32:605–44.
15. Doll R, Peto R. The causes of cancer: quantitative estimates of avoidable risks of cancer in the United States today. J Natl Cancer Inst 1981;66:1191–308.
16. President's cancer panel. 2008–2009 annual report. Reducing environmental cancer risk: what we can do now. Bethesda (MD): National Cancer Institute, National Institutes of Health, U.S. Department of Health and Human Services; 2010. Available at: http://deainfo.nci.nih.gov/advisory/pcp/annualReports/pcp08-09rpt/PCP_Report_08-09_508.pdf. Accessed April 5, 2012.
17. Harvard Center for Cancer Prevention, Harvard School of Public Health. Harvard Report on Cancer Prevention. Vol. 1: human causes of cancer. Cancer Causes Control 1996;7(1):S3–4. Available at: http://www.hsph.harvard.edu/cancer/resources_materials/reports.index.htm. Accessed June 1, 2012.
18. Doll R. Epidemiological evidence of the effects of behavior and the environment on the risk of human cancer. Recent Results Cancer Res 1998;154:3–21.
19. Travis LB, Gospodarowicz M, Curtis RE, et al. Lung cancer following chemotherapy and radiotherapy for Hodgkin's disease. J Natl Cancer Inst 2002;94:182–92.

20. Herbst RS, Heymach JV, Lippman SM. Lung cancer. N Engl J Med 2008;359(13):1367–80.

21. El Ghissassi F, Baan R, Straif K, et al. A review of human carcinogens–part D: radiation. Lancet Oncol 2009;10(8):751–2.

22. National Council on Radiation Protection and Measurement. Ionizing radiation exposure of the population of the United States. Report No. 160, Figure 1–1. Bethesda (MD): NCRP; 2009.

23. IARC Monographs on the Evaluation of Carcinogenic Risks to Humans. A review of human carcinogens: Radiation. vol. 100D; 2012. p. 341. Available at: http://monographs.iarc.fr/ENG/Monographs/vol100D/mono100D-9.pdf. Accessed May 15, 2012.

24. Zhou H, Randers-Pehrson G, Suzuki M, et al. Genotoxic damage in non-irradiated cells: contribution from the bystander effect. Radiat Prot Dosimetry 2002;99(1–4):227–32.

25. National Research Council. Health effects of exposure to radon: BEIR VI. Committee on the health risks of exposure to radon. Washington, DC: National Academy Press; 1999.

26. Agricola G. 1556. De Re Metallica. New York: Dover Publications Inc; 1950. p. 638. [Hoover HC, Hoover LH].

27. Schefflers CL. Abhandlung von der Gesundheit der Bergleute. Chemnitz (Germany): Strossel; 1770. p. 274.

28. Hesse W. Das Vorkommen von primärem Lungenkrebs bei den Bergleuten der consortschaftlichen Gruben in Schneeberg. Archiv der Heilkunde 1878;19:160–2 [in German].

29. Harting FH, Hesse W. Der Lungenkrebs, die bergkrankheit in den schneeberger gruben. Viertel Gerichtl Med Oeff Sanitaetswes 1879;31:102–32 [in German].

30. Field RW. Radon: an overview of health effects. In: Nriagu JO, editor. Encyclopedia of environmental health, vol. 4. Burlington (Ontario): Elsevier; 2011. p. 745–53.

31. Lubin JH. Environmental factors in cancer: radon. Rev Environ Health 2010;25(1):33–8.

32. International Commission on Radiological Protection. ICRP Publication 115: lung cancer risk from radon and progeny. Ann ICRP 2012;40(1). Available at: http://www.icrp.org/publication.asp?id=ICRP_Publication_115.

33. National Research Council, National Academy of Science. Uranium mining in Virginia: scientific, technical, environmental, human health and safety, and regulatory aspects of uranium mining and processing in Virginia, Prepublication, 2011. Available at: http://dels.nas.edu/Report/Uranium-Mining-Virginia-Scientific-Technical/13266. Accessed April 20, 2012.

34. Schubauer-Berigan MK, Daniels RD, Pinkerton LE. Radon exposure and mortality among white and American Indian uranium miners: an update of the Colorado Plateau cohort. Am J Epidemiol 2009;169(6):718–30.

35. Rage E, Vacquier B, Blanchardon E, et al. Risk of lung cancer mortality in relation to lung doses among French uranium miners: follow-up 1956-1999. Radiat Res 2012;177(3):288–97.

36. Lane RS, Frost SE, Howe GR, et al. Mortality (1950-1999) and cancer incidence (1969-1999) in the cohort of Eldorado uranium workers. Radiat Res 2010;174(6):773–85.

37. Kreuzer M, Schnelzer M, Tschense A, et al. Cohort profile: the German uranium miners cohort study (WISMUT cohort), 1946-2003. Int J Epidemiol 2010;39(4):980–7.

38. U.S. EPA. EPA assessment of risks from radon in homes. Washington, DC: U.S. Environmental Protection Agency, Office of Radiation and Indoor Air; 2003. Available at: http://www.epa.gov/radiation/docs/assessment/402-r-03-003.pdf. Accessed April 15, 2012.

39. Lubin JH, Wang ZY, Boice JD, et al. Risk of lung cancer and residential radon in China: pooled results of two studies. Int J Cancer 2004;109(1):132–7.

40. Darby S, Hill D, Deo H, et al. Residential radon and lung cancer—detailed results of a collaborative analysis of individual data on 7148 persons with lung cancer and 14208 persons without lung cancer from 13 epidemiologic studies in Europe. Scand J Work Environ Health 2006;32:1–84.

41. Krewski D, Lubin JH, Zielinski JM, et al. Residential radon and risk of lung cancer—a combined analysis of 7 north American case-control studies. Epidemiology 2005;16(2):137–45.

42. Field RW, Smith BJ, Lynch CF, et al. Intercomparison of radon exposure assessment methods: implications for residential radon risk assessment. J Expo Anal Environ Epidemiol 2002;12(3):197–203.

43. US Environmental Protection Agency, US Department of Health and Human Services, US Department of Agriculture, US Department of Defense, US Department of Energy, US Department of Housing and Urban Development, US Department of Interior, US Department Veterans Affairs, and US General Services Administration. Protecting people and families from radon, a federal action plan for saving lives. 2011. Available at: http://www.epa.gov/radon/pdfs/Federal_Radon_Action_Plan.pdf. Accessed April 3, 2012.

44. Agency for Toxic Substances and Disease Registry (ATSDR). Toxicological profile for plutonium. Atlanta (GA): U.S. Department of Health and Human Services, Public Health Services; 2010. Available at: http://www.atsdr.cdc.gov/toxprofiles/tp.asp?id=648&tid=119. Accessed April 15, 2012.

45. IARC, Ionizing radiation, Part 2: some internally deposited radionuclides. IARC Monogr Eval Carcinog Risks Hum 2001;78:1–559.
46. Wing S, Richardson D, Wolf S, et al. Plutonium-related work and cause-specific mortality at the United States Department of Energy Hanford Site. Am J Ind Med 2004;45:153–64.
47. Brown SC, Ruttenber AJ. Lung cancer and plutonium exposure in Rocky Flat waters. Radiat Res 2005;163:696–7.
48. Brown SC, Schonbeck MF, McClure D, et al. Lung cancer and internal lung doses among plutonium workers at the Rocky Flats Plant: a case-control study. Am J Epidemiol 2004;160:163–72.
49. Kreisheimer M, Sokolnikov ME, Koshurnikova NA, et al. Lung cancer mortality among nuclear workers of the Mayak facilities in the former Soviet Union. An updated analysis considering smoking as the main confounding factor. Radiat Environ Biophys 2003;42:129–35.
50. Shilnikova NS, Preston DL, Ron E, et al. Cancer mortality risk among workers at the Mayak nuclear complex. Radiat Res 2003;159:787–98.
51. Jacob V, Jacob P, Meckbach R, et al. Lung cancer in Mayak workers: interaction of smoking and plutonium exposure. Radiat Environ Biophys 2005;44:119–29.
52. Gilbert ES, Koshurnikova NA, Sokolnikov ME, et al. Lung cancer in Mayak workers. Radiat Res 2004;162:505–16.
53. Sokolnikov ME, Gilbert ES, Preston DL, et al. Lung, liver and bone cancer mortality in Mayak workers. Int J Cancer 2008;123:905–11.
54. UNSCEAR; United Nations Scientific Committee on the Effects of Atomic Radiation. Report. Annex A. Epidemiological studies of radiation and cancer. New York: United Nations; 2008.
55. National Research Council, Committee to Assess Health Risks from Exposure to Low Levels of Ionizing Radiation, Board on Radiation Effects. Health risks from exposure to low levels of ionizing radiation: BEIR VII, Phase 2. Washington, DC: National Academies Press; 2006.
56. Preston DL, Shimizu Y, Pierce DA, et al. Studies of mortality of atomic bomb survivors. Report 13: solid cancer and noncancer disease mortality: 1950-1997. Radiat Res 2003;160:381–407.
57. Preston DL, Ron E, Tokuoka S, et al. Solid cancer incidence in atomic bomb survivors: 1958-1998. Radiat Res 2007;168:1–64.
58. Gilbert ES, Stovall M, Gospodarowicz M, et al. Lung cancer after treatment for Hodgkin's disease: focus on radiation effects. Radiat Res 2003;159:161–73.
59. Furukawa K, Preston DL, Lonn S, et al. Radiation and smoking effects on lung cancer incidence among atomic bomb survivors. Radiat Res 2010;174:72–82.
60. HSDB. Hazardous Substances Data Bank. National Library of Medicine. 2012. Available at: http://toxnet.nlm.nih.gov/cgi-bin/sis/search/f?./temp/~ZkJdFQ:1. Accessed April 20, 2012.
61. NIOSH. National occupational exposure survey (1981-83). National Institute for Occupational Safety and Health; 1990. Available at: http://www.cdc.gov/noes/noes1/x6315sic.html. Accessed April 21, 2012.
62. Krieger RI, Dinoff TM, Zhang X. Octachlorodipropyl ether (s-2) mosquito coils are inadequately studied for residential use in Asia and illegal in the United States. Environ Health Perspect 2003;111(12):1439–42.
63. Pauluhn J. Overview of inhalation exposure techniques: strengths and weaknesses. Exp Toxicol Pathol 2005;57(1):111–28.
64. IARC Monographs on the Evaluation of Carcinogenic Risks to Humans. A review of human carcinogens: chemical agents and related occupations, bis(chloromethyl)ether. vol. 100F; 2012. Available at: http://monographs.iarc.fr/ENG/Monographs/vol100F/mono100F-25.pdf. Accessed April 25, 2012.
65. Weiss W, Boucot KR. The respiratory effects of chloromethyl methyl ether. JAMA 1975;234:1139–42.
66. IARC Monographs on the Evaluation of Carcinogenic Risks to Humans. A review of human carcinogens: chemical agents and related occupations, sulfur mustard. vol. 100F; 2012. Available at: http://monographs.iarc.fr/ENG/Monographs/vol100F/mono100F-30.pdf. Accessed April 25, 2012.
67. IARC. Genetic and related effects: an updating of selected IARC monographs from Volumes 1 to 42. IARC Monogr Eval Carcinog Risks Hum Suppl 1987;6:1–729.
68. National Toxicology Program. Report on carcinogens, 2011, coal tars and coal-tar pitches. 12th edition. US Department of Health and Human Services, Public Health Service. p. 111–3. Available at: http://ntp.niehs.nih.gov/ntp/roc/twelfth/profiles/CoalTars.pdf. Accessed April 20, 2012.
69. IARC. Some non-heterocyclic polycyclic aromatic hydrocarbons and some related exposures. IARC Monogr Eval Carcinog Risks Hum 2010;92:1–853. Available at: http://monographs.iarc.fr/ENG/Monographs/vol92/mono92.pdf. Accessed May 1, 2012.
70. Boffetta PI, Burstyn T, Partanen H, et al. Cancer mortality among European asphalt workers: an international epidemiological study, results of the analysis based on job titles. Am J Ind Med 2003;43:18–27.
71. Olsson A, Kromhout H, Agostini M, et al. A case-control study of lung cancer nested in a cohort of European asphalt workers. Environ Health Perspect 2010;118(10):1418–24.

72. National Toxicology Program. Report on carcinogens, 2011, soots. 12th edition. US Department of Health and Human Services, Public Health Service. p. 379–80. Available at: http://ntp.niehs.nih.gov/ntp/roc/twelfth/profiles/Soots.pdf. Accessed April 20, 2012.

73. National Chimney Sweep Guild. Available at: http://www.ncsg.org/. Accessed April 15, 2012.

74. IARC Monographs on the Evaluation of Carcinogenic Risks to Humans. A review of human carcinogens: chemical agents and related occupations, soot, as found in occupational exposures of chimney-sweeps. vol. 100F; 2012. Available at: http://monographs.iarc.fr/ENG/Monographs/vol100F/mono100F-21.pdf. Accessed April 25, 2012.

75. Pukkala E, Martinsen JI, Lynge E, et al. Occupation and cancer—follow-up of 15 million people in five Nordic countries. Acta Oncol 2009;48:646–790.

76. McDonald JD, Campen MJ, Harrod KS, et al. Engine-operating load influences diesel exhaust composition and cardiopulmonary and immune responses. Environ Health Perspect 2011;119(8):1136–41.

77. Pronk A, Coble J, Stewart PA. Occupational exposure to diesel exhaust: a literature review. J Expo Sci Environ Epidemiol 2009;19:443–57.

78. IARC Monographs on the Evaluation of the Carcinogenic Risks of Chemicals to Humans. Diesel and Gasoline Engine Exhausts and Some Nitroarenes. Volume 46. Lyon (France): International Agency for Research on Cancer; 1989. Available at: http://monographs.iarc.fr/ENG/Monographs/vol46/index.php. Accessed June 10, 2012.

79. International Agency for Research on Cancer. Monographs on the Evaluation of Carcinogenic Risks to Humans. Diesel and gasoline engine exhausts and some nitroarenes. Lyon (France): vol. 105; 2012. p. 5–12. Available at: http://www.iarc.fr/en/media-centre/iarcnews/2012/mono105-info.php. Accessed June 12, 2012.

80. International Agency for Research on Cancer. Diesel engine exhaust carcinogenic. Press release. Available at: http://press.iarc.fr/pr213_E.pdf. Accessed June 12, 2012.

81. National Toxicology Program, Department of Health and Human Services. Diesel exhaust particulates report on carcinogens. 12th Edition. 2011. Available at: http://ntp.niehs.nih.gov/ntp/roc/twelfth/profiles/DieselExhaustParticulates.pdf. Accessed June 12, 2012.

82. Silverman DT, Samanic CM, Lubin JH, et al. The diesel exhaust in miners study: a nested case–control study of lung cancer and diesel exhaust. J Natl Cancer Inst 2012;104(11):855–68.

83. IARC Monographs on the Evaluation of Carcinogenic Risks to Humans. A review of human carcinogens: chemical agents and related occupations. vol. 100F; 2012. Available at: http://monographs.iarc.fr/ENG/Monographs/vol100F/index.php. Accessed April 15, 2012.

84. Bosetti C, Boffetta P, La Vecchia C. Occupational exposures to polycyclic aromatic hydrocarbons, and respiratory and urinary tract cancers: a quantitative review to 2005. Ann Oncol 2007;18:431–46.

85. IARC Monographs on the Evaluation of Carcinogenic Risks to Humans. A review of human carcinogens: chemical agents and related occupations, occupational exposure as a painter. vol. 100F; 2012. Available at: http://monographs.iarc.fr/ENG/Monographs/vol100F/mono100F-35.pdf. Accessed April 15, 2012.

86. Bachand A, Mundt KA, Mundt DJ, et al. Meta-analyses of occupational exposure as a painter and lung and bladder cancer morbidity and mortality 1950-2008. Crit Rev Toxicol 2010;40(2):101–25.

87. Guha N, Merletti F, Steenland NK. Lung cancer risk in painters: a meta-analysis. Environ Health Perspect 2010;118:303–12.

88. IARC Monographs on the Evaluation of Carcinogenic Risks to Humans. Occupational exposure in the rubber-manufacturing industry. vol. 100F; 2012. Available at: http://monographs.iarc.fr/ENG/Monographs/vol100F/mono100F-36.pdf. Accessed April 15, 2012.

89. Fajen JM, Carson GA, Rounbehler DP, et al. N-nitrosamines in the rubber and tire industry. Science 1979;205:1262–4.

90. International Agency for Research on Cancer. Printing processes, printing inks, carbon blacks and some nitro compounds, vol. 65. Lyon (France): International Agency for Research on Cancer; 1996.

91. Straif K, Keil U, Taeger D, et al. Exposure to nitrosamines, carbon black, asbestos, and talc and mortality from stomach, lung, and laryngeal cancer in a cohort of rubber workers. Am J Epidemiol 2000;152(4):297–306.

92. Alder N, Fenty J, Warren F, et al. Meta-analysis of mortality and cancer incidence among workers in the synthetic rubber-producing industry. Am J Epidemiol 2006;164:405–20.

93. Taeger D, Weiland SK, Sun Y, et al. Cancer and non-cancer mortality in a cohort of recent entrants (1981–2000) to the German rubber industry. Occup Environ Med 2007;64:560–1.

94. Dost A, Straughan J, Sorahan T. A cohort mortality and cancer incidence survey of recent entrants (1982–91) to the UK rubber industry: findings for 1983–2004. Occup Med (Lond) 2007;57:186–90.

95. Pira E, Pelucchi C, Romano C. Mortality from cancer and other causes in an Italian cohort of male rubber tire workers. J Occup Environ Med 2012;54(3):345–9.

96. Winder C, Stacey NH, editors. Toxicity of metals, occupational toxicology. 2nd edition. Boca Raton (FL): CRC Press; 2004.

97. IARC Monographs on the Evaluation of Carcinogenic Risks to Humans. A review of human carcinogens: arsenic, metals, fibres, and dusts, arsenic and arsenic compounds. vol. 100C; 2012. Available at: http://monographs.iarc.fr/ENG/Monographs/vol100C/mono100C-6.pdf. Accessed April 25, 2012.

98. Lubin JH, Moore LE, Fraumeni JF Jr, et al. Respiratory cancer and inhaled inorganic arsenic in copper smelter workers: a linear relationship with cumulative exposure that increases with concentration. Environ Health Perspect 2008;116(12):1661–5 Epidemiology 2000;11(6):673–79.

99. Ferreccio C, González C, Milosavjlevic V, et al. Lung cancer and arsenic concentrations in drinking water in Chile. Epidemiology 2000;11:673–9.

100. Cantor KP, Lubin JH. Arsenic, internal cancers, and issues in inference from studies of low level exposures in human populations. Toxicol Appl Pharmacol 2007;222(3):252–7.

101. McCleskey TM, Buchner V, Field RW, et al. Recent advances in understanding the biomolecular basis of chronic beryllium disease: a review. Rev Environ Health 2009;24(2):75–115.

102. IARC Monographs on the Evaluation of Carcinogenic Risks to Humans. A review of human carcinogens: arsenic, metals, fibres, and dusts, beryllium and beryllium compounds. vol. 100C; 2012. Available at: http://monographs.iarc.fr/ENG/Monographs/vol100C/mono100C-7.pdf. Accessed April 25, 2012.

103. United States General Accounting Office. Report to Congressional Requesters, Occupational Safety and Health, Government responses to beryllium uses and risks, GAO/OCG-00–6. 2000. Available at: http://www.dau.mil/educdept/mm_dept_resources/reports/Government-responses-to-Beryllium.pdf. Accessed May 1, 2012.

104. Materion Brush Inc. Sources of beryllium. Available at: http://www.beryllium.com/sources-beryllium. Accessed May 17, 2012.

105. Kreiss K, Day GA, Schuler CR. Beryllium: a modern industrial hazard. Annu Rev Public Health 2007;28:259–77.

106. Agency for Toxic Substances and Disease Registry (ATSDR). Toxicological profile for beryllium. Atlanta (GA): U.S. Department of Health and Human Services, Public Health Service; 2002.

107. NIOSH, Comments of the National Institute for Occupational Safety and Health on the Department of Energy. Request for information on Chronic Beryllium Disease Prevention Program. Docket No. HS-RM-1 0-CBDPP RIN 1992-AA39, 2/22/11. Cincinnati (OH): Department of Health and Human Services, Centers for Disease Control and Prevention; 2011.

108. IARC. Beryllium, cadmium, mercury, and exposures in the glass manufacturing industry. IARC Monogr Eval Carcinog Risks Hum 1993;58:1–415.

109. Schubauer-Berigan MK, Deddens JA, Steenland K, et al. Adjustment for temporal confounders in a re-analysis of a case-control study of beryllium and lung cancer. Occup Environ Med 2008;65:379–83.

110. Deubner DC, Roth HD. Rejoinder: progress in understanding the relationship between beryllium exposure and lung cancer. Epidemiology 2009;20:341–3.

111. Schubauer-Berigan MK, Couch JR, Petersen MR, et al. Cohort mortality study of workers at seven beryllium processing plants: update and associations with cumulative and maximum exposure. Occup Environ Med 2011;68(5):345–53.

112. Schubauer-Berigan MK, Deddens JA, Couch JR, et al. Risk of lung cancer associated with quantitative beryllium exposure metrics within an occupational cohort. Occup Environ Med 2011;68(5):354–60.

113. Boffetta P, Fryzek JP, Mandel J. Occupational exposure to beryllium and cancer risk: a review of the epidemiologic evidence. Crit Rev Toxicol 2012;42(2):107–18.

114. USGS Commodity Report. Cadmium. United States Geological Survey, Cadmium Statistics and Information. Available at: http://minerals.usgs.gov/minerals/pubs/commodity/cadmium/. Accessed May 18, 2012.

115. Agency for Toxic Substances and Disease Registry, US Department of Health and Human Services, Public Health Service. Draft toxicological profile for cadmium. 2008. Available at: http://www.atsdr.cdc.gov/toxprofiles/tp5.pdf. Accessed April 25, 2012.

116. National Toxicology Program, Department of Health and Human Services. Report on carcinogens. 12th edition (2011). Cadmium and cadmium compounds. CAS No. 7440-43-9 (Cadmium). Available at: http://ntp.niehs.nih.gov/ntp/roc/twelfth/profiles/Cadmium.pdf. Accessed May 18, 2012.

117. US Geological Survey. Minerals yearbook. US Department of the Interior. Cadmium, by Amy C. Tolcin. 2010. Available at: http://minerals.usgs.gov/minerals/pubs/commodity/cadmium/myb1-2010-cadmi.pdf. Accessed May 18, 2012.

118. IARC Monographs on the Evaluation of Carcinogenic Risks to Humans. A review of human carcinogens: arsenic, metals, fibres, and dusts, beryllium and beryllium compounds, cadmium and cadmium compounds. vol. 100C; 2012. Available at: http://monographs.iarc.fr/ENG/Monographs/vol100C/mono100C-8.pdf. Accessed April 25, 2012.

119. Beveridge R, Pintos J, Parent ME, et al. Lung cancer risk associated with occupational exposure to nickel, chromium VI, and cadmium in two population-based case-control studies in Montreal. Am J Ind Med 2010;53(5):476–85.

120. Park RM, Stayner LT, Petersen MR, et al. Cadmium and lung cancer mortality accounting for simultaneous arsenic exposure. Occup Environ Med 2012;69(5):303–9.

121. Occupational Safety and Health Administration. Department of Labor. Occupational exposure to hexavalent chromium. Final rule. Fed Regist 2006; 71:10099–385.

122. Agency for Toxic Substances and Disease Registry. Toxicological profile for chromium. (Draft for public comment). Atlanta (GA): U.S. Department of Health and Human Services, Public Health Service; 2008.

123. Luo J, Hendryx M, Ducatman A. Association between six environmental chemicals and lung cancer incidence in the United States. J Environ Public Health 2011;2011. Article ID 463701. Available at: http://www.hindawi.com/journals/jeph/2011/463701/. Accessed May 18, 2012.

124. NIOSH. Hexavalent chromium, criteria document update, external review draft, occupational exposure to hexavalent chromium. Department of Health and Human Services, Centers for Disease Control and Prevention, National Institute for Occupational Safety and Health. 2008.

125. IARC Monographs on the Evaluation of Carcinogenic Risks to Humans. A review of human carcinogens: arsenic, metals, fibres, and dusts, chromium (VI) compounds. vol. 100C; 2012. Available at: http://monographs.iarc.fr/ENG/Monographs/vol100C/mono100C-9.pdf. Accessed April 25, 2012.

126. USGS. 2009 Minerals yearbook, nickel (advance release). US Department of the Interior, US Geological Survey. Available at: http://minerals.usgs.gov/minerals/pubs/commodity/nickel/myb1-2009-nicke.pdf. Accessed April 25, 2012.

127. National Toxicology Program. Nickel compounds and metallic nickel substance profiles. Report on Carcinogens. 12th edition. US Department of Health and Human Services, Public Health Service; 2011. Available at: http://ntp.niehs.nih.gov/ntp/roc/twelfth/roc12.pdf. Accessed May 18, 2012.

128. Davis JR. Uses of nickel. ASM specialty handbook: nickel, cobalt, and their alloys. ASM International 2000;7–13. Available at: http://www.knovel.com/web/portal/browse/display?_EXT_KNOVEL_DISPLAY_bookid=3142&VerticalID=0. Accessed April 25, 2012.

129. IARC Monographs on the Evaluation of Carcinogenic Risks to Humans. A review of human carcinogens: arsenic, metals, fibres, and dusts, nickel and nickel compounds. vol. 100C; 2012. Available at: http://monographs.iarc.fr/ENG/Monographs/vol100C/mono100C-8.pdf. Accessed April 25, 2012.

130. Agency for Toxic Substances and Disease Registry. Toxicological profile for nickel. Atlanta (GA): U.S. Department of Health and Human Services, Public Health Service; 2005.

131. Grimsrud TK, Berge SR, Martinsen JI, et al. Lung cancer incidence among Norwegian nickel-refinery workers 1953–2000. J Environ Monit 2003;5:190–7.

132. Grimsrud TK, Berge SR, Haldorsen T, et al. Can lung cancer risk among nickel refinery workers be explained by occupational exposures other than nickel? Epidemiology 2005;16:146–54.

133. Andersen A, Berge SR, Engeland A, et al. Exposure to nickel compounds and smoking in relation to incidence of lung and nasal cancer among nickel refinery workers. Occup Environ Med 1996; 53:708–13.

134. Grimsrud TK, Berge SR, Haldorsen T, et al. Exposure to different forms of nickel and risk of lung cancer. Am J Epidemiol 2002;156:1123–32.

135. Goodman JE, Prueitt RL, Dodge DG, et al. Carcinogenicity assessment of water-soluble nickel compounds. Crit Rev Toxicol 2009;39(5):365–417.

136. IARC Monographs on the Evaluation of Carcinogenic Risks to Humans. A review of human carcinogens: arsenic, metals, fibres, and dusts, nickel and nickel compounds. vol. 100C; 2012. Available at: http://monographs.iarc.fr/ENG/Monographs/vol100C/100C-05-Table2.3.pdf. Accessed April 25, 2012.

137. Grimsrud TK, Andersen A. Unrecognized risks of nickel-related respiratory cancer among Canadian electrolysis workers. Scand J Work Environ Health 2012 [Epub ahead of print].

138. De Matteis S, Consonni D, Lubin JH, et al. Impact of occupational carcinogens on lung cancer risk in a general population. Int J Epidemiol 2012; 41(3):711–21.

139. National Toxicology Program. Asbestos, Department of Health and Human Services report on carcinogens. 12th edition. 2011. Available at: http://ntp.niehs.nih.gov/ntp/roc/twelfth/profiles/Asbestos.pdf. Accessed May 27, 2012.

140. US EPA. Asbestos ban and phase out. US Environmental Protection Agency. Available at: http://www.epa.gov/asbestos/pubs/ban.html. Accessed May 27, 2012.

141. US Geological Survey. Mineral commodity summaries, asbestos. 2012. Available at: http://minerals.usgs.gov/minerals/pubs/commodity/asbestos/mcs-2012-asbes.pdf. Accessed May 27, 2012.

142. ATSDR. Toxicological profile for asbestos. Agency for Toxic Substances and Disease Registry. 2001. Available at: http://www.atsdr.cdc.gov/toxprofiles/tp61.pdf. Accessed May 15, 2012.

143. Suvatne J, Browning RF. Asbestos and lung cancer. Dis Mon 2011;57:55–68.

144. IARC Monographs on the Evaluation of Carcinogenic Risks to Humans. A review of human carcinogens: arsenic, metals, fibres, and dusts, asbestos (chrysotile, amosite, crocidolite, tremolite,

actinolite, and anthophyllite). vol. 100C; 2012. Available at: http://monographs.iarc.fr/ENG/Monographs/vol100C/mono100C-11.pdf. Accessed May 25, 2012.

145. Yarborough CM. Chrysotile as a cause of mesothelioma: an assessment based on epidemiology. Crit Rev Toxicol 2006;36:165–87.

146. Hodgson JT, Darnton A. The quantitative risks of mesothelioma and lung cancer in relation to asbestos exposure. Ann Occup Hyg 2000;44: 565–601.

147. Stayner LT, Dankovic DA, Lemen RA. Occupational exposure to chrysotile asbestos and cancer risk: a review of the amphibole hypothesis. Am J Public Health 1996;86(2):179–86.

148. Berman DW, Crump KS. Update of potency factors for asbestos-related lung cancer and mesothelioma. Crit Rev Toxicol 2008;38(Suppl):11–47.

149. Stayner L, Kuempel E, Gilbert S, et al. An epidemiological study of the role of chrysotile asbestos fibre dimensions in determining respiratory disease risk in exposed workers. Occup Environ Med 2008; 65:613–9.

150. Lenters V, Vermeulen R, Dogger S. A meta-analysis of asbestos and lung cancer: is better quality exposure assessment associated with steeper slopes of the exposure–response relationships? Environ Health Perspect 2011;119:1547–55.

151. Loomis D, Dement JM, Richardson D, et al. Asbestos fibre dimensions and lung cancer mortality among workers exposed to chrysotile. Occup Environ Med 2009;67:580–4.

152. Mirabelli D, Calisti R, Barone-Adesi F, et al. Excess of mesotheliomas after exposure to chrysotile in Balangero, Italy. Occup Environ Med 2008;65: 815–9.

153. Loomis D, Dement JM, Wolf SH, et al. Lung cancer mortality and fibre exposures among North Carolina asbestos textile workers. Occup Environ Med 2009;66(8):535–42.

154. Elliott L, Loomis D, Dement J, et al. Lung cancer mortality in North Carolina and South Carolina chrysotile asbestos textile workers. Occup Environ Med 2012;69(6):385–90.

155. Loomis D, Dement JM, Elliott L, et al. Increased lung cancer mortality among chrysotile asbestos textile workers is more strongly associated with exposure to long thin fibres. Occup Med 2012; 69(8):564–8.

156. US Department of the Interior, US Bureau of Mines, US Geological Survey, staff, Branch of Industrial Minerals. Crystalline silica primer. Available at: http://minerals.er.usgs.gov/minerals/pubs/commodity/silica/780292.pdf. Accessed June 3, 2012.

157. National Institute for Occupational Safety and Health, Department of Health and Human Services, Centers for Disease Control and Prevention. NIOSH Hazard review, health effects of occupational exposure to respirable crystalline silica. Cincinnati (OH): DHHS (NIOSH); 2002. Publication No. 2002–129.

158. Esswein E, Kiefer MS, Snawder J, et al. Worker exposure to crystalline silica during hydraulic fracturing. NIOSH Science Blog, Safer Healthier Workers, Centers for Disease Control and Prevention. Available at: http://blogs.cdc.gov/niosh-science-blog/2012/05/silica-fracking/. Accessed June 4, 2012.

159. IARC Monographs on the Evaluation of Carcinogenic Risks to Humans. A review of human carcinogens: silica dust, crystalline, in the form of quartz or cristobalite. vol. 100C; 2012. Available at: http://monographs.iarc.fr/ENG/Monographs/vol100C/mono100C-14.pdf. Accessed May 1, 2012.

160. Steenland K, Sanderson W. Lung cancer among industrial sand workers exposed to crystalline silica. Am J Epidemiol 2001;153:695–703.

161. Lacasse Y, Martin S, Gagné D, et al. Dose response meta-analysis of silica and lung cancer. Cancer Causes Control 2009;20:925–33.

162. Erren TC, Glende CB, Morfeld P, et al. Is exposure to silica associated with lung cancer in the absence of silicosis? A meta-analytical approach to an important public health question. Int Arch Occup Environ Health 2009;82:997–1004.

163. Pelucchi C, Pira E, Piolatto G, et al. Occupational silica exposure and lung cancer risk: a review of epidemiological studies 1996–2005. Ann Oncol 2006;17:1039–50.

164. Borm PJ, Tran L, Donaldson K. The carcinogenic action of crystalline silica: a review of the evidence supporting secondary inflammation-driven genotoxicity as a principal mechanism. Crit Rev Toxicol 2011;9:756–70.

165. Checkoway H, Franzblau A. Is silicosis required for silica-associated lung cancer? Am J Ind Med 2000; 37:252–9.

166. Stayner L. Silica and lung cancer: when is enough evidence enough? Epidemiology 2007;18:23–4.

167. Mannetje A, Brennan P, Zaridze D, et al. Welding and lung cancer in Central and Eastern Europe and the United Kingdom. Am J Epidemiol 2012; 175(7):706–14.

168. IARC Monographs on the Evaluation of Carcinogenic Risk to Humans. Priority agents for future IARC Monographs. Available at: http://monographs.iarc.fr/ENG/Meetings/PriorityAgents.pdf. Accessed June 12, 2012.

Military Service and Lung Disease

Cecile S. Rose, MD, MPH[a,b,*]

KEYWORDS

- Military • Iraq • Afghanistan • Lung disease • Asthma • Bronchiolitis
- Acute eosinophilic pneumonia • Inhalational exposures

KEY POINTS

- Military personnel can be exposed to unusual inhalational toxicants and extreme conditions that can contribute to lung diseases.
- This article describes what is known about the inhalational exposures and lung diseases associated with military service, focusing on the recent Iraq and Afghanistan wars.
- Inhalational exposures of concern during military service in Iraq and Afghanistan include desert dusts and related particulates, numerous combustion products from burning of waste, hydrogen sulfide, blast exposures, and metal fragments.

Lung illnesses from military service, although overlapping with those faced in civilian workplaces, may arise from unusual exposures in extreme circumstances and create particular challenges in diagnosis, management, and prevention. Respiratory toxicants such as chemical and biologic warfare agents, common respiratory infectious agents, general and specific air pollutants (eg, desert dusts, burn pit smoke, oil well fires, and local industrial pollutants), extreme physical demands and settings (including extremes of topography and weather), explosive blasts (sometimes with retained metal fragments) and other diverse exposures in adverse and unfamiliar environments (**Box 1**) have contributed to the risk for lung disease associated with military service since recorded history. Such service-related exposures have become a growing concern among veterans and their health care providers.[1,2]

There are a number of features that distinguish military occupational health risks. Compared with the civilian work force, military recruits as a whole are younger, more athletic, and have been regularly exercising. Army recruits must be able to pass a 2-mile physical fitness test run (similar to the Air Force physical readiness test) without difficulty. These requirements vary with age, ranging from a minimum time for a 2-mile run of 16.5 minutes for soldiers who are 23 years old to 19.5 minutes for those who are 48 years of age. In addition to strenuous physical demands, military personnel are often subjected to crowded living conditions, increased exposure to respiratory disease agents, and high levels of stress.[3] Deployment to a battle site creates a different spectrum of duty positions and exposures (eg, oil well fires, depleted uranium, tainted water, sand flies, and preventive medications and vaccinations).

Research on exposure-related lung disease among military personnel is hampered by difficulties with characterizing and measuring exposures in combat settings, the lack of baseline lung health

---

Funding Sources: Department of Defense.
Conflict of Interest: None.
[a] Division of Environmental and Occupational Health Sciences, National Jewish Health, 1400 Jackson Street, Denver, CO 80206, USA; [b] Division of Pulmonary Sciences and Critical Care, University of Colorado Denver, Aurora, CO, USA
* Division of Environmental and Occupational Health Sciences, National Jewish Health, 1400 Jackson Street, Denver, CO 80206.
E-mail address: rosec@njhealth.org

Box 1
Spectrum of military deployment exposures with potential adverse respiratory effects

1. Environmental
   a. Outdoor
      i. Particulate matter/desert dusts
      ii. Pollutants from local industries
      iii. Burn pit smoke
      iv. Vehicular exhaust
      v. JP8 and other jet fuels
      vi. Smoke from oil well fires
   b. Indoor
      i. Second-hand smoke
      ii. Poor indoor air quality (eg, tent heater smoke)
      iii. Close proximity – risk for infectious agent spread
      iv. Chemicals used in usual job tasks (paints, solvents, pesticides)
2. Combat related
   a. Blasts from explosive devices
   b. Embedded shrapnel
   c. Chemical and biologic warfare agents

---

information on combatants before deployment, and the variability and unpredictability of occupational exposures associated with particular job titles and duties in theater. Despite these challenges, historic and more recent studies have found associations between exposures during military service and adverse health outcomes. This article focuses mainly on inhalational exposures and lung diseases associated with the 2 most recent US wars, those in Iraq and Afghanistan.

HISTORICAL OVERVIEW

The earliest recorded use of gas warfare in the West dates back to the 5th century BCE, during the Peloponnesian War between Athens and Sparta. Spartan forces placed a lighted mixture of wood, pitch, and sulfur under the walls of the enemy city, hoping that the noxious smoke would incapacitate the Athenians and diminish their resistance to the assault that followed. Many other historical examples of use of toxic inhalants during war have been reported.[4] The first major use of chemical warfare agents occurred in World War I. Over 50,000 tons of pulmonary, lachrymatory, and vesicant agents were deployed by both sides in this conflict, including chlorine, phosgene, and mustard

gas. Official figures estimate 1,176,500 nonfatal casualties and 85,000 fatalities directly caused by chemical warfare agents during the course of the war.[5] Chlorine and phosgene gas were first used in 1915. Sulfur mustard, commonly known as mustard gas, was introduced as a war agent toward the end of World War I in July 1917. Thousands of soldiers were exposed to sulfur mustard, a vesicant that was dispersed as a liquid aerosol, causing skin sloughing, corneal damage, upper airway injury, and tracheitis. Those who survived were often disabled by severe breathlessness and cough, with chest radiographic findings of air trapping that suggest chronic large and small airway injuries.

Since World War I, mustard gas has been used in several wars and conflicts, sometimes against civilians, most recently during the last years of the Iraq–Iran war (1984–1988). Chronic lung sequelae from sulfur mustard exposure have been described, including asthma, bronchiectasis, tracheal stenosis, tracheobronchomalacia, obliterative bronchiolitis, and pulmonary fibrosis.[6,7] Use of chemical warfare agents was prohibited by the 1925 Geneva Protocol and in 1993 by the Chemical Weapons Convention. The latter agreement also prohibited the development, production, stockpiling, and sale of such weapons.

Concern for the long-term health consequences of exposures during military service have emerged after more recent conflicts. In a retrospective survey of 1500 Vietnam veterans who sprayed phenoxyherbicides (resulting in exposure to Agent Orange and its dioxin contaminants), odds ratios were increased for chronic nonmalignant respiratory conditions (odds ratio, 1.62; 95% confidence interval, 1.28–2.05), but not for those who served in Vietnam without such exposures.[8]

In August 1990, in response to the Iraqi invasion of Kuwait, the United States and several other countries sent military service members to the Saudi Arabian peninsula in an effort referred to as Operation Desert Shield/Desert Storm. The United States deployed nearly 700,000 service members, 83% of whom were active duty and 17% National Guard/Reserves. In early 1991, shortly before the start of the ground phase of the Persian Gulf War, Iraqi forces set fire to more than 600 oil wells, exposing thousands of troops to oil well fire smoke. Those in the Army and Marine Corps were stationed most frequently in the vicinity of oil well fires. Most of those exposed were later included in a registry of at-risk military personnel containing information on respiratory symptoms, unit location, and exposure. A case-control study found significant associations between asthma and oil fire smoke exposure based on both self-reported and modeled exposures.[9] Concern about exposure to environmental toxins and potential health outcomes was a defining feature of the first Persian Gulf War.

The 2 most recent conflicts involving US military deployments began after September 11, 2001. In Iraq, Operation Iraqi Freedom (OIF) began in March 2003 and ended in August 2010. In Afghanistan, Operation Enduring Freedom (OEF) began in October 2001 and continues to the present. More than 2 million Americans have been deployed to these areas of conflict, and approximately 1.4 million have separated from the military and become veterans. Based on responses to a survey completed within 3 to 6 months of returning from these deployment areas, 20% to 33% of US service members have concerns about hazardous exposures during deployment.[1] Among the top 5 health concerns reported by nearly 119,000 returning service members between September 2005 and August 2006, 4 involved inhalational exposures including desert sand, burn pit smoke from burning trash and feces, vehicle exhaust, and jet fuels.[1] Follow-up analysis in a sample of 469 OIF/OEF veterans showed high levels of concern about exposures, the most prevalent being air pollution (reported by 94%), vaccines (86%), and petrochemicals (81%).[2]

HAZARDOUS INHALATIONAL EXPOSURES AND RECENT MILITARY SERVICE IN IRAQ AND AFGHANISTAN
Desert Dusts and Other Geogenic Sources of Particulate Matter Exposure During Military Service

Geogenic dust inhalation in Southwest Asia may occur from frequent exposure to low to moderately high levels of particulate matter (PM) during windy conditions; as a result of activity-related exposure to dusts generated by military operations such as traffic on dirt roads leading to re-suspension of settled dusts; and from acute high exposures to extreme dust loads during severe dust storms, sometimes lasting for days and often intense enough to obscure visibility. Geogenic dusts elsewhere in the world have been shown to contain elevated levels of both natural and anthropogenic toxicants and pathogens, and long-term exposures have been linked with risk for pneumoconioses and other lung diseases in local populations. For example, dust from the Owens dry lake area in California contains high levels of arsenic; dust from the Aral Sea in Asia contains increased concentrations of pesticides and other chemicals; and dusts from the US desert southwest contains spores of the soil fungus

Coccidioides immitis that can cause lung infection owing to Valley Fever. Limited environmental sampling from Middle East deployment sites have identified bacterial, fungal, and other pathogens in Iraq soils and settled dusts. The military's Enhanced Particulate Matter Surveillance Program collected more than 3000 filter samples along with bulk dust and soil samples from 15 deployment sites (2 in Afghanistan and 6 in Iraq).[10] All sites exceeded the 1-year Military Exposures Guidelines value of 15 $\mu g/m^3$ for PM2.5, the fraction in which trace metal concentrations of lead, arsenic, cadmium, antimony, and zinc were concentrated. Exposure to geogenic dust was a major source of PM exposure in these settings.

Burn Pits

The open air burning of trash and other waste, often in close proximity to military quarters and work sites, has generated concern about risk for lung disease from deployment exposure to "burn pits." Pollutants including volatile organic compounds, dioxins and respirable PM may be generated in such circumstances, with potential acute respiratory irritant effects as well as concerns about long-term lung and other health risks.

A 2011 Institute of Medicine (IOM) report focused on potential exposure to burn pit emissions at Joint Base Balad (JBB) and other US military bases in Iraq and Afghanistan and potential health effects of these exposures.[11] The IOM committee found that military personnel were exposed to a mixture of burn pit combustion products and other air pollutants from local and regional sources, including wind-blown soils and local industrial PM. This PM, from both geogenic and anthropogenic sources, contained substantial amounts of windblown dust combined with elemental carbon and metals that arise from transportation and industrial activities. Both PM and acrolein were detected in air samples at JBB at average concentrations exceeding US air pollution standards. The committee commented that increased respiratory morbidity and mortality have been observed in numerous epidemiologic studies of PM exposure at lower concentrations, and noted that susceptibility to respiratory and cardiovascular PM health effects could be exacerbated by other military service exposures including stress, smoking, and climatic conditions.[11]

The IOM committee noted substantial limitations in available air monitoring data, including inadequate information on concentration, composition, frequency, and duration of smoke episodes at the site. As a result, the committee was unable to conclude whether exposures to burn pit emissions at JBB increased the risks for long-term health effects. The report suggested that "service in Iraq or Afghanistan might be associated with long-term health effects, particularly in susceptible (for example, those who have asthma) or highly exposed subpopulations (such as those who worked at the burn pit)."[11]

In follow-up to the IOM committee report, several epidemiologic investigations were undertaken by scientists with the US Army Public Health Command. One study[12] used a case-crossover design to estimate the short-term relative risk of acute cardiovascular and respiratory outcomes (based on analysis of in-theater respiratory health encounters at JBB) associated with measured levels of PM2.5 ($\leq$2.5 microns in aerodynamic diameter) and PM10. Although no effect was found, the authors reflect that study design limitations, including the short study duration (1 year), small study population, limited PM sampling, and incomplete data in the electronic medical record, may have hampered their results.

The Al-Mishraq Sulfur Fire and Other Industrial Sources of Hazardous Inhalation Exposures

In June 2004, a large fire began at the state-run Al-Mishraq sulfur plant near Mosul, Iraq, creating a dense plume of smoke containing sulfurous compounds that persisted over the next month despite efforts to extinguish the blaze. At the time, thousands of US military men and women were in the area in support of OIF. Some were mobilized to assist in firefighting efforts, and others helped evacuate local residents; most continued usual military missions and transport operations at Q-West base camp, 25 km southwest of the fire, and at Mosul Airfield, located 50 km north.

Burning sulfur emits a number of known respiratory hazards including sulfur dioxide (SO_2) and hydrogen sulfide (H_2S). SO_2 is a respiratory irritant that can cause symptoms of rhinorrhea, cough, sputum production, and dyspnea. Depending on exposure dose, SO_2-related lung injury may lead to irritant-induced asthma with bronchoconstriction, chronic bronchitis, or constrictive bronchiolitis (CB).[13] Similar pulmonary effects can occur with exposure to high concentrations of H_2S. Limited environmental sampling for H_2S and SO_2 showed that the military population was potentially exposed to levels associated with lung health effects.[14] A retrospective cohort study examined the post-deployment respiratory health status of active-duty US Army personnel potentially exposed to sulfur emissions from the Al-Mishraq fire.[15] The cohort included 191 exposed fire

fighters and 6341 other potentially exposed personnel within a 50 km radius of the fire. Findings from standardized post-deployment health assessment questionnaires, along with analysis of ICD-9-CM diagnosis codes for chronic obstructive pulmonary disease, asthma, chronic bronchitis, and other respiratory outcomes, were analyzed in exposed deployed personnel. The findings were compared with 2 "control" cohorts: One whose tour to the same area began after the fire was extinguished and the second a contemporaneous cohort from other deployment sites. The study found a significant increase in respiratory symptoms in those exposed to the sulfur fire.[15] It also found increased rates of respiratory-related medical encounters from the pre-deployment to the post-deployment period for all of the study cohorts (including both comparison groups). The authors conclude that there was no definitive link between sulfur fire exposure in Iraq and respiratory disease.

Air pollutants from local industries contribute in variable degrees to the inhalational risks faced by troops serving in deployed areas. Lead–zinc and battery-processing industries were identified as 1 of the 3 major sources of PM exposure based on environmental sampling from 15 Middle East deployment sites.[16]

Blasts and Explosions

Blast exposure emanates from improvised explosive devices, rocket-propelled or hand-held grenades, or land mines. In a study of 805 enlisted Army National Guard and Reserve soldiers deployed to Iraq or Afghanistan,[2] reported rates of blast exposure were higher than any other environmental hazard, with 15.2% reporting exposure to 1 blast, 9.4% to 2, 7.7% to 3, and 28.5% to 5 or more blasts. Although body armor may protect personnel from most ballistic projectiles, it does not protect against the primary blast injury.

The lung is highly susceptible to primary blast injury, the most common critical injury to people in close proximity to a blast center.[17] The temporal sequence of injuries from blast explosions include tissue damage from the blast short wave (primary blast injury); material propelled into the casualty; the casualty propelled against other objects; heat, chemicals, and toxins delivered by the explosive device; and the systemic inflammatory response to the injury.[17] Fatal blast lung injury can occur without signs of external trauma. The mechanism of damage to the lung involves dynamic pressure changes (stress and shear waves) at the alveolar–capillary membrane causing pulmonary hemorrhage and contusion. Pulmonary injuries, if severe, can be rapidly fatal. Individuals who survive the acute injury may develop progressive respiratory failure and require mechanical ventilation for acute respiratory distress syndrome, with a mortality rate of up to 50%.[18] Symptoms and signs may include respiratory distress, restlessness, hemoptysis, cyanosis, and hypoxemia. Imaging features include unilateral or bilateral focal opacities and loss of lung translucency. Evidence of barotrauma from blast lung injury may include pneumothorax, pneumomediastinum, pneumopericardium, subcutaneous emphysema and hemothorax owing to pulmonary parenchymal lacerations. In an analysis of 1151 post-mortem chest radiographs, tension pneumothorax was the cause of death in 3% to 4% of fatally wounded combat casualties.[19]

Embedded Metal Fragments

Concern about systemic effects from embedded metals prompted the US Department of Veterans Affairs to establish a special registry in 2008 for medical surveillance and management of veterans with retained metal fragments from improvised explosive devices used in Iraq and Afghanistan. Some of the embedded metal contaminants, including aluminum, arsenic, cobalt, chromium, and nickel, may have immunogenic respiratory health effects. In a recent report from the Toxic Embedded Fragment Surveillance Center, of 89 urine samples tested, 47% exceeded the reference value for aluminum and 31% for tungsten.[20] However, no clinically significant respiratory health effects have been detected to date. An unusual case report of chronic beryllium disease was described in a 41-year-old Israeli soldier who suffered a mortar shell injury with retained shrapnel in the chest wall.[21] The patient was initially diagnosed with sarcoidosis after presenting with cough, dyspnea, bilateral mediastinal and hilar lymphadenopathy, and restrictive pulmonary function abnormalities with a diminished diffusion capacity. After the patient raised the possibility of a link between his war wound and his lung disease, blood lymphocyte proliferation testing was positive to beryllium salts, and beryllium in the shrapnel matrix was confirmed. Because removal carries risk of surgical morbidity, careful consideration of risk versus benefit must be based on the size, shape, composition, location, accessibility, and stability of the embedded metal fragment in situ.

Infectious Agents

Respiratory pathogens have been a major source of respiratory disease-related morbidity and mortality in the US military since its inception.[22]

During the Revolutionary and Civil Wars, 90% of casualties occurred owing to non-battle injuries, including respiratory illness such as measles, whooping cough, and pneumonia. Periodic infectious respiratory illnesses, mainly pharyngitis and tonsillitis, accounted for 8% to 20% of military illnesses through the late 1880s.[23] The devastating impact of the influenza A pandemic on the military population at the end of World War I, with high mortality rates from complicating pneumonia, led to the creation of the Pneumonia Commission in 1918, the Army Epidemiological Board in 1941, and its post-war successor, the tri-service Armed Forces Epidemiological Board, focused on research and prevention of military infectious disease outbreaks.

Contemporary military life, beginning with basic training, often results in large numbers of young recruits arriving from geographically disperse locations for training in close quarters. Such circumstances can provide the perfect setting for respiratory infectious disease transmission.[24] Perhaps because of high rates of indoor air recirculation, rates of acute febrile respiratory illness were found to be higher in military trainees housed in new, energy-efficient, tight barracks compared with those living in older buildings.[25] The impact of acute respiratory infections on troops deployed to Iraq and Afghanistan is unclear. In 1 study,[26] the rate of respiratory system encounters decreased by 8% from before deployment to after deployment, a finding driven largely by a significant drop in acute respiratory infections.

Cigarette Smoking and Environmental Tobacco Smoke

Smoking rates among military personnel are high, damaging health, affecting troop readiness, and costing the Department of Defense an estimated $564 million per year for medical care associated with tobacco use.[27] Recently, the military has seen an increase in tobacco use among young enlisted military members.[28] The military is an important market for the tobacco industry, having long been the target of cigarette promotional advertisements.[29] Smoking during military service has been historically encouraged through liberal smoking breaks, social interaction in designated smoking areas, and cheap and convenient tobacco products sold on military bases, including aboard ship.[30] Moreover, smoking is often seen as a method to combat the stress and boredom of military life and to avoid weight gain. In addition to cigarettes, there is a high prevalence of alternative forms of tobacco use in young military recruits, including cigars (12.3%), pipes (1.1%), bidis (2.0%), and kreteks (clove cigarettes; 3.0%).[31] A number of studies have examined prevalence of smoking and use of tobacco products in active-duty US military personnel. Based on a 2008 Department of Defense Survey of 28,546 service members, 41.2% reportedly used 1 or more forms of tobacco in the previous month, with 21.3% reporting cigarette smoking.[32] Two thirds were daily cigarette smokers, and the majority smoked 15 or fewer cigarettes per day. Current smokers were more likely that nonsmokers to be enlisted, younger, and have lower body mass index measurements.[33] More than half of active smokers increased their tobacco consumption during deployment. Rates of cigarette smoking among active duty US military personnel ranged from 23% among Air Force to 38% among Army personnel. Based on data from the 21 year longitudinal Millennium Cohort study,[34] smoking initiation was found in 1.3% of non-deployed personnel and 2.3% of deployed personnel who were former never smokers. Smoking resumption in ex-smokers occurred in 28.7% of non-deployed and 39.4% of deployed personnel. Deployed personnel who reported combat exposures had a 1.6 times greater odds of initiating smoking among baseline never smokers (95% confidence interval, 1.2–2.3), and a 1.3 times greater odds of resuming smoking among baseline past smokers, compared with those not reporting combat exposures. Multiple deployments and deployment duration exceeding 9 months were independently associated with post deployment smoking recidivism.

SPECTRUM OF LUNG ILLNESSES ASSOCIATED WITH RECENT US COMBAT OPERATIONS
Increased Rates of Respiratory Symptoms

Respiratory symptoms have been commonly reported among soldiers who served in the Middle East, including those participating in Desert Storm and more recently in those returning from Afghanistan and Iraq.

Reports of dyspnea were found in more than 20% of veterans returning from Operation Desert Storm.[35] Concerns about the impact of respiratory disease prompted a questionnaire-based investigation of nearly 2600 combat troops stationed for a mean of 102 days in northeastern Saudi Arabia during Operation Desert Shield before the oil fires in Kuwait occurred.[3] A high prevalence of respiratory complaints was found including 43% with cough, 34% with sore throat, and 15% with chronic rhinorrhea; 1.8% reported being unable to perform routine duties owing to respiratory symptoms. Frequency of respiratory symptoms was associated with longer duration of deployment,

smoking status (37% of population), and prior history of respiratory disease (primarily mild asthma). Troops who slept in air-conditioned buildings were more likely to report sore throat and cough than those who slept in tents and warehouses with more outdoor exposures, who were more likely to report rhinorrhea. In a retrospective exposure and symptom survey of military personnel 5 years after the Persian Gulf War, Lange and colleagues[36] found a modest correlation between self-reported and modeled exposures to oil well fires ($r = 0.48$; $P<.05$). Odds ratios for asthma, bronchitis, and major depression increased with increasing self-reported exposure, although there was no association between these outcomes and modeled exposures (based on spatial and temporal records of smoke concentrations with troop movements). Findings did not support an association between oil fire smoke exposure and respiratory symptoms among Gulf War veterans.

Several investigations have shown that OEF/OIF deployed military personnel report increased rates of respiratory symptoms. In a large survey of troops deployed to Iraq and Afghanistan, Roop and colleagues[37] found that both asthmatic and non-asthmatic patients reported significantly increased respiratory symptoms during deployment compared with pre-deployment symptom prevalence. Sanders and colleagues[38] reported that 69% of military personnel deployed to OEF/OIF reported in-theater respiratory illnesses, of which 17% required medical care. In those survey respondents deployed to Iraq, respiratory illnesses doubled in prevalence from pre-combat compared with combat periods. Subsequent investigation[39] showed that deployers (defined as those remaining in country for at least 30 days) had higher rates of newly reported respiratory symptoms than non-deployers (14% vs 10%), although rates of physician-diagnosed asthma and bronchitis were not increased. In this study, deployment was associated with increased reports of respiratory symptoms in Army and Marine Corps personnel, independent of smoking status. Moreover, a linear dose–response relation between length of deployment and respiratory symptoms was found for Army (but not Navy, Air Force, or Marine) personnel, suggesting a different exposure risk for land-based service members. The authors suggest that specific environmental exposures, rather than deployment in general, are determinants of post-deployment respiratory illness.

Asthma

Although preexisting asthma historically has been a disqualifying condition for entrance into the US military, asthma—either newly diagnosed or previously unrecognized—remains a significant cause of respiratory symptoms in the military population.[37] New recruits may be reluctant to report ongoing respiratory symptoms or a history of asthma, and may begin military service undiagnosed. The circumstances of military duty, including strenuous physical exertion often while wearing helmet and body armor, extended exposure to outdoor environmental extremes during deployment to austere locations, exposure to high levels of dusts, fumes, and smoke, and more limited access to medications and medical care, may contribute to higher asthma prevalence or unmask subclinical asthma in deployers. In a 1991 survey of soldiers deployed to Kuwait during the oil fires, those with self-reported asthma or allergies were more likely to report cough (27.8 vs 18.8%) and shortness of breath (17.6 vs 8.6%).[40]

Psychological stress may also contribute to asthma risk. The link between combat exposure, asthma, and posttraumatic stress disorder has been investigated. In a study of male veteran twin pairs who served during the Vietnam era, symptoms of posttraumatic stress disorder were associated with a significantly increased prevalence of physician-diagnosed asthma, even after adjusting for familial/genetic and other potentially confounding factors, such as cigarette smoking, educational attainment, body mass index, and depression.[41]

In 2002, the US Army issued new medical standards for asthma, allowing soldiers who can perform their duties on maintenance therapy to remain in active service, provided they do not require either chronic corticosteroid use or hospitalization because of asthma exacerbations. With this change, more soldiers with asthma are deploying and performing strenuous military tasks in challenging operational environments. In a survey of 1250 active-duty soldiers and Department of Defense contractors returning from deployment in Iraq and Afghanistan, 5% reported a previous diagnosis of asthma. Both asthmatics and non-asthmatics were found to have increased respiratory symptoms of wheezing, cough, sputum production, chest tightness, and allergy symptoms during deployment compared with pre-deployment ($P < .05$ for all). In a retrospective review of more than 6000 medical records from OIF/OEF veterans evaluated between March 2004 and May 2007, Szema and colleagues[42] found increased rates of new-onset asthma compared with military personnel who had not been deployed (6.6% vs 4.3%; odds ratio, 1.58; 95% confidence interval, 1.18–2.11). Concurrent rhinitis was also more likely to be diagnosed in the Iraq-deployed patients. Other upper airway effects from deployment may include laryngotracheitis and associated variable extra-thoracic airway obstruction.[43]

Bronchiolitis

Constrictive/obliterative bronchiolitis was among the lung sequelae in survivors of sulfur mustard gas exposure in World War I, and more recently in the 1980s Iran–Iraq conflict.[44] In 2011, investigators from Vanderbilt University[45] published a case series of soldiers referred for evaluation of unexplained dyspnea on exertion, frequently manifested by post-deployment inability to complete the physical fitness test requirements for active duty. Eighty soldiers with unexplained respiratory symptoms underwent extensive diagnostic lung evaluation, including high-resolution chest imaging as well as rest and exercise pulmonary function testing. Of 49 who underwent surgical lung biopsy, 38 (35 men and 3 women) had histologic findings of CB; peribronchiolar pigment deposition was also commonly described. Most (31 [81.5%]) were never or former smokers. Chest radiographs were normal in all those with CB, and only 25% had high-resolution chest computed tomographic findings of mosaic air trapping or centrilobular nodules. Pulmonary function trended toward the lower limits of normal and was significantly lower compared with a group of historical military controls. Of those with CB, the majority (28 [74%]) had served in northern Iraq near Mosul in 2003 and reported exposure to the smoke plume from the nearby Al-Mishraq sulfur plant fire. Notably, 11 with biopsy-proven CB reported no sulfur mine fire exposure, suggesting that risk for lung disease was not limited to those with an occupational history of exposure to a specific event. Longitudinal follow-up of soldiers with CB is planned.

Chronic Obstructive Pulmonary Disease

Based on the spectrum of in-theater inhalational exposures associated with deployment to Iraq and Afghanistan, risk for long-term chronic obstructive lung disease remains a concern. In a nested case-control study of more than 50,000 military personnel deployed to Iraq and Afghanistan,[26] significant increases in both respiratory symptom rates and in encounters for obstructive lung disease (predominantly asthma [46%] and bronchitis [50%]) were found after deployment. Female gender, enlisted personnel, and Army personnel (but not age or combat occupation) were independent predictors of new pulmonary disease encounters. Neither multiple deployments nor extended cumulative time of deployment was associated with obstructive lung disease encounters. The study was limited by the short follow-up time (as low as 6 months), and the authors acknowledge that longer latency diseases such as emphysema would not be detected in this analysis.

Acute Eosinophilic Pneumonia and Other Interstitial Diseases

Acute eosinophilic pneumonia is a rare, idiopathic lung disease characterized by acute onset of fever and chest symptoms accompanied by diffuse infiltrates on chest imaging and eosinophilia in bronchoalveolar lavage and/or lung biopsy. In 2004, 18 cases of acute eosinophilic pneumonia (including 2 fatalities) were reported among 183,000 troops deployed to Iraq between March 2003 and March 2004.[46] All of the cases were cigarette smokers, with 78% reporting new onset smoking; all but 1 reported exposure to airborne dust during deployment. Investigation showed no common source exposure, temporal or geographic clustering of cases, association with recent vaccination, or person-to-person transmission. The authors suggest that "recent exposure to tobacco may prime the lung in some way such that a second exposure or injury, eg, in the form of dust, triggers a cascade of events that culminates in [acute eosinophilic pneumonia]."

Deployment-related exposure to respirable silica and to soil contaminants having inflammatory or immunogenic properties may confer risk for interstitial lung diseases. Desert Storm pneumonitis, or Al Eskan disease, is a term coined to describe a spectrum of respiratory problems observed in Al Eskan village, near Riyadh. Although the clinical features of the condition have not been clearly characterized, the authors suggested that inhalation of fine calcium-rich sand, possibly aggravated by co-exposure to infectious or irritant agents, may be causally important.[47] Whether exposures during OIF/OEF deployment increase the risk for interstitial lung diseases with longer latency awaits further study.

SUMMARY

Military men and women deployed to OIF and OEF are exposed to high levels of airborne PM from a number of sources that can exceed environmental, occupational, and military exposure guidelines. The spectrum of potential adverse lung health outcomes associated with military service is broad; however, the prevalence of these conditions is uncertain, as are the causative exposures. Most studies of lung conditions associated with OIF/OEF deployment are limited by lack of deployment-specific exposure assessment. Deployment is generally used as a rough proxy for environmental exposures, limiting analysis of the effects of exposures such as PM, burn pit smoke, and combat-related exposures. The large-scale epidemiologic studies of OIF/OEF lung health outcomes, based mainly on analysis of respiratory diagnostic codes and symptom reports, are hampered by multiple deployments and exposures, short follow-up times, and lack of correlation with medical test findings, including pulmonary function testing and lung imaging. Prospective study of risks from exposure to burn pits at JBB, as recommended by the IOM committee,[11] may be helpful in clarifying possible associated lung health risks. However, burn pit exposures were one of many deployment-related exposures. Given the large numbers of OIF/OEF US veterans and concerns regarding long-term health consequences, longitudinal studies in these veterans, including algorithms to estimate past deployment related exposures, could help to assess potential chronic effects, and associated risk factors.

Recent discussions have focused on the addition of baseline spirometry to current military accession procedures, particularly for those facing deployment,[48] to enable a baseline for comparison with post-deployment or development of respiratory symptoms or illnesses. Spirometry testing pre-deployment and over time might help to clarify post-deployment chest symptoms, identify those for whom further diagnostic testing is warranted, and provide insight into possible deployment-related exposure risks. Those with obstruction on spirometry before deployment could be considered for more complete pulmonary evaluation to determine fitness for duty. Whether the challenges and costs of high quality spirometry over time or other lung-focused medical surveillance for US troops is warranted remains uncertain.[49] Such medical surveillance data would be best incorporated into epidemiology studies to assess potential chronic health effects related to deployment, including accelerated loss of lung function.

In addition to epidemiologic and clinicopathologic studies, further investigation of the content, pathogenicity and toxicity of PM from areas of combat operations may shed light on short- and long-term exposure risks.

Respiratory illnesses affect mission readiness, burden active duty military and veterans' health care systems, and may lead to significant morbidity and mortality. Primary preventive strategies such as the elimination of open-air burn pits as well as education and enforcement for what cannot be burned in open settings will be important in minimizing future exposure risks. Additionally, targeted smoking cessation programs would likely help to reduce respiratory symptoms and their functional effects before and during deployment. Preventing adverse lung health consequences of deployment-related exposures as well as lowering military smoking rates will require high levels of command support.[50,51]

REFERENCES

1. McAndrew LM, Teichman RF, Osinubi OY, et al. Environmental exposure and health of Operation Enduring Freedom/Operation Iraqi Freedom veterans. J Occup Environ Med 2012;54(6):665–9.

2. Quigley KS, McAndrew LM, Almeida L, et al. Prevalence of environmental and other military exposure concerns in Operation Enduring Freedom and Operation Iraqi Freedom veterans. J Occup Environ Med 2012;54(6):659–64.

3. Richards AL, Hyams KC, Watts DM, et al. Respiratory disease among military personnel in Saudi Arabia during operation Desert Shield. Am J Public Health 1993;83(9):1326–9.

4. Mayor A. Greek fire, poison arrows & scorpion bombs: biological and chemical warfare in the ancient world. London: Over-Duckworth; 2003.

5. Heller CE. Chemical warfare in World War I: the American experience, 1917-1918. Fort Leavenworth, KA: US Army Command and General Staff College; 1984.

6. Emad A, Rezainin R. The diversity of the effects of sulfur mustard gas inhalation on respiratory system 10 years after a single heavy exposure. Chest 1997;112:734–8.

7. Thomason JW, Rice TW, Milstone AP. Bronchiolitis obliterans in a survivor of a chemical weapons attack. JAMA 2003;290(5):598–9.

8. Kang HK, Dalager NA, Needham LL, et al. Health status of army chemical corps Vietnam veterans who sprayed defoliant in Vietnam. Am J Ind Med 2006;49(11):875–84.

9. Cowan DN, Lange JL, Heller J, et al. A case-control study of asthma among U.S. Army Gulf War veterans and modeled exposure to oil well fire smoke. Mil Med 2002;167(9):777–82.

10. Engelbrecht JP, McDonald EV, Gillies JA, et al. Department of defense Enhanced particulate matter surveillance program (EPMSP). Final report. Reno, NV: Department of Defense, Desert Research Institute; 2008.

11. Institute of Medicine. Long-term health consequences of exposure to burn pits in Iraq and Afghanistan. Washington, DC: National Academies Press; 2011.

12. Abraham JH, Baird CP. A case-crossover study of ambient particulate matter and cardiovascular and respiratory medical encounters among US military personnel deployed to Southwest Asia. J Occup Environ Med 2012;54(6):733–9.

13. Charan NB, Myers CG, Lakshminarayan S, et al. Pulmonary injuries associated with acute sulfur dioxide inhalation. Am Rev Respir Dis 1979;119(4):555–60.

14. Carn S, Krueger A, Krotkov N, et al. Fire at Iraqi sulfur plant emits SO_2 clouds detected by Earth Probe TOMS. Geophysical Res Lett 2004;31:1–4.

15. Baird CP, Debakey S, Reid L, et al. Respiratory health status of US army personnel potentially exposed to smoke from 2003 Al-Mishraq Sulfur Plant Fire. J Occup Environ Med 2012;54(6):717–23.

16. Engelbrecht JP, McDonald EV, Gillies JA, et al. Characterizing mineral dusts and other aerosols from the Middle East–Part 1: ambient sampling. Inhal Toxicol 2009;21(4):297–326.

17. Mackenzie IM, Tunnicliffe B. Blast injuries to the lung: epidemiology and management. Philos Trans R Soc Lond B Biol Sci 2011;366(1562):295–9.

18. Morris MJ. Acute respiratory distress syndrome in combat casualties: military medicine and advances in mechanical ventilation. Mil Med 2006;171(11):1039–44.

19. McPherson JJ, Feigin DS, Bellamy RF. Prevalence of tension pneumothorax in fatally wounded combat casualties. J Trauma 2006;60(3):573–8.

20. Squibb KS, Gaitens JM, Engelhardt S, et al. Surveillance for long-term health effects associated with depleted uranium exposure and retained embedded fragments in US veterans. J Occup Environ Med 2012;54(6):724–32.

21. Fireman E, Bar Shai A, Lerman Y, et al. Chest wall shrapnel-induced beryllium-sensitization and associated pulmonary disease. Sarcoidosis Vasc Diffuse Lung Dis, in press.

22. Ottolini MG, Burnett MW. History of U.S. military contributions to the study of respiratory infections. Mil Med 2005;170(Suppl. 4):66–70.

23. Gray GC, Blankenship TL, Gackstetter G. History of respiratory illness at the U.S. Naval Academy. Mil Med 2001;166(7):581–6.

24. Denny FW, Wannamaker LW, Brink WR, et al. Prevention of rheumatic fever; treatment of the preceding streptococcic infection. JAMA 1950;143(2):151–3.

25. Brundage JF, Scott RM, Lednar WM, et al. Building-associated risk of febrile acute respiratory diseases in Army trainees. JAMA 1988;259(14):2108–12.

26. Abraham JH, Debakey SF, Reid L, et al. Does deployment to Iraq and Afghanistan affect respiratory health of US military personnel? J Occup Environ Med 2012;54(6):740–5.

27. Dall TM, Zhang Y, Chen YJ, et al. Cost associated with being overweight and with obesity, high alcohol consumption, and tobacco use within the military health system's TRICARE prime-enrolled population. Am J Health Promot 2007;22(2):120–39.

28. Owers RC, Ballard KD. "What else is there to do?" A qualitative study of the barriers to soldiers stopping smoking. J R Army Med Corps 2008;154(3):152–5.

29. Smith EA, Malone RE. Tobacco promotion to military personnel: "the plums are here to be plucked". Mil Med 2009;174(8):797–806.

30. Haddock CK, Taylor JE, Hoffman KM, et al. Factors which influence tobacco use among junior enlisted personnel in the United States Army and Air Force: a formative research study. Am J Health Promot 2009;23(4):241–6.

31. Klesges RC, DeBon M, Vander Weg MW, et al. Efficacy of a tailored tobacco control program on long-term use in a population of U.S. military troops. J Consult Clin Psychol 2006;74(2):295–306.

32. Olmsted KL, Bray RM, Reyes-Guzman CM, et al. Overlap in use of different types of tobacco among active duty military personnel. Nicotine Tob Res 2011;13(8):691–8.

33. Macera CA, Aralis H, MacGregor A, et al. Weight changes among male Navy personnel deployed to Iraq or Kuwait in 2005-2008. Mil Med 2011;176(5):500–6.

34. Smith B, Ryan MA, Wingard DL, et al. Cigarette smoking and military deployment: a prospective evaluation. Am J Prev Med 2008;35(6):539–46.

35. Kroenke K, Koslowe P, Roy M. Symptoms in 18,495 Persian Gulf war veterans. Latency of onset and lack of association with self-reported exposures. J Occup Environ Med 1998;40(6):520–8.

36. Lange JL, Schwartz DA, Doebbeling BN, et al. Exposures to the Kuwait oil fires and their association with asthma and bronchitis among gulf war veterans. Environ Health Perspect 2002;110(11):1141–6.

37. Roop SA, Niven AS, Calvin BE, et al. The prevalence and impact of respiratory symptoms in asthmatics and nonasthmatics during deployment. Mil Med 2007;172(12):1264–9.

38. Sanders JW, Putnam SD, Frankart C, et al. Impact of illness and non-combat injury during operations Iraqi freedom and enduring freedom (Afghanistan). Am J Trop Med Hyg 2005;73(4):713–9.

39. Smith B, Wong CA, Smith TC, et al. Newly reported respiratory symptoms and conditions among military personnel deployed to Iraq and Afghanistan: a prospective population-based study. Am J Epidemiol 2009;170(11):1433–42.

40. Petruccelli BP, Goldenbaum M, Scott B, et al. Health effects of the 1991 Kuwait oil fires: a survey of US army troops. J Occup Environ Med 1999;41(6):433–9.

41. Goodwin RD, Fischer ME, Goldberg J. A twin study of post-traumatic stress disorder symptoms and asthma. Am J Respir Crit Care Med 2007;176(10):983–7.

42. Szema AM, Peters MC, Weissinger KM, et al. New-onset asthma among soldiers serving in Iraq and Afghanistan. Allergy Asthma Proc 2010;31(5):67–71.

43. Das AK, Davanzo LD, Poiani GJ, et al. Variable extrathoracic airflow obstruction and chronic laryngotracheitis in Gulf War veterans. Chest 1999;115(1):97–101.

44. Ghanei M, Harandi AA. Long term consequences from exposure to sulfur mustard: a review. Inhal Toxicol 2007;19(5):451–6.

45. King MS, Eisenberg R, Newman JH, et al. Constrictive bronchiolitis in soldiers returning from Iraq and Afghanistan. N Engl J Med 2011;365(3):222–30.

46. Shorr AF, Scoville SL, Cersovsky SB, et al. Acute eosinophilic pneumonia among US Military personnel deployed in or near Iraq. JAMA 2004;292(24):2997–3005.

47. Korenyi-Both AL, Korenyi-Both AL, Juncer DJ. Al Eskan disease: Persian Gulf syndrome. Mil Med 1997;162(1):1–13.

48. Rose C, Abraham J, Harkins D, et al. Overview and recommendations for medical screening and diagnostic evaluation for postdeployment lung disease in returning US warfighters. J Occup Environ Med 2012;54(6):746–51.

49. Zacher LL, Browning R, Bisnett T, et al. Clarifications from representatives of the department of defense regarding the article "recommendations for medical screening and diagnostic evaluation for postdeployment lung disease in returning US warfighters". J Occup Environ Med 2012;54(6):760–1.

50. Chretien JP. Protecting service members in war–non-battle morbidity and command responsibility. N Engl J Med 2012;366(8):677–9.

51. Arvey SR, Malone RE. Advance and retreat: tobacco control policy in the U.S. military. Mil Med 2008;173(10):985–91.

Respiratory Health in Home and Leisure Pursuits

Lawrence A. Ho, MD*, Ware G. Kuschner, MD

KEYWORDS

- Asthma • Respiratory adverse health effects • Household • Cleaning • Dust • Vapors • Hobbies
- Pets

KEY POINTS

- A diverse array of home-based and leisure activities may generate hazardous respirable exposures.
- Routine domestic activities such as cooking and cleaning, heating systems, and a variety of hobbies, avocations, and leisure pursuits have been associated with a spectrum of respiratory tract disorders, including acute irritation or lung injury, rhinitis, asthma, and chronic obstructive lung disease.
- The home environment – where people spend as much as 50% of their life – and leisure activities – where certain particularly hazardous exposures could be avoided – present special health risks that should be part of the health assessment of individuals across all demographic groups.

INTRODUCTION

A diverse array of home-based and leisure activities may generate hazardous respirable exposures (**Fig. 1**). Because these activities are extensive, so, too, are the adverse respiratory effects that may be associated with them. Adverse respiratory effects associated with home and leisure activities include both upper and lower airway conditions and parenchymal diseases. Respiratory tract disorders potentially attributable to home-based and leisure activities–associated exposures include respiratory tract irritant effects, asthma, chronic obstructive lung disease, rhinitis, malignancy, and selected interstitial lung diseases. Although numerous reports have established causal relationships between a spectrum of exposures and adverse health effects, significant knowledge gaps persist regarding the epidemiology of home and leisure exposures, exposure–response relationships, and adverse health outcomes. Selected exposures covered in this review include some that present major worldwide public health challenges (eg, cooking and heating with biomass fuels), others that are sporadic yet notable (eg, bird fancying), and still others that are mainly of historical interest (eg, certain photographic processing exposures), but nonetheless they all serve to illustrate important principles of environmental respiratory health. An encyclopedic cataloging of all possible home-based and leisure activity exposures and their adverse health effects is beyond the scope of this review, but the subject matter covered should provide a context and framework for approaching this diversity of topics.

HOME ENVIRONMENT
General Considerations

In post industrial societies, people spend approximately 90% of their time indoors. More than half of this time is spent at home.[1] Advances in home construction and building insulation have led to improved mechanical air conditioning and heating efficiency, but typically at the cost of diminished air exchange between the indoor and outdoor

Veterans Affairs Palo Alto Health Care System, Stanford University School of Medicine, Division of Pulmonary and Critical Care Medicine, 3801 Miranda Avenue, MC 111P, Palo Alto, CA 94304, USA
* Corresponding author.
E-mail address: laho@stanford.edu

Clin Chest Med 33 (2012) 715–729
http://dx.doi.org/10.1016/j.ccm.2012.08.001
0272-5231/12/$ – see front matter © 2012 Elsevier Inc. All rights reserved.

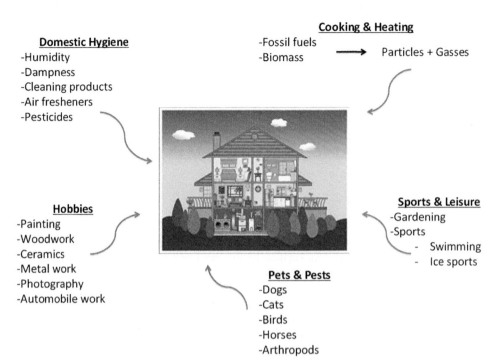

Domestic Hygiene
-Humidity
-Dampness
-Cleaning products
-Air fresheners
-Pesticides

Cooking & Heating
-Fossil fuels
-Biomass   → Particles + Gasses

Hobbies
-Painting
-Woodwork
-Ceramics
-Metal work
-Photography
-Automobile work

Sports & Leisure
-Gardening
-Sports
  - Swimming
  - Ice sports

Pets & Pests
-Dogs
-Cats
-Birds
-Horses
-Arthropods

Fig. 1. Home and leisure based activities that may cause respiratory disease.

environments. Diminished indoor–outdoor air exchange rates can result in the accumulation of indoor air pollutants.[2] Although the relationships among air exchange rates, indoor air quality, and adverse health effects are complex, high concentrations of respirable contaminants, including combustion byproducts, mineral dusts, or aeroallergens, are widely appreciated to cause irritant effects in exposed individuals or trigger exacerbations of asthma in susceptible or sensitized individuals.

Humidity can be another important factor that influences the air quality in the home.[3] Most modern buildings experience some kind of water damage during their life span. Water damage can result from ground penetration or leaks in windows, roofs, and pipes.[4] Other activities, such as showering or bathing, humidifier use, and cooking, further contribute to indoor moisture. Drywall is a favorite construction material for interior walls but it can easily absorb water and moisture. Leaks into a wall or ceiling constructed with drywall, even from a single event, can initiate significant mold growth within days. Modern construction techniques include the use of drywall treated with antifungal agents such as sodium pyrithione and the use of antimildew products such as tributyltin. Although these agents are effective in preventing mold growth, they may have their own adverse effects. For instance, tributyltin can cause eye and throat irritant effects.[5]

Humid and damp environments are ideal for the growth of molds, fungi, bacteria, mites, and insects.[1,6] A spectrum of respiratory and nonrespiratory complaints have been described among building occupants exposed to mold and fungal spores. Mold spores produce mycotoxins and glucans that may be associated with respiratory effects, although there is contentious mechanistic debate over the role of specific mediators of such effects in humans.[7] Respiratory disorders attributed to indoor fungi include new onset asthma,[8–12] exacerbations of asthma,[13,14] hypersensitivity pneumonitis,[15,16] and a spectrum of symptoms including cough, dyspnea, and wheeze.[17] Upper respiratory tract symptoms and respiratory infections have also been attributed to indoor mold exposure.[18] A recent report found a relationship between building-related rhinosinusitis in water-damaged buildings and the subsequent development of asthma.[19] Although more commonly considered an outdoor mold, positive skin prick tests for the mold genus *Alternaria* have been associated with asthma and hypersensitivity pneumonitis.[20] By promoting the proliferation of mold and other microorganisms, dampness can synergistically increase the eosinophilic inflammation in airways by inducing adjuvant-like activities of allergens.[21]

Unusually wet weather patterns may lead to changes in indoor ecology resulting in respiratory disease. During the winter of 1997–1998, a weather phenomenon known as El Niño resulted in extensive flooding in the western region of the United States. Flood damage to one residence during this period was reported to lead to biopsy-proved hypersensitivity pneumonitis in a previously healthy woman. Home inspection revealed an unusual mushroom growing in the basement of the patient's residence. Air sampling and serum precipitans testing established the etiologic exposure as the fungus *Pezizia domiciliana*. Investigators labeled this a case of "El Niño lung."[22]

Cleaning

Cleaning in the home environment is a routine activity. Hazardous respiratory exposures can result from mobilization of substances during cleaning activities, because asthma exacerbations have been linked to mobilization of particles such as animal dander, house dust, mites, and microbes. More important, however, are direct exposures to toxic cleaning products.[23,24] There is a large body of literature relating professional cleaning to asthma and other respiratory disorders.[23–27] Homemakers have also been found to have an increased risk of asthma,[26] which is not surprising because similar chemical products are used in both the professional and the home environment.[26,27] In the home environment, both the individual(s) performing the cleaning task and bystanders (ie, other household members) may be at risk for significant respiratory exposure and associated health effects.

Cleaning agents

There are numerous cleaning agents intended for use on multiple surfaces. These agents consist of many different chemicals to serve 4 main purposes: removal of surface contaminants, surface maintenance, disinfection, and fragrance.[28] Common components of cleaning products include alkaline agents, acids, disinfectants, detergents, solvents, corrosion inhibitors, polishers, and perfume or scents.[29] Respiratory exposure occurs with evaporation of volatile components, aerosolization of droplets, or scattering particulate (eg, with scouring powders). The amount of exposure depends on the amount and concentration of product used, as well as the method of delivery.[28] Some products, such as butoxyethanol (a common component of window cleaners liquid, soaps, cosmetics, varnishes, and latex paints), can cause sensory irritation at the relatively low concentration of 2 ppm (10 mg/m^3).[30] Products used in spray form are more easily inhaled than are products in pure liquid form.[27] Irritant-induced asthma is commonly associated with cleaning products, specifically hypochlorite bleach and mixing bleach with other products such as acids or ammonia.[29] Ammonia itself can cause rhinitis.[28] Respiratory sensitization can also occur with exposure to several cleaning products, such as with exposure to limonene, which is a terpene-related scent.[29]

Laundry products

Laundry products, including detergents, fabric softeners, and dryer sheets, can contain encapsulated enzymes (previously, nonencapsulated formulations were marketed), soaps, and fragrances. The encapsulated enzymes include amylases and lipases. These have been labeled as potential respiratory sensitizers and, following significant exposure, allergic asthma can develop.[29] This is mainly found in manufacturing workers because there is a 10-fold lowering of the concentration of these enzymes in household products, reducing typical household exposures.[29] Nonetheless, enzyme-associated asthma in homemakers has been reported.[31]

Air fresheners

By design, air fresheners release airborne perfume or fragrance that is easily inhaled and can be sensed via odor-detecting pathways.[27] Such products typically contain deodorizers and other volatile organic compounds (VOCs). Some of the VOCs found in common household fragranced products have been labeled by the US Environmental Protection Agency (EPA) as "hazardous air pollutants."[32] Common VOCs include limonene (already noted), ethanol, linalool, β-phenethyl alcohol, and β-myrcene.[33] Common respiratory tract symptoms associated with air fresheners can include chest tightness, wheezing, asthma, decreased pulmonary function, and rhinitis.[34–36]

Household pesticides

Pesticides are commonly used in domestic settings. These products can be delivered in multiple routes, including spray cans, combustible coils releasing airborne repellants, and slow-release vaporizing systems.[28] The composition of products varies depending on the route of administration. Common constituents of insecticides include irritant combustion gases, VOCs, particulates, organophosphates, carbamates, and pyrethrins.[28,37,38] Pyrethrins are perhaps the most important common component of household pesticides. They are derived from ground and dried flowers of *Chrysanthemum cinerariaefolium* or from synthetic analogs of this naturally occurring substance and have been reported to cause adverse respiratory symptoms.[38] Respiratory responses to pesticides depend on both the administration route and the composition of the product. For example, mosquito coils may carry the additional exposure of irritant incomplete combustion gasses.[39]

Cooking and Home Heating

Cooking and heating are universal sources of indoor pollutants in domestic settings.[40] There may be multiple sources of pollutants attributable to cooking and heating in the home. The combustion of fossil fuels used in gas cooking produces mixtures of particles including VOCs, sulfur dioxide, carbon dioxide, carbon monoxide (CO), and nitrogen dioxide (NO_2). Cooking also produces small particulates and water vapor that can also affect respiratory health. Food preparation itself can cause significant aerosolization leading to inhalational exposure. For example, asparagus is documented to cause IgE-mediated asthma, and garlic-induced asthma has been reported to cause occupational asthma.[41,42] Extensive documentation of potential foodstuff-related asthma is beyond the scope of this review, but it merits emphasis that asthma exacerbation from preparing any material to which an individual has become sensitized is a potential hazard of the home environment.

Exposure to emissions from cooking and heating depends on the fuel used, ventilation, time spent in the area of the cooking, and ergonomic factors (eg, proximity to the source of combustion). Adverse health effects are believed to be mediated by multiple mechanisms broadly defined, including (1) increasing susceptibility to airway infections, (2) promotion of airway inflammation from oxidative damage, and (3) enhanced responses to inhaled allergens.[29] These responses may have a role in the initiation or exacerbation of asthma or chronic obstructive pulmonary disease (COPD). There are data linking adverse respiratory health effects, including a reduction in forced expiratory volume in 1 second, to gas cooking.[43,44] Exposure to coal emissions in the domestic environment has been linked with the development of COPD in nonsmokers in China.[45]

A widely studied emission produced by gas cooking is NO_2. Concentrations of NO_2 in kitchens with gas stoves should typically be low. NO_2 concentrations, however, have been found to exceed the World Health Organization's outdoor air quality standard in poorly ventilated environments.[30,46,47] High-intensity exposure to NO_2 is associated with the development of pulmonary edema, but the health effects of short-term exposure to NO_2 are less well established.[48] Selected reports have demonstrated an association between NO_2 and respiratory symptoms, including sore throats, colds, nasal symptoms, and decreased forced vital capacity.[49,50]

In less-developed economic settings, solid fuels, including biomass (crop residues, animal dung, and wood) and coal and peat, are commonly used for domestic cooking and heating and are the most important source of domestic indoor air pollution in such settings.[46] Approximately 3 billion people use biomass fuels or coal for home heating, not simply for cooking.[51] Exposure to biomass smoke can increase the risk of respiratory tract infections in children and lead to poor lung growth.[51,52] Among adults, prolonged exposure to biomass smoke is associated with increased risk of COPD, asthma, lung cancer, and respiratory tract infections.[51,52] Emissions from the combustion of biomass and kerosene have been associated with tuberculosis in women.[53] Biomass smoke exposure is not limited to developing economies. Wood-burning stoves used for heating in post industrial nations have been linked to increased subjective symptoms including cough and wheezing and to increased respiratory tract infections.[54]

LEISURE PURSUITS
Pets and Other Animals Including Household Arthropods

Pets are a common household source of exposure, animals kept for other purposes (eg, livestock) can be another major exposure factor, and household arthropods are ubiquitous. The Humane Society of the United States has estimated 39% of US households own at least one dog and 33% of households keep at least one cat. The potential relevance of a pet exposure depends on the types of pets in the household and the age of individuals in the household. As opposed to pets that are an intentional part of the household, undesired animals, including pests, may also be present in the home environment.

Dogs and cats
Dogs and cats produce multiple allergens that are measurable in the home environment. These allergens are ubiquitous, being found in the air, in settled dust, and contaminating the surfaces of sofas, carpets, buses, and cars.[55] Dog and cat allergens have also been found in households that do not own dogs or cats.[55] Dog allergens *can f 1* and *can f 2* are produced by tongue epithelia tissues and parotid glands. IgE reactivity is found in about 80% of patients with allergies to dogs.[55,56] *Fel d 1, fel d 3*, and *fel d 4* are the major cat allergens. *Fel d 1* is produced by salivary, anal, and sebaceous glands in cats, and IgE reactivity is

found in about 80% of patients with cat allergies.[55–57]

Previously, it was thought that young children were at risk for sensitization when exposed at an early age to dogs and cats, but recent data on this topic are conflicting. Birth cohort studies have found no increase in sensitivity among young children (aged 0–7 years) exposed to cats or dogs.[58–60] In fact, dog ownership may reduce the risk of sensitivity in children of this age group.[61] Young children in high-risk populations, however (defined as exposure to cats with high levels of *fel d 1*), manifested an increased risk of sensitization.[59,60] Another study found that of the 287 children studied with cat sensitivity, 237 had never owned a cat.[62] Data for older children and adults are equally unclear. Studies in Sweden have found that cat ownership seems to be associated with decreased sensitization to cats, whereas dog ownership was found to have either no association with sensitization or reduced sensitization among high-risk dog owners.[62–64] In contrast, a German analysis found an increased sensitization to cats among owners of this pet.[65] Overall, there are more studies reporting an association between cat ownership and sensitization to cats than there are for dog ownership and sensitization to dogs.[66]

Birds

Birds can carry approximately 22 zoonotic organisms; of these, 7 affect the human respiratory system.[67] Exposure to birds can be relatively intense, as they are often housed within human living quarters or in close proximity.[68] The risk of acquiring avian influenza (H5N1) from pet birds is low because they have minimal to no contact with the principal reservoirs, including poultry or waterfowl.[67] Instead, the 3 main diseases associated with pet birds are asthma, hypersensitivity pneumoconiosis (HP), and psittacosis. Pigeons, parakeets, and parrots have received the most attention with respect to the development of HP. Bird fancier's lung is a type of HP that is associated with inhalation of avian antigens. Avian antigens are complex high and low molecular weight molecules found in bird droppings, serum, feathers, and "bloom." Bloom is the waxy, fine, keratinous dust that coats bird's feathers for waterproofing. The bloom of pigeons and parakeets is frequently implicated in HP.[67,69] Exposure to live birds is not required to develop HP, as it has also been associated with duvets and feather pillows.[70] Feather duvet lung (FDL) is a rare subgroup of bird fancier's lung. It is caused by inhalation of organic dust originating from goose or duck feathers in duvets or pillows. A retrospective review of the medical records of 13 patients with FDL found that 4 had been exposed to duvets or pillows filled with raw goose feathers from their own farms. In all patients, specific IgG antibodies to goose and/or duck feathers were detected. High-resolution computed tomography was performed in 11 patients and demonstrated ground-glass opacities in 10 and fibrosis in 6.[71] Other case series have described presentations of both acute and chronic forms of FDL.[72] Exposure to feather duvets can exacerbate chronic bird fancier's lung. In one case, a man who had been diagnosed with chronic bird fancier's lung based on a positive peripheral lymphocyte proliferation to pigeon serum had been stable for 6 years when he became a daily user of a feather duvet. A chest computed tomography scan showed newly developed peribronchial ground-glass opacities and preexisting honeycombing, and an inhalation provocation test was positive.[73]

Psittacosis is a bacterial infection caused by *Chlamydophilia psittaci*. Psittacosis is also known as parrot fever, parrot disease, and ornithosis. The disease is manifested as conjunctivitis diarrhea, apathy, anorexia, and nasal discharge in birds.[67] Although the disease can be transmitted via feathers or eggs, it is most commonly spread from dried fecal matter, as *C psittaci* is found in high concentrations in bird droppings.[74] The organisms can stay viable in the environment for long periods of time.[75] In humans, symptoms can vary from mild symptoms to severe pneumonia. The symptoms typically include respiratory distress, myalgias, severe headaches, and conjunctivitis.[74] The typical incubation period for human illness is 4 to 14 days.[75]

Horses

An estimated 4.6 million Americans are involved in the equine industry.[76] Respiratory exposures in relation to horses stem from both the horses themselves and the barns in which horses are housed.[77] Sensitization to horse dander is well established in occupational exposures, but recent literature also suggests that around 3% of an atopic urban population without direct exposure to horses demonstrated allergic sensitization.[78,79] Case reports have attributed exposure to horses with the development of sudden onset of rhinorrhea, wheezing, sneezing, erythematous skin reaction, and lip swelling in young children.[77] Given the relatively high prevalence of sensitization to horse dander, it is recommended that highly atopic individuals undergo skin prick testing with evaluation of serum specific IgE before beginning any activity with close interactions with horses.[79]

High levels of endotoxin and organic dust (including molds, hay, horse dander, and other animal proteins) have been found in equine barns, which contribute to inflammatory airway disease in horses; this disease in horses is known as heaves.[80] Heaves, a chronic disorder characterized by airway hyperresponsiveness and inflammation, is similar in presentation, pathologic symptoms, and physiologic changes to human response to the same substances.[81,82] Compared with other farm environments, horse barn exposure is also associated with higher prevalence rates of chronic bronchitis, dyspnea, organic dust toxic syndrome (ODTS), and farmer's lung (a form of HP).[83]

Household Arthropods

Exposure to other "animals" encountered in the home environment, that is, various arthropods, is usually associated with asthma and rhinitis.[68] Sensitization to house dust mites is a major risk factor for the development of asthma, rhinitis, and dermatitis.[84,85] House dust mites are arthropods in the class Arachnidae; there are 13 different mite species found in house dust.[55] The most common species in house dust are *Dermatophagoides farinae* and *Dermatophagoides pteronyssinus*.[55,86] Allergens stem from the mite bodies and feces. *Der p 1* is the major group of allergens from dust mites, but there are many other minor allergens.[55] Humidity and temperature greatly influence mite growth, because the ideal climate for house dust mites are high temperature humidity environments.[86] Modern insulation and heating practices have aided the proliferation of house dust mites. House dust mites are found on many objects but are mostly linked to upholstered furniture, carpets, and bedding.

Like house dust mites, cockroach allergens are an important component of house dust. Also, like house dust mites, cockroaches thrive in higher temperature climates. House dust mites, though, are ubiquitous across many housing environments, whereas cockroaches are found more often in the highest concentrations in inner-city low-income housing.[87] Cockroaches have been found to be one of the most important risk factors for children in inner-city homes and developing asthma.[88] One study has found that children with asthma exposed to greater than 2 U/g of cockroach allergens were admitted to the hospital 4 to 5 times more often than children who were not exposed to cockroach allergens.[89] Cockroach allergens originate from saliva, feces, secretions, and cast skin.[55] There are several known allergens from cockroaches, and it is estimated that 60% to 70% of cockroach-sensitive individuals have IgE antibodies to allergens *bla g 4* and *bla g 5*.[55]

Prevention against exposure to cockroach allergens includes eradication of home cockroaches. Eradication can put home residents at risk for pesticide exposures as discussed in previous sections; however, eradication methods such as the use of cockroach bait generally do not contain pyrethrins.[90]

Gardening

Exposures from gardening vary depending on the specific type of plants and soils used. There are few reports that address respiratory disorders specifically attributable to the avocation of gardening, although the respiratory health hazards associated with commercial agriculture have received substantial attention.[91] Some of the diseases associated with the agricultural industry might theoretically also affect the gardening hobbyist.

Farmer's lung, already noted in regard to horse barns, is a common form of HP. Classically, farmer's lung has been described with exposure to moldy hay contaminated by *Thermophilic actinomycetes*. HP has been associated with many other agricultural exposures, however, including, but not limited to, mold on grapes (wine maker's lung), mushrooms (mushroom worker's lung), and sugar cane (bagassosis).[92] Acute cases of farmer's lung can present with the abrupt onset of influenza-like respiratory and constitutional symptoms including cough, dyspnea, chest tightness, fevers, chills, headaches, malaise, and myalgia, but often the disease is far more indolent.

ODTS is an influenza-like illness that may develop after exposures to heavy concentrations of organic dust contaminated with microorganisms. Unlike HP, ODTS has been documented in landscapers and gardening hobbyists.[93] Exposures occur in the setting of shoveling or moving organic materials such as oats, wood chips, composted leaves, and silage. The condition is characterized by influenza-like symptoms including fever, cough, malaise, and a leukocytosis and sometimes dyspnea. Headache, rhinitis, and conjunctivitis may also develop. Symptoms develop abruptly, usually within 12 hours after exposure to an organic dust, and may last up to 5 days.[93]

In contrast with farmer's lung, ODTS does not involve an anamnestic response. Thus, prior sensitization is relevant to the development of ODTS in exposed individuals. Reports of clusters of cases with high attack rates among the exposed also suggest individual susceptibility is not an important for disease risk.[92–94] Cases of ODTS typically follow high-intensity dust exposure consistent with a heavy exposure burden being required to cause disease. This contrasts with HP, for which even modest antigen exposure can precipitate illness as an anamnestic response in a person who has already become sensitized (consistent with the scenario of an "acute" episode of HO as previously delineated).

Arts and Crafts

Numerous reports have associated adverse respiratory effects with various arts and crafts activities, including painting, photography, ceramic work, weaving, woodworking, metalworking, jewelry making, and glass working.[68] On the commercial level, there is evidence linking most of these activities to occupational asthma.[95–97] Many chemicals and substances found in products used for commercial applications are also found in consumer home products. In the industrial setting, exposures to potentially harmful substances are theoretically controlled to conform to occupational safety and health regulations. In contradistinction, unsalaried hobbies in the home environment may be conducted where ventilation is inadequate compared with what can be expected in a regulated commercial setting. **Table 1** shows examples of common home art and craft activities and their effect on respiratory health.

Painting

Paints include film formers, solvents, additives, pigments, and polyurethanes.[95] Pigments present in paints may carry the risk of metal-related respiratory tract toxicity. In regard to paint pigments, even though lead is the most well known as a health hazard, its toxicity beyond route of exposure is not relevant to the respiratory tract.[98] More relevant to respiratory health is exposure to polyurethanes found in paints and in a variety of other products. Polyurethanes are based on diisocyanates, a group of chemicals that have been

Table 1
Exposures and adverse respiratory effects potentially associated with hobbies, avocations, and select leisure activities

Hobby	Exposure	Respiratory Health Effects	Comments
Painting	Polyurethanes, diisocyanates	Airway obstruction, bronchospasm	Inhalation and dermal exposure
Painting	Metallic pigments	Sensitization	Aerosolization is uncommon
Wood working	Wood dust	Sensitization	Specifically exotic woods
Wood working	Wood dust	Sinonasal carcinoma	Mostly industrial wood work
Photography	Developers	Sensitization	Photographic processing
Photography	Carbon fumes	Rare earth pneumoconiosis	Carbon-arc lighting
Photography	Platinum salts	Asthma	Platinotype prints
Metal work	Asbestos	Asbestos-related lung disease	Protective equipment – asbestos blankets
Metal work	Cutting	Pneumonitis	Cadmium, phosgene
Metal work	Welding	Fume fever, acute lung injury	Galvanized metal
Metal work	Sand casting	Silicosis	Mostly in foundry work
Ceramics	Metallic glaze	Sensitization	Exposure while mixing slurry
Ceramics	Irritant gas exposure	Irritation	Kiln fumes
Ceramics	Particulate byproducts	COPD	Raku – Japanese pottery
Ceramics	silica	Silicosis	More relevant in industrial ceramics
Automobile work	Asbestos	Asbestos-related lung disease	Clutch and brake repair
Automobile work	CO, NO_2, VOCs	Asthma, bronchitis	Exhaust fumes
Automobile work	Metal fumes	Asthma, toxic pneumonitis, metal fume fever	Cutting, grinding, and welding auto parts
Automobile work	Polyurethanes, diisocyanates	Airway obstruction, bronchospasm	Automotive painting

well studied and are among the more commonly reported causes of sensitizer occupational asthma.[96] In workers who have become sensitized to isocyanates, recurrent exposures are notorious for causing respiratory symptoms at low exposures. However, their role in nonoccupational asthma may be overlooked. Diisocyanates are found in many polyurethane-containing products used specifically for arts and crafts and home repairs including adhesives, sealants, paints, and foams.[96,98] Application of such products, which can also contain solvents, amines, polyols and other hazardous chemicals, can cause respiratory symptoms even though such consumer products might be presumed to be nontoxic.[97,99] The precise mechanism by which diisocyanates cause sensitization and asthma has yet to be elucidated. Exposure to diisocyanates can occur via inhalation or dermal contact. Recent studies have suggested that dermal exposures may also be important in regard to developing sensitization and asthma.[98,100] This is relevant because diisocyanates are able to break through protective equipment such as latex gloves.[101]

Woodwork

Amateur woodworking presents the risk of exposure to airborne wood dust that may cause asthma symptoms.[102] The mechanism by which wood dust contributes to asthma may be mediated by 2 mechanisms: (1) bronchial responsiveness caused by terpenes in pines and other coniferous trees[103] and (2) lytic damage to bronchial epithelial cells from abietic acid in tree resin.[104] Woodworking hobbyists engaged in fine wood working (including musical instrument making and cabinet production) can be exposed to more exotic types of woods than commercial woodworkers.[103] These woods may include African cherry, zebrawood, and iroko, all of which are all known to cause rhinitis and asthma.[68] Wood dust has also been associated with sinonasal adenocarcinoma, albeit it has only been observed in industrial settings.[105] The average time between first exposure to wood dust and development of cancer is about 40 years.[106] Finally, woodworkers are also exposed to adhesives and sealants containing polyurethane, as described previously, as well as glues and epoxies that also have been associated with asthma and rhinitis.[107]

Photography

In the not too distant past, a large portion of amateur photography included chemical-based photographic processing. Photographic processing is the means by which photographic film is treated to develop a positive or negative image and then this image is printed. With the advent of digital photography, these skills and procedures are becoming less and less common. There are several significant exposures encountered in photographic processing that may soon be of historical interest only. Photographic processing involves treating the film and paper in several chemical baths. The chemicals are usually nonbiodegradable compounds that can act as respiratory sensitizers.[68] Carbon-arc lighting had been used as a lighting source in photographic processing (albeit more commonly in film projection); the fumes produced by carbon-arc lighting have been reported to cause rare earth pneumoconiosis.[108] Finally, there are specific types of photographic printing techniques that are associated with specific exposures such as platinotypes. This process, also known as platinum printing, is a monochrome print that gives a wide tonal range. Platinotypes use platinum salts that are a well-known cause of occupational asthma.[109]

Metal work

Metal sculpting, blacksmithing, and various metal-repairing techniques (such as might be used in car body repair or other garage activities) can be associated with respiratory symptoms as a result of the manipulation of metal by welding, flame cutting, or brazing. Previously, other exposures included protective equipment such as fire mitts and fire blankets because they were made from asbestos. The type of symptoms caused by metal work depends on the form of manipulation and the type of metal being worked on. For example, welding galvanized materials can cause metal fume fever; flame cutting sheet metal can cause cadmium pneumonitis; and working on newly degreased metals can cause phosgene acute lung injury.[68] Metal fume fever develops after inhalation of metal oxide fume, specifically zinc oxide. Flulike symptoms develop and are usually self-limited with resolution around 48 hours. There have been rare cases of purported zinc oxide exposure associated with lung injury but these may have involved other concomitant exposures.[110] Mixed exposures are important because cadmium pneumonitis can have an overlapping exposure history (flame cutting metal) and clinical presentation (onset of systemic symptoms) as zinc oxide–caused metal fume fever, but the former syndrome is not self-limited and can progress to severe acute lung injury.[111] Phosgene acute lung injury occurs after inhalation of phosgene generated from the breakdown of chlorinated solvents via heat or ultraviolet light exposure, which can occur if solvent contaminated metals are welded or flame-cut.[112] Symptoms of phosgene acute lung injury depend on the vapor concentration and usually include an acute and delayed phase. The acute phase occurs immediately after inhalation. At low concentrations, eye and throat irritations are the usual symptoms, and at higher doses, cough and chest tightness prevail. The delayed phase occurs around 48 hours after exposure. Pulmonary edema develops, causing dyspnea, cough, tachypnea, and respiratory distress.[112]

Ceramics

Respiratory exposures surrounding ceramics usually occur during the firing process with irritant gas exposure from the kiln fumes. There are also specific forms of firing that can produce more particulate byproducts. Raku, a type of Japanese pottery, is one of these forms and has been linked to the development of COPD.[68] Before the firing phase, when the dried pottery is manipulated, there is also a risk of silica exposure that can lead to silicosis.[113] Exposure to various metal pigments (eg, cobalt or chromium) can also occur in mixing or applying glazes before firing.[114]

Automobile work

Exposures related to amateur automobile work depends on the specific task being performed and the specific car part that is being worked on. Car painting is a major source of respiratory exposure and has respiratory consequences detailed in the section on painting as a result of the diisocyanate composition of car paint; use of welding and flame-cutting has also been alluded to previously. Clutch and brake repair carries the risk of solvent and asbestos exposure.[115] Asbestos exposure (which can result from working with brake linings) can lead to asbestos-related lung disease, most saliently mesothelioma, for which no threshold of effect in believed to exist.[116]

Another important respiratory exposure during automobile work includes exhaust fumes. Motor vehicle emissions are widely accepted as causing or aggravating symptoms of obstructive airway disease, including bronchitis.[117] Among the potentially toxic components of motor vehicle emissions are particulate matter, VOCs, oxides of nitrogen (NO_x), and carbon monoxide (CO).[118] The most dangerous component of vehicle emissions is likely particulate matter that is formed by incomplete combustion. Particulate matter includes soot, dust, and smoke that are easily inhaled into the airways. Once in the airways, the particulate matter can either accumulate or be absorbed into the bloodstream.[117,119] VOCs from motor vehicle exhaust include benzene, ethylbenzene, formaldehyde, toluene, and xylenes. These VOCs and NO_x are important components of ground level ozone.[117] Ground level ozone can exacerbate asthma and has been shown to lead to reductions in forced expiratory volume in 1 second and forced vital capacity.[120] Diesel exhaust has been recently recognized by the International Agency for Research on Cancer as a human lung carcinogen.[121]

Indoor Sports

These leisure activities do not occur typically in the residential home environment, but their indoor nature is a common link with the subject at hand. The most widely associated respiratory disease with sports is exercise-induced asthma or exercise-induced bronchospasm (EIB).[122] EIB is an acute and temporary airway narrowing that occurs during or shortly after exercise. Exercise is a frequent trigger for asthmatics and EIB also occurs in 10% of patients who otherwise do not have known asthma.[123,124] EIB can occur in any athlete, from the recreational athlete to the professional.[125] EIB can be triggered by sport specific conditions or locations (eg, turf fields, chlorinated swimming pools, ice arenas, and athletic fields in an urban or high vehicle traffic area, or indoor home exercise [for example, a stationary bicycle or treadmill]).[126]

Ice sports

Ice sports including figure skating, hockey, curling, speed skating, and recreational skating are typically performed in an ice arena. Temperatures in ice arenas must be kept lower to prevent the ice from melting, and cold air is a well-known trigger for asthma. Besides the cold air, there are other known respiratory irritants in ice arena air circulation, including NO_x, VOCs, aldehydes, and particulate matter.[77] The most important source of these pollutants in ice arenas are ice resurfacing machines, which produce exhaust (ie, "Zamboni machines"), although other sources include food preparation stations.[127] Levels of these irritants can be particularly high in poorly ventilated arenas. The concentration of airborne pollutants is, in part, a function of the amount of use of these machines, particularly the number of times the machines are turned on and off.[127] The onset of symptoms is typically rapid as symptoms develop from minutes to hours after exposure and usually abates after cessation of the exposure. The health effects of long-term exposure to indoor ice arenas are not well established.[77]

Water sports

Water sports are extremely common, with practitioners ranging from leisure pool loungers to professional athletes. In 2005, an estimated 16 million Americans swam for fitness activities.[77] As with ice sports, indoor swimming carries the risk of poor ventilation. The literature pertaining to asthma and swimming is mixed. Swimming is often a recommended sport for asthmatics because inhaling moist air is thought to be less of an asthmatic trigger.[128] However, chronic exposure to swimming pools has been shown to cause increased respiratory symptoms in lifeguards, and elite swimmers have higher rates of asthma compared with elite athletes who perform other sports.[127,129,130]

Common irritants stem from disinfection of the water source. There are several different chemicals used for disinfection, but the most common are chlorine-based products.[131] Respiratory effects of inhalation of high levels of chlorine are well known and include laryngeal edema, chemical burns, and asthma attacks. Effects of lower levels or intermittent exposures are not as well established.[132]

Chlorine products contain hypochlorite, chlorine gas, and isocyanurates.[77] These chemicals react with ammonia and amino-compounds from by-products of swimmers (particularly sweat and urine) to produce monochloramine, dichloarmine, and tricholoramine.[131] These chloramines are particularly volatile and can cause mucous membrane irritation with ocular and respiratory symptoms.

Besides asthma, water sports have been linked to HP. This is also relevant to one major home indoor water "sport" exposure (casting this broadly): the recreational use of home spas and hot tubs. Although many different microbial agents found in the pool and spa environment can cause HP, the most well-known form, in fact, is widely known as "hot tub lung." In selected populations, hot tub lung may be one of the second most common types of HP.[133] Hot tub lung refers to HP caused by inhalational exposure to *Mycobacterium avium* complex.[134] Like other forms of acute HP, symptoms of dyspnea and cough and nonspecific constitutional symptoms resolve with avoidance of the inciting irritant.

Other, less common respiratory effects of water sports and home spas can include infections and pulmonary edema. Infections include both upper and lower respiratory tract infections. Common pathogens for upper respiratory tract infections can include *Pseudomonas* spp and *Adenovirus*, whereas lower respiratory tract infections include *Legionella*, nontuberculous *Mycobacteria*, and *Staphylococcus aureus*.[77] Pulmonary edema is rare and occurs mainly with strenuous swimming or deep breath-hold diving.[135]

SUMMARY

People spend approximately 50% of their life in the home. Many routine activities performed at home, such as cooking, cleaning, and laundering, may result in airborne exposures that cause or contribute to respiratory disease. Worldwide, cooking and heating with biomass fuels are important contributors to the total public health burden of lung disease. Respiratory exposures can also occur from leisure activities such as arts and crafts, gardening, and sports (many of which occur indoor, albeit not in the home). Airborne mold and aeroallergens from animals, including pets and arthropods, may contribute to poor indoor air quality and associated adverse health effects that include cough, asthma, rhinitis, and HP. Irritant effects may result from a spectrum of vapors, gases, dusts, and particulates, and misadventures with cleaning products. COPD attributable to long-term exposure to poor indoor air quality, including biomass fuel smoke, develops in an insidious manner, resulting in underrecognition of this exposure–effect relationship. Many hazardous exposures can be avoided or mitigated, underscoring the potential value of identifying unhealthy domestic environments. Assessment of home and leisure exposures should be part of the health assessment of individuals across all demographic groups presenting with respiratory disorders.

REFERENCES

1. Richardson G, Eick S, Jones R. How is the indoor environment related to asthma? literature review. J Adv Nurs 2005;52:328–39.
2. Heinrich J. Influence of indoor factors in dwellings on the development of childhood asthma. Int J Hyg Environ Health 2011;214:1–25.
3. Billings CG, Howard P. Damp housing and asthma. Monaldi Arch Chest Dis 1998;53:43–9.
4. Hakkola JK, Quansah R. Building materials and furnishings. In: Tarlo SM, Cullinan P, Nemery B, editors. Occupational and environmental lung disease. 1st edition. West Sussex (United Kingdom): Wiley-Blackwell; 2010. p. 69–80.
5. Tributyltin hydride material safety data sheet. 2010. Available at: http://www.sciencelab.com/msds.php?msdsId=9925303. Accessed July August 10, 2012.
6. Park JH, Cox-Ganser JM. Mold exposure and respiratory health in damp indoor environments. Front Biosci (Elite Ed) 2011;3:757–71.
7. Jarvis BB, Miller JD. Mycotoxins as harmful indoor air contaminants. Appl Microbiol Biotechnol 2005;66:367–72.

8. Cox-Ganser JM, White SK, Jones R, et al. Respiratory morbidity in office workers in a water-damaged building. Environ Health Perspect 2005;113:485–90.

9. Jaakkola JJ, Hwang BF, Jaakol N. Home dampness and molds, parental atopy, and asthma in childhood: a six-year population-based cohort study. Environ Health Perspect 2005;113:357–61.

10. Matheson MD, Abramson MD, Dharmage SC, et al. Changes in indoor allergen and fungal levels predict changes in asthma activity among young adults. Clin Exp Allergy 2005;35:907–13.

11. Jaakkola JJ, Ieromnimon A, Jaakkola MS. Interior surface materials and asthma in adults: a population based incident case-control study. Am J Epidemiol 2006;164:742–9.

12. Park JH, Cox-Ganser JM, Kreiss K, et al. Hydrophilic fungi and ergosterol associated with respiratory illness in a water-damaged building. Environ Health Perspect 2008;116:45–50.

13. Committee on Damp Indoor Spaces and Health. "Front matter." Damp indoor spaces and health. Washington, DC: The National Academies Press; 2004.

14. Institute of Medicine. Dampness moisture and flooding. In: Climate Change, the Indoor Environment, and Health. p. 137-56. Available at: http://213.55.83.52/ebooks/URBAN_ENVIRONMENT_AND_CLIMATE_CHANGE/Climate_Change_the_Indoor_Environment_and_Health-ebook.pdf. Accessed September 12, 2012.

15. Ando M, Arima K, Yoneda R, et al. Japanese summer-type hypersensitivity pneumonitis. Geographic distribution, home environment, and clinical characteristics of 621 cases. Am Rev Respir Dis 1991;144:765–9.

16. Flannigan B, McCabe EM, McGarry F. Allergenic and toxigenic micro-organisms in houses. Soc Appl Bacteriol Symp Ser 1991;20:61S–73S.

17. Fisk WJ, Lei-Gomez Q, Mendell MJ. Meta-analyses of the associations of respiratory health effects with dampness and mold in homes. Indoor Air 2007;17:284–96.

18. Mendell MJ, Mirer AG, Cheung K, et al. Respiratory and allergic health effects of dampness, mold, and dampness-related agents: a review of the epidemiologic evidence. Environ Health Perspect 2011;119:748–56.

19. Park JH, Kreiss K, Cox-Ganser JM. Rhinosinusitis and mold as risk factors for asthma symptoms in occupants of a water-damaged building. Indoor Air 2012. http://dx.doi.org/10.1111/j.1600-0668.2012.00775.x.

20. Custovic A, Woodcock A. Clinical effects of allergen avoidance. Clin Rev Allergy Immunol 2000;18:397–419.

21. Goplen N, Karim Z, Liang Q, et al. Combined sensitization of mice to extracts of dust mites, ragweed and Aspergillus species breaks through tolerance and establishes chronic features of asthma. J Allergy Clin Immunol 2009;123:925–32.

22. Wright RS, Dyer Z, Liebhaber MI, et al. Hypersensitivity pneumonitis from Pezizia domiciliana. A case of El Niño lung. Am J Respir Crit Care Med 1999;160:1758–61.

23. Wolkoff P, Schneider T, Kildeso J, et al. Risk in cleaning: chemical and physical exposure. Sci Total Environ 1998;215:135–56.

24. Medina-Ramon M, Zock JP, Kogevinas M, et al. Asthma, chronic bronchitis and exposure to irritant agents in occupational domestic cleaning: a nested case-control study. Occup Environ Med 2005;62:598–606.

25. Rosenman KD, Reilly MJ, Schill DP, et al. Cleaning products and work-related asthma. J Occup Environ Med 2003;45:556–63.

26. Kogevinas M, Anto JM, Sunyer J, et al. Occupational asthma in Europe and other industrialized areas: a population based study. Lancet 1999;353:1750–4.

27. Zock JP, Plana E, Jarvis D, et al. The use of household cleaning sprays and adult asthma. Am J Respir Crit Care Med 2007;176:735–41.

28. Zock JP. Cleaning and other household products. In: Tarlo SM, Cullinan P, Nemery B, editors. Occupational and environmental lung disease. 1st edition. West Sussex (United Kingdom): Wiley-Blackwell; 2010. p. 55–68.

29. Quirce S, Barranco P. Cleaning agents and asthma. J Investig Allergol Clin Immunol 2010;20:542–50.

30. Bello A, Quinn MM, Pery MR. Characterization of occupational exposures to cleaning products used for common cleaning task – a pilot study of hospital cleaners. Environ Health 2009;27:8–11.

31. Basketter DA, English JS, Wakelin SH, et al. Enzymes, detergents and skin: facts and fantasies. Br J Dermatol 2008;158:1177–81.

32. Steinemann AC, MacGregor IC, Gordon SM, et al. Fragranced consumer products: chemicals emitted, ingredients unlisted. Environ Impact Asses Rev 2009;29:32–8.

33. Cooper SD, Raymer JH, Pellizzari ED, et al. Polar organic compounds in fragrances of consumer products. (Final report, contract 68-02-4544.). Research Triangle Park (NC): US EPA; 1992.

34. Kumar P, Caradonna-Graham VM, Gupta S, et al. Inhalation challenge effects of perfume scent strips in patients with asthma. Ann Allergy Asthma Immunol 1995;75:429–33.

35. Elliott L, Longnecker MP, Kissling GE, et al. Volatile organic compounds and pulmonary function. In the Third National Health and Nutrition Examination Survey, 1988-1994. Environ Health Perspect 2006;114:1210–4.

36. Larson ML, Frisk M, Hallstrom J, et al. Environmental tobacco smoke exposure during childhood is associated with increased prevalence of asthma in adults. Chest 2001;120:711–7.

37. Achmadi UF, Pauluhn J. Household insecticides: evaluation and assessment of inhalation toxicity: a workshop summary. Exp Toxicol Pathol 1998;50: 67–72.

38. Osimitz TG, Sommers N, Kingston R. Human exposure to insecticide products containing pyrethrins and piperonyl butoxide (2001-2003). Food Chem Toxicol 2009;47:1406–15.

39. Liu WK, Zhang J, Hashim JH, et al. Mosquito coil emissions and health implications. Environ Health Perspect 2003;111:1454–60.

40. Jarvis D. Emissions related to cooking and heating. In: Tarlo SM, Cullinan P, Nemery B, editors. Occupational and environmental lung disease. 1st edition. West Sussex (United Kingdom): Wiley-Blackwell; 2010. p. 45–54.

41. Eng PA, Yman L, Maaninen E, et al. Inhalant allergy to fresh asparagus. Clin Exp Allergy 1996;26: 330–4.

42. Felleroni AE, Zeiss CR, Levits D. Occupational asthma secondary to inhalation of garlic dust. J Allergy Clin Immunol 1981;68:156–60.

43. Chauhan AH. Gas cooking appliances and indoor pollution. Clin Exp Allergy 1999;29:1009–13.

44. Comstock GW, Meyer MD, Helsing KJ. Respiratory effects of household exposures to tobaccos smoke and gas cooking. Am J Epidemiol 2008; 168:810–5.

45. Zhou Y, Wang C, Yao W. COPD in Chinese nonsmokers. Eur Respir J 2009;33:509–18.

46. Lambach RJ, Kipen HM. Respiratory health effects of air pollution: update on biomass smoke and traffic pollution. J Allergy Clin Immunol 2012;129: 3–11.

47. Moran SE, Strachan DP, Johnston ID, et al. Effects of exposure to gas cooking in childhood and adulthood on respiratory symptoms, allergic sensitisation and lung function in young British adults. Clin Exp Allergy 1999;29:1033–41.

48. Ekwo EE, Weinberger MM, Lachenbruch PA, et al. Relationship of parental smoking and gas cooking to respiratory disease in children. Chest 1983;84: 662–8.

49. Pilotto LS, Douglas RM, Attewell RG, et al. Respiratory effects associated with indoor nitrogen dioxide exposure in children. Int J Epidemiol 1997;26: 788–96.

50. Schindler C, Ackermann-Liebrich U, Leuenberger P, et al. Associations between lung function and estimated average exposure to NO2 in eight areas of Switzerland. The SAPALDIA Team. Swiss Study of Air Pollution and Lung Diseases in Adults. Epidemiology 1998;9:405–11.

51. Kodgule R, Slavi S. Exposure to biomass smoke as a cause for airway disease in women and children. Curr Opin Allergy Clin Immunol 2012;12:82–90.

52. Laumach RJ, Kipen HM. Respiratory health effects of air pollution: update on biomass smoke and traffic pollution. J Allergy Clin Immunol 2012;129: 3–11.

53. Pokhrel AK, Bates MN, Verma SC. Tuberculosis and indoor biomass and kerosene use in Nepal: a case-control study. Environ Health Perspect 2010;118(4):558–64.

54. Levesque B, Allaire S, Gauvin D, et al. Wood-burning appliances and indoor air quality. Sci Total Environ 2001;281:47–62.

55. Blay FD, Posa M, Pauli G, et al. Mites, pets, fungi and rare allergens. In: Tarlo SM, Cullinan P, Nemery B, editors. Occupational and environmental lung disease. 1st edition. West Sussex (United Kingdom): Wiley-Blackwell; 2010. p. 81–93.

56. Erwin EA, Woodfolk JA, Custis N, et al. Animal danders. Immunol Allergy Clin North Am 2003;23: 469–81.

57. Kelly LA, Erwin EA, Platts-Mills TA. The indoor air and asthma: the role of cat allergens. Curr Opin Pulm Med 2012;18:29–34.

58. Arshad SH, Tariq SM, Matthews S, et al. Sensitisation to common allergens and its association with allergic disorders at age 4 years: a whole population birth cohort study. Pediatrics 2001;108:E33.

59. Lau S, Illi S, Sommerfeld C, et al. Early exposure to house dust mite and cat allergens and development of childhood asthma: a cohort study. Lancet 2000;356:1392–7.

60. Custovic A, Simpson BM, Simpson A, et al. Effect of environmental manipulation in pregnancy and early life on respiratory symptoms and atopy during first year of life: a randomized trial. Lancet 2001;358:188–93.

61. Ownby DR, Johnson CC, Peterson EL. Exposure to dogs and cats in the first year of life and risk of allergic sensitisation at age 6 to 7 years. JAMA 2002;288:963–72.

62. Perzanowski MS, Ronmark E, Platts-Mills TA, et al. Effect of cat and dog ownership on sensitization and development of asthma among preteenage children. Am J Respir Crit Care Med 2002;166: 696–702.

63. Hesselmar B, Aberg N, Aberg B, et al. Does early exposure to cat or dog protect against later allergy development. Clin Exp Allergy 1999;29:611–7.

64. Braback L, Kjellman NI, Sandin A, et al. Atopy among school children in northern and southern Sweden in relation to pet ownership and early life events. Pediatr Allergy Immunol 2001;12:4–10.

65. Holscher B, Frye C, Wichmann HE, et al. Exposure to pets and allergies in children. Pediatr Allergy Immunol 2002;13:334–41.

66. Simpson A, Custovic A. Pets and the development of allergic sensitization. Curr Allergy Asthma Rep 2005;5:212–20.

67. Gorman J, Cook A, Ferguson C, et al. Pet birds and risks of respiratory disease in Australia: a review. Aust N Z J Public Health 2009;33:167–72.

68. Blanc PD. Hobby pursuits. In: Tarlo SM, Cullinan P, Nemery B, editors. Occupational and environmental lung disease. 1st edition. West Sussex (United Kingdom): Wiley-Blackwell; 2010. p. 95–105.

69. Longbottom JL. Pigeon breeder's disease: quantitative immunoelectrophorectic studies of pigeon bloom antigen. Clin Exp Allergy 1989;32:517–21.

70. Haitjema T, van Velzen-Blad H, van den Bosch JM. Extrinsic allergic alveolitis caused by goose feathers in a duvet. Thorax 1992;47:990–1.

71. Koschel D, Wittstruck H, Renck T, et al. Presenting features of feather duvet lung. Int Arch Allergy Immunol 2010;152:264–70.

72. Inase N, Ohtani R, Sumi Y, et al. A clinical study of hypersensitivity pneumonitis presumable caused by feather duvets. Ann Allergy Asthma Immunol 2006;96:98–104.

73. Inase N, Sakashita H, Ohtani Y, et al. Chronic bird fancier's lung presenting with acute exacerbation due to use of a feather duvet. Intern Med 2004; 43:835–7.

74. Telfer BL, Moberley SA, Hort KP, et al. Probable psittacosis outbreak linked to wild birds. Emerg Infect Dis 2005;11:391–7.

75. Butler JC. Emerging and under-recognized respiratory infections in children. Semin Pediatr Infect Dis 1995;6:201–8.

76. Mazan MR, Svatek J, Maranda L, et al. Questionnaire assessment of airway disease symptoms in equine barn personnel. Occup Med (Lond) 2009; 59:220–5.

77. Paintal HS, Kuschner WG. Indoor sports. In: Tarlo SM, Cullinan P, Nemery B, editors. Occupational and environmental lung disease. 1st edition. West Sussex (United Kingdom): Wiley-Blackwell; 2010. p. 137–57.

78. Tutluoglu B, Atis S, Anakkaya AN, et al. Sensitization to horse hair, symptoms and lung function in grooms. Clin Exp Allergy 2002;32:1170–3.

79. Liccardi G, Salzillo A, Dente B, et al. Horse allergens: an underestimated risk for allergic sensitization in an urban atopic population without occupational exposure. Respir Med 2009;103: 414–20.

80. Pirie RS, Dixon PM, Colliee DD, et al. Pulmonary and systemic effects of inhaled endotoxin in control and heaves horses. Equine Vet J 2001; 33:311–8.

81. Ghio AJ, Mazan MR, Hoffman AM, et al. Correlates between human lung injury after particle exposure and recurrent airway obstruction in the horse. Equine Vet J 2006;38:362–7.

82. Leclere M, Lavoie-Lamoureux A, Lavoie JP. Heaves, an asthma-like disease of horses. Respirology 2011;16:1027–46.

83. Kimbell-Dunn MR, Fishwick RD, Bradshaw L, et al. Work-related respiratory symptoms in New Zealand farmers. Am J Ind Med 2001;39: 292–300.

84. Tupker RA, De Monchy JG, Coenraads PJ. House-dust mite hypersensitivity, eczema, and other non-pulmonary manifestations of allergy. Allergy 1998; 53:92–6.

85. Platts-Mills TA, Sporik RB, Wheatley LM, et al. Is there a dose-response relationship between exposure to indoor allergens and symptoms of asthma? J Allergy Clin Immunol 1995;96:435–40.

86. Roche N, Chinet TC, Huchon GJ. Allergic and nonallergic interactions between house dust mite allergens and airway mucosa. Eur Respir J 1997; 10:719–26.

87. Gelber LE, Seltzer LH, Bouzoukis JK, et al. Sensitization and exposure to indoor allergens as risk factors for asthma among patients presenting to hospital. Am Rev Respir Dis 1993;147: 573–8.

88. Huss K, Naumann PL, Mason PJ, et al. Asthma severity, atopic status, allergen exposure and quality of life in elderly persons. Ann Allergy Asthma Immunol 2001;86:524–30.

89. Rabito FA, Carlson J, Holt EW, et al. Coackroach exposure in dependent of sensitization status and association with hospitalizations for asthma in inner-city children. Ann Allergy Asthma Immunol 2011;106:103–9.

90. Wang C, El-Nour MM, Bennett GW. Survey of pest infestation, asthma and allergy in low-incoming housing. J Community Health 2008;33:31–9.

91. Spurzem JR, Romberg DJ, Von Essen SG. Agricultural lung disease. Clin Chest Med 2002;23: 795–810.

92. Rose CS, Lara AR. Hypersensitivity pneumonitis. In: Mason RJ, Murray JF, Broaddus VC, et al, editors. Murray and Nadel's textbook of respiratory medicine. 5th edition. Philadelphia: Saunders Elsevier; 2010. p. 1587–600.

93. Boehmer TK, Jones TS, Ghosh TS, et al. Cluster of presumed organic dust toxic syndrome cases among urban landscape workers-Colorado, 2007. Am J Ind Med 2009;52:534–8.

94. Brinton WT, Vastbinder EE, Greene JW. An outbreak of organic dust toxic syndrome in a college fraternity. JAMA 1987;258:1210–2.

95. Estalnder T, Jolanki R, Kanerva L. Paints, lacquers and varnishes. In: Kanerva L, Elsner P, Wahlberg J, et al, editors. Handbook of occupational dermatology. Berlin: Springer; 2000. p. 662–78.

96. Tarlo SM, Liss GM. Diisocyanate-induced asthma: diagnosis, prognosis and effects of medical surveillance measures. Appl Occup Environ Hyg 2002;17:902–8.

97. Rosenstock L, Cullen MR, editors. Textbook of clinical, occupational and environmental medicine. Philadelphia: WB Saunders; 1994. p. 794–6.

98. Krone CA. Diisocyanates and nonoccupational disease: a review. Arch Environ Health 2004;59: 306–16.

99. Wirpsza Z. Polyurethanes: chemistry, technology and applications. New York: Ellis Horwood Publishers; 1993. p. 517.

100. Littorin M, Rylander L, Skarping G, et al. Exposure bio-markers and risk from gluing and heating of polyurethane: a cross sectional study of respiratory symptoms. Occup Environ Med 2000;57:396–405.

101. Liu Y, Stow MH, Bello D, et al. Respiratory protection from isocyanate exposure in the autobody repair and refinishing industry. J Occup Environ Hyg 2006;3:234–9.

102. Perez-Rios M, Ruano-Ravina A, Etmian M, et al. A meta-analysis on wood dust exposure and risk of asthma. Allergy 2010;65:467–73.

103. Ayars GH, Altman LC, Frazier CE, et al. The toxicity of constituents of cedar and pine woods to pulmonary epithelium. J Allergy Clin Immunol 1989;83: 610–8.

104. Schlunssen V, Schaumburg I, Heederik D, et al. Indices of asthma atopic and non-atopic woodworkers. Occup Environ Med 2004;61:504–11.

105. Innocenti A, Ciapini C, Natale D, et al. Longitudinal changes of pulmonary function in workers with high wood dust levels. Med Lav 2006;97: 30–5.

106. Nylander LA, Dement JM. Carcinogenic effects of wood dust: review and discussion. Am J Ind Med 1993;24:619–47.

107. Kopp SK, McKay RT, Moller DR, et al. Asthma and rhinitis due to ethylcyanocarcylate instant glue. Ann Intern Med 1985;102:613–5.

108. Waring PM, Watling RJ. Rare earth deposits in a deceased movie projectionist. A new case of rare earth pneumoconiosis? Med J Aust 1990; 153:726–30.

109. Merget R, Caspari C, Dierkes-Globisch A, et al. Effectiveness of a medical surveillance program for the prevention of occupational asthma caused by platinum salts: a nested case-control study. J Allergy Clin Immunol 2001;107: 707–12.

110. Bydash J, Kasmani R, Naraharisetty K. Metal fume-induced diffuse alveolar damage. J Thorac Imaging 2010;25:W27–9.

111. Barnhart S, Rosenstock L. Cadmium chemical pneumonitis. Chest 1984;86:789–91.

112. Grainge C, Rice P. Management of phosgene-induced acute lung injury. Clin Toxicol 2010;48: 497–508.

113. Ulm K, Waschulzik B, Ehnes H, et al. Silica dust and lung cancer in the German stone, quarrying, and ceramics industries: results of a case control study. Thorax 1999;54:347–51.

114. Krecisz B, Kiec-Swiercynska M, Krawczyk P, et al. Cobalt-induced anaphylaxis, contact urticarial, and delayed allergy in a ceramics decorator. Contact Derm 2009;60:173–4.

115. Stowe MH, Redlich CA. Automobile maintenance, repair and refinishing. In: Tarlo SM, Cullinan P, Nemery B, editors. Occupational and environmental lung disease. 1st edition. West Sussex (United Kingdom): Wiley-Blackwell; 2010. p. 203–15.

116. Finklestein MM. Asbestos fibre concentrations in the lungs of brake workers: another look. Ann Occup Hyg 2008;52:455–61.

117. Orru H, Rain J, Marko K, et al. Chronic traffic-induced PM exposure and self-reported respiratory and cardiovascular health in the RHINE Tartu cohort. Int J Environ Res Public Health 2009;6: 2740–51.

118. Burr ML, Karani G, Davies B, et al. Effects on respiratory health of a reduction in air pollution from vehicle exhaust emissions. Occup Environ Med 2004;61:212–8.

119. Chan CC. Driver exposure to volatile organic compounds, CO, ozone and NO2 under different driving conditions. Environ Sci Technol 1991;25: 964–72.

120. Kim BJ, Kwon JW, Seo JH, et al. Association of ozone exposure with asthma, allergic rhinitis, and allergic sensitization. Ann Allergy Asthma Immunol 2011;107:214–9.

121. International Agency for Research on Cancer. IARC: diesel engine exhaust carcinogenic. (Press release No. 213.) 2012. Available at: http://press.iarc.fr/pr213_E.pdf. Accessed July 27, 2012.

122. Carlsen KH. Outdoor sports. In: Tarlo SM, Cullinan P, Nemery B, editors. Occupational and environmental lung disease. 1st edition. West Sussex (United Kingdom): Wiley-Blackwell; 2010. p. 445–56.

123. Parson JP, Mastronarde JG. Exercise-induced bronchoconstriction in athletes. Chest 2005;128: 3966–74.

124. Randolph C. An update on exercise-induced bronchoconstriction with and without asthma. Curr Allergy Asthma Rep 2009;9:433–8.

125. Anderson SD, Holzer K. Exercise-induced asthma: is it the right diagnosis in elite athletes? J Allergy Clin Immunol 2000;106:419–28.

126. Rundell KW, Caviston R, Hollenbach AM, et al. Vehicular air pollution, playgrounds and youth athletic fields. Inhal Toxicol 2006;18:541–7.

127. Pelham TW, Holt LE, Moss MA. Exposure to carbon monoxide and nitrogen dioxide in enclosed ice arenas. Occup Environ Med 2002;59:224–33.

128. Goodman M, Hays S. Asthma and swimming: a meta-analysis. J Asthma 2008;45:639–47.

129. Massin N, Bohadan AB, Wild P, et al. Respiratory symptoms and bronchial responsiveness in lifeguards exposed to nitrogen trichloride in indoor swimming pools. Occup Environ Med 1998;55:258–63.

130. Levesque B, Duchesne JF, Ginras S, et al. The determinants of prevalence of health complaints among young competitive swimmers. Int Arch Occup Environ Health 2006;80:32–9.

131. Nemery B, Hoet PH, Nowak D. Indoor swimming pools, water chlorination and respiratory health. Eur Respir J 2002;19:790–3.

132. Das R, Blanc PD. Chlorine gas exposure and the lung: a review. Toxicol Ind Health 1993;9:439–55.

133. Hanak V, Golbin JM, Ryu JH. Causes and presenting features in 85 consecutive patients with hypersensitivity pneumonitis. Mayo Clin Proc 2007;82:812–6.

134. Hanak V, Kalra V, Aksamit TR, et al. Hot tub lung: presenting features and clinical course of 21 patients. Repir Med 2006;100:610–5.

135. Pollocj NW. Breath-hold diving: performance and safety. Diving Hyperb Med 2008;38:79–86.

Implications of OSA on Work and Work Disability Including Drivers

Ann Y. Teng, DO[a],*, Christine Won, MD, MS[b]

KEYWORDS

- OSA • Disability • Drivers • Sleep • Apnea • Impairment • Snoring • SDB

KEY POINTS

- This article illustrates the impact of obstructive sleep apnea (OSA) on the work force.
- Specifics of OSA impact on individuals are discussed with regard to veterans, first responders, farmers, and pilots, with a special concentration on commercial vehicle drivers.
- The pathophysiology of the disease as well as the consequence of impairment and disability due to OSA on work capacity is introduced.
- Federal guidelines for occupational specific recommendations are presented. Importance is placed on the health care provider's role in identifying and incorporating effective screening and treatment strategies for workers with sleep apnea.

Obstructive sleep apnea (OSA) is a common and debilitating disease characterized by repetitive upper airway obstruction associated with sleep disruption, oxygen desaturation, and exaggerated sympathetic tone. OSA is associated with significant medical diseases such as increased cardiovascular morbidity and cognitive and psychological limitations. With respect to the workplace, there is increasing recognition that untreated and ineffectively treated OSA has adverse effects on individual performance as well as the overall safety for workers and, in certain circumstances, the general public **Fig. 1**.

The prevalence of OSA (defined by an apnea–hypopnea index [AHI] $\geq$5) in the middle-aged adult population has been estimated to be up to 24% in men and 9% in women.[1] The National Commission on Sleep Disorders Research estimates that OSA affects 7 million to 18 million people in the United States and that OSA remains undiagnosed in approximately 92% of affected women and 80% of affected men.[2] Given such a high prevalence, untreated OSA becomes a significant burden on the entire workforce. At the individual level, treatment of OSA and its associated comorbities can contribute to increasing health care costs for employers, increased absenteeism, and alterations in job performance. The consequence of OSA poses a danger to public safety not only for workers but also for those whom they serve.

Several risk factors for OSA such as male gender, obesity, and increasing age influence the growing impact and presentation of OSA in the workplace. The current obesity epidemic in the general population could lead to the increasing presence of OSA in the workplace. More than half of morbidly obese

Disclosure: No relationships to disclose for both authors.
[a] Occupational Environmental Medicine, Yale School of Medicine, 135 College Street, 3rd Floor, New Haven, CT 06515, USA; [b] Pulmonary and Critical Care Medicine, Yale School of Medicine, 300 Cedar Street, New Haven, CT 06520-8057, USA
* Corresponding author.
E-mail address: ann.teng@yale.edu

Screening Recommendation for CMV Drivers With Possible or Probable Sleep Apnea

Medically Qualified To Drive Commercial Vehicles if Driver Meets Either of the Following:	In-Service Evaluation Recommended if Driver Falls Into Any One of the Following Five Major Categories (3-mo Maximum Certification):	Out-of-Service Immediate Evaluation Recommended if Driver Meets Any One of the Following Factors:
1. No positive findings or any of the numbered in-service evaluation factors	1. Sleep history suggestive of OSA (snoring, excessive daytime sleepiness, witnessed apneas)	1. Observed unexplained excessive daytime sleepiness (sleeping in examination or waiting room) or confessed excessive sleepiness
2. Diagnosis of OSA with continuous positive airway pressure compliance documented	2. Two or more of the following (1) body mass index > 35 kg/m^2; (2) neck circumference > 17 inches in men and 16 inches in women; (3) hypertension (new, uncontrolled, or unable to control with fewer than two medications)	2. Motor vehicle accident (run off road, at fault, rear-end collision) likely related to sleep disturbance unless evaluated for sleep disorder in the interim.
	3. Epworth sleepiness scale score > 10	3. Epworth sleepiness scale score ≥ 16 or functional outcomes of sleep questionnaire score < 18
	4. Previously diagnosed sleep disorder; compliance claimed, but no recent medical visits/compliance data available for immediate review (must be reviewed within 3-month period); if found not to be compliant, should be removed from service (includes surgical treatment)	4. Previously diagnosed sleep disorder (1) noncompliant (continuous positive airway pressure treatment not tolerated); (2) no recent follow-up (within recommended time frame); (3) any surgical approach with no objective follow-up
	5. Apnea-hypopnea index > 5 but < 30 in a prior sleep study or polysomnography and no excessive daytime somnolence (Epworth sleepiness scale score < 11); no motor vehicle accidents; no hypertension requiring two or more agents to control	5. Apnea hypopnea index > 30.

Fig. 1. Screening recommendations for CMV drivers with possible or probable sleep apnea. (*From* Hartenbaum N, Callop N, Rosen IM, et al. Sleep apnea and commercial motor vehicle operators. Chest 2006;130(3):902; with permission.)

Recommendation Regarding the Evaluation for Fitness for Duty for Commercial Drivers With Possible or Probable Sleep Apnea

Categories	Recommendations
Diagnosis	1. Diagnosis should be determined by a physician and confirmed by polysomnography, preferably in an accredited sleep laboratory or by a certified sleep specialist.
	2. A full-night study should be done unless a split-night study is indicated (severe OSA identified after at least 2 h of sleep).
Treatment	1. First-line treatment for CMV drivers with OSA should be delivered via positive airway pressure (continuous positive airway pressure, bilevel positive airway pressure).
	2. All CMV drivers receiving positive airway pressure must use a machine that is able to measure time on pressure.
	3. A minimum acceptable average use of continuous positive airway pressure is 4 h within a 24-h period, but drivers should be advised that longer treatment would be more beneficial.
	4. Treatment should be started as soon as possible, but within 2 wk of the sleep study.
	5. Follow-up by a sleep specialist should be done after 2 to 4 wk of treatment.
Return to work after treatment (treatment with positive airway pressure)	1. After approximately 1 wk of treatment there contact between the patient and personnel from either the durable medical equipment supplier, treating provider, or sleep specialist.
	2. An apnea-hypopnea index < 5 is documented with continuous positive airway pressure at initial titration (full night or split night) or after surgery or with use of oral appliance; apnea hypopnea index is ≦ 10 depending on clinical findings.
	3. Query the driver about mask fit and compliance, and remind him/her to bring card (if used) or machine to next session.
	4. At a minimum of 2 wk after initiating therapy, but within 4 wk, the driver should be re-evaluated by the sleep specialist, and compliance and BP assessed.
	5. If the driver is compliant and BP is improving (must meet FMCSA criteria), the driver can return to work but should be certified for no longer than 3 mo.
Return to work after treatment (treatment with oral appliances)	1. Oral appliances should only be used as a primary therapy if the apnea-hypopnea index is < 30.
	2. Prior to returning to service, the driver must have a follow-up sleep study demonstrating an apnea-hypopnea index < 5, but ≦ 10 while wearing an oral appliance.
	3. All reported symptoms of sleepiness must be resolved, and BP must be controlled or improving (must meet FMCSA criteria).
Return to work after treatment (treatment with surgery or weight loss)	The driver should have a follow-up sleep study; the apnea-hypopnea index is ideally < 5, but ≦ 10 required to document efficacy.

Fig. 1. (continued)

persons are reported to have OSA, and it is 50% more prevalent in persons with cardiac or metabolic disorders.[2] There is evidence that obese employees have "presenteeism" and are less productive while on the job.[3] OSA itself contributes to increased fatigue and cognitive decline. Based on trends observed from NHANES studies from 1976 to 2004 it is projected that, by the year 2030, 86.3% of all American adults will be overweight or obese and 51.1% of them will be obese.[4] Therefore, the direct and indirect financial cost of obesity in the US workforce would be astronomical if this current trend continues.

With the aging of the workforce, the prevalence of OSA in the older population prompts an additional concern for the workforce. It has been projected that the American workforce is aging and that between the years of 2006 and 2016, the number of workers 55 to –64 years of age will increase by 36.5%, whereas the number of workers older than 65 years will increase by 80%.[3] It is anticipated that in 2015, 1 in 5 workers will be 55 years of age or older.[5] Studies have shown that absence of chronic illness and good mental health are the factors that have been scientifically observed to be associated with low occupational injury rates.[5] An older working population complicated by additional chronic illnesses could incur more workplace injuries and impairment.

This article explores the impact of OSA on the workplace. The neurocognitive limitations and comorbidities such as increased cardiovascular morbidity associated with OSA are reviewed. The presentation of OSA among specific working populations including commercial vehicle drivers, first responders, and veterans is discussed. The regulations, recommendations, and policies set forth by specific agencies for the screening, management, and treatment of OSA and the definitions of impairment and disability with regard to OSA are described.

IMPACT OF OSA ON NEUROCOGNITION

Multiple studies suggest neurocognitive defects that contribute to the decrements in workplace performance seen in workers with OSA. The exact pathophysiological mechanisms that cause neurocognitive defects in patients with OSA are not completely clear. Some studies have observed that OSA is related to changes in cognition, including impaired memory, attention, vigilance, executive function, and psychomotor deficits.[6,7] A meta-analysis of the neuropsychological effects of OSA revealed a decline in vigilance, executive functioning, and coordination, but not in intelligence, verbal functioning, or visual perception.[6] In a small

cohort study by Nagele and colleagues,[7] it was found that patients with OSA had a significantly decreased ability to initiate new mental processes and to inhibit automatic ones. Frontal lobe dysfunction was found to be correlated most significantly with the severity of hypoxemia, whereas memory deficits were correlated with the number of apneic episodes per hour of sleep.[7] In a cross-sectional study of the cohorts from the Apnea Positive Pressure Long-term Efficacy Study (APPLES), no association was found between AHI and neurocognitive performance. The severity of oxygen desaturation was only found to be weakly associated with worse neurocognitive performance.[8]

Although there is variability in study results regarding OSA's impact on neurocognition, it is consistently demonstrated that OSA causes chronic sleepiness and affects a patient's quality of life. OSA has been found to significantly affect a patient's moods, specifically including increased irritability, fatigue, depression, and anxiety.[6,7] One study incorporated the Short Form (36) questionnaire to test the impact of sleep disruption on patients. It found that patients with OSA scored lower on all 8 dimensions thought to reflect the psychological well-being and performance status of individuals.[9] When the same questionnaire was implemented in another study, quality of life in the mental domain was significantly affected, revealing that depression was highly correlated with OSA.[10] It was observed that patients who had neurocognitive deficits, assessed by a psychomotor vigilance test, had greater impairments in the physical domain (physical functioning, general health perceptions, bodily pain, role limitations because of physical health) in assessment of quality of life.[10]

The influences of comorbidities associated with OSA are quite pertinent. Patients with hypertension, diabetes, and stroke have been found to have cognitive impairments from neurovascular changes.[11] Studies of neuroimaging done on patients with OSA have reflected vasculature changes and unique cerebral alterations.[10,12] Neuroimaging techniques using structural magnetic resonance imaging and proton magnetic resonance spectroscopy have exhibited changes to brain structure and metabolism. Neuronal cell damage was seen in both gray and white matter, resulting in reduced prefrontal activation during working memory task in patients with OSA.[12]

Patients with OSA often experience performance deficits in the workplace with regard to productivity and reaction time. In a small crossover study, subjects with OSA were less aware of their impairment caused by sleep deprivation. After a sleep deprivation experiment was imposed, those with OSA showed a longer reaction time than those without it.[13] In addition, for blue-collar workers, significant differences have been observed between patients with mild OSA (AHI 5–15/h) and those with severe OSA (AHI >30/h) on a validated work limitation questionnaire.[14] It seems that blue-collar workers with severe OSA were approximately 2 times more likely to report limitations at work stemming from time management and mental interpersonal demands.[14] These differences were not observed in white-collar workers. In general, subjects without excessive daytime sleepiness (EDS) were not found to have significant changes in work productivity, whereas those with OSA who reported EDS indicated decreased level of productivity.[15]

IMPACT OF OSA ON DRIVING

The impact of OSA on driving has been thoroughly studied. The contribution of sleep disorders such as OSA to fatal motor vehicle accidents has been increasingly recognized in the past few decades, given the threat posed by commercial vehicle drivers with OSA.[16] It has been observed that driving performance consistently worsens in sleep loss states, resulting in more crashes. Sleep loss states affect a driver's maintenance of lane positions, reaction time, and steering in simulation.[17] A retrospective study found that after adjustment for potential confounders, such as alcohol consumption, visual refraction disorders, body mass index (BMI), years of driving, age, history with respects to traffic accidents, use of medications causing drowsiness, and sleep schedule, subjects with sleep apnea had traffic accident rates that were 2 to 15 times higher than that of the general population.[18] A sleep apneic patient with an AHI of 10 or more was found to have 6.3 (95% confidence interval [CI] 2.4–16.2) times the risk of having a traffic accident than the general public.[18]

Simulation studies have shown that patients with OSA demonstrate slower reaction times, incur increased steering errors, have an increased time to target acquisition, and have more off-road incidents.[17] According to a study on alcohol use and sleep restrictions, patients with OSA demonstrated an increased steering deviation of 50.5 cm (95% CI 46.1–54.9 cm) as compared with 38.4 cm (95% CI 32.4–44.4 cm) for controls.[19] The deviation was 40% greater with sleep restriction and alcohol compared with the controls with the same interventions.[19] In the simulation, patients with OSA experienced a greater number of microsleeps and prolonged eye closures than the controls, thereby crashing more frequently (odds ratio [OR] = 25.4).[19] Sleep restriction and alcohol have

been demonstrated to have a profound impact on patients with OSA. In a study of truck drivers, sleep latency was related to severity of OSA: those with moderate or severe OSA had a mean sleep latency of 4.36 minutes as opposed to 7.9 minutes in drivers without OSA.[11]

IMPACT OF OSA IN SPECIFIC WORKFORCES
Commercial Motor Vehicle Drivers

The prevalence of OSA on commercial motor vehicle (CMV) operators contributes to significant safety and health risks. CMV operators are also likely to be subject to sleep-related issues from shift work and sleep deprivation. Studies have suggested that CMV operators have a higher prevalence of OSA than the general population.[20] In a study of Belgian truck drivers, 26% of commercial drivers were at high risk for OSA, based on the Berlin questionnaire, compared with 21% of the general population.[21] It has been hypothesized that truck drivers often exhibit more risk factors for developing OSA because of poor dietary habits, lack of exercise, and prevalent obesity. A higher prevalence of smoking within this population also constitutes an additional risk factor for OSA.[22]

Acknowledging the implications of health and safety risk, the US Department of Transportation's Task Force on Pulmonary Disorders and Commercial Drivers has determined that untreated OSA is an important and preventable cause of motor vehicle accidents, and new regulations are potentially forthcoming.[23]

Pilots

OSA in pilots is of great concern to the Federal Aviation Administration (FAA) and the National Transportation Safety Board (NTSB). In 2 isolated incidents in 2008 and 2009, aircraft overflew destination points in Minnesota and Hawaii. These incidents prompted investigation into pilot fatigue and led to increased awareness of the impact of OSA. Information obtained by the FAA noted that people with mild-to-moderate OSA can show performance degradation equivalent to 0.06% to 0.08% blood alcohol level, a level greater than that of legal intoxication in many states.[24] The NTSB cites that OSA is responsible for a 6-fold increased risk of aviation crashes.[25]

Inconsistent sleep times and sleep/wake cycles, time zone changes, and long flights are problematic and exacerbate the symptoms of OSA. The insufficient supply of pilots coupled with longer flight hours prompted by the automation of cockpit technology further contributed to pilot fatigue.[26] Studies of airline pilots show an increased risk of crashes or near misses because of sleep deprivation.[27]

Police Officers and First Responders

There have been limited studies to address sleep apnea in police officers. A cross-sectional and prospective cohort study done on North American police officers indicated that sleep disorders led to increased risk of errors, unintended injuries, motor vehicle crashes, administrative errors, and even uncontrolled anger toward subjects.[28] Within one cohort of 4957 police officers, 40.4% screened positive for a sleep disorder and 33.6% were positive for OSA.[28] A synopsis of the results is shown in **Table 1** and demonstrates the increased risk of certain tasks performed by police officers with OSA over that of controls.[28]

The frequency of extended shifts, shift work, and long work hours accompanying the occupation enhances the effects of OSA. Circadian rhythm disruptions of sleep deprivation, deficits, and fragmentation are all important consequences of the altered work schedules.[29] Accordingly, although the line-of-duty deaths rates in police have decreased significantly since the 1970s, the proportion of deaths due to unintentional injuries have shown little change, and in 2003, it even exceeded that of felonious death.[28] One-third of line-of-duty deaths were related to motor vehicle accidents, and because OSA contributes significantly to increased sleepiness and vehicle accidents, it has been speculated that several accidents that were prevented were related to OSA appropriately diagnosed and treated.[28]

OSA has been additionally identified as a potential consequence of responders at the World Trade Center (WTC) worksite. A study by Sunderram and colleagues[30] found that there was a high prevalence of OSA in WTC responders that did not match the general population. In the responder sample, the lack of association between BMI or weight and AHI is suggestive of mechanisms other than obesity that contribute to the development of OSA. The authors postulated new-onset upper airway inflammation as a factor in the pathogenesis of OSA in these individuals. It was also found that 36.5% of 11,701 male WTC first responders scored "high risk" for OSA on the modified Berlin questionnaire. The incidence of converting to "high risk" for OSA among the 4576 WTC first responders who did not initially score "high risk" was 16.9% over an average duration of 1.4 years. It should be noted that although the Berlin questionnaire is a validated tool for identifying those at risk for OSA, an overnight polysomnogram is required to confirm a diagnosis of sleep apnea.[31]

Farmers

More than half of the nation's principal farm operators hold concurrent off-farm jobs.[32] The demands of the concurrent job combined with the high-demand seasonality of production increases the risk of injury to workers.[32] Inadequate amounts of sleep, erratic sleep patterns, and the use of sleep medications and stimulants are believed to contribute to injury rates. A greater number of injuries and fatalities on the farm in older farmers has been linked to snoring and sleep disorders, although not specifically to OSA.[33] In 1994, the National Institute for Occupational Safety and Health funded a project of Farm Family Health and Hazard Surveillance. A telephone interview examining 3 separate signs of sleep apnea in male farmers (snoring, gasping/snorting, and stopping breathing) demonstrated that in the previous year farmers with these signs were 2 times as likely to report injuries as those who did not have them.[32]

Veterans

A recent study has shown that US veterans are 4 times as likely as other Americans to have sleep apnea.[34] With more than 63,000 veterans receiving benefits for sleep apnea, the benefits now cost tax payers more than $500 million per year.[34] Along with increased screening, the prevalence can be associated with exposures to dust, sand, and grit from deployment that may contribute to airway inflammation.

In addition, some research has shown that post-traumatic stress disorder may be associated with increased OSA.[35] Data show that psychosis is significantly more common in veterans diagnosed with sleep apnea than those not diagnosed with sleep apnea and that these psychotic symptoms may be improved with the treatment of the sleep apnea.[35] OSA accompanied by comorbid conditions of stress and hypertension has been shown

Table 1	
Odds ratios of specific tasks in police officers with OSA	

Odds Ratio	Task
1.43	Administrative error
1.51	Falling asleep while driving
1.63	Error or safety violation related to fatigue
1.25	Adverse work-related outcome (includes uncontrolled anger toward subjects)
1.23	Absenteeism
1.95	Falling asleep during meetings

to affect cognitive impairment, including deficits in auditory and verbal memory as well as executive function.[36]

TREATING OSA AND PERFORMANCE OUTCOME

It is often acknowledged that the economic cost of screening and testing underlying sleep disorders is reasonable.[22] Studies have indicated that appropriate treatment of OSA, such as nasal positive airway pressure, can reduce the risk of traffic accidents.[37] Simulated driving measures improved after 3 months of continuous positive airway pressure (CPAP) treatment in patients with severe OSA, whereas cognitive performance continued to be impaired when compared with controls.[38] Despite this fact, it is estimated that 38,800 accidents involving drivers with sleep apnea could be prevented annually if these drivers were treated.[38]

Some neurobehavorial deficits found in patients with sleep apnea may not fully recover after CPAP treatment.[19] One study showed that after 15 days of CPAP treatment, attention, visuospatial learning, and motor performances returned to normal, whereas complex executive functions, semantic memorization, and visuoconstructive abilities remained impaired.[39,40] The long-term effects of regular CPAP use on neurocognitive function are not well studied. Although some impairments resulting from chronic untreated OSA may not be fully reversible with OSA treatment, the impact of CPAP therapy may be appreciable through its ability to prevent further degradation of neurocognitive performance in the workplace.

LAWS AND POLICIES
The Federal Motor Carrier Safety Administration (FMSCA)

As previously noted, the prevalence of OSA is greater in the commercial vehicle operators than the general population.[20] The Federal Motor Carrier Safety Administration (FMCSA) is the government agency entrusted with setting regulations for the physical fitness of truck and bus drivers. FMCSA projects that as many 28% of commercial driver license holders have sleep apnea.[41] With an estimated 14 million commercial drivers' license holders in the United States, this estimate means that there are up to 3.9 million professional drivers with OSA.[42] According to 49 CFR 391.41 of the federal safety regulations, a driver must have "no established medical history or clinical diagnosis of a respiratory dysfunction likely to interfere with his/her ability to control and drive a commercial motor vehicle safely."[43] With the growing recognition of

the impact of OSA on driving performance, recent revisions to the regulation cite sleep apnea as an example of respiratory dysfunction that may interfere with a driver's ability to safely control and drive commercial vehicles.

Although mentioned in the regulations, management and qualification standards for sleep apnea are not specifically provided. Federal medical examiners are responsible for determining the fitness of duty of drivers with sleep apnea, but the regulations are open ended and variable. Moderate-to-severe sleep apnea interferes with safe driving and is considered a disqualifying condition, but no definition of moderate-to-severe sleep apnea is given.[41] Because medical certification is generally for 2 years, if a driver develops new conditions or impairment that may be disqualifying before the next medical examination, it is the legal responsibility of the driver to obtain recertification from a qualified medical examiner before resuming operations as a CMV driver.[44] In addition, each state may have its own medical standards for driving a CMV in intrastate commerce.[41] This, coupled with the fact that many states have adopted a medical regulation indicating that sleep apnea is a disqualifying condition, forces medical examiners to consult with local departments of motor vehicles.[45]

Commercial drivers follow the so-called Hours of Services (HOS) regulations while driving a CMV. This federal regulation is meant to reduce driver fatigue and decrease the likelihood of an accident. Although changes may still be made, at present, the new HOS "final rule" (effective February 27, 2012, implemented by July 1, 2013) limits a driver's workweek to 70 hours (decreased from 82 hours). For every 8 hours of work, drivers must take a minimum of 30 minutes of break. If a driver works the maximum 70 hours in a week, the driver must rest from 1:00 AM to 5:00 AM at least twice that week and must take a minimum of 34 hours off duty before beginning the next workweek. In addition, this "final rule" maintains the prior daily driving maximum of 11 hours until the FMCSA is able to conduct further research examining the benefits of a lesser limit.[46]

In a clerical error, the FMCSA had accidentally published proposed recommendations on sleep apnea on April 20, 2012 in the Federal Register, only to have it withdrawn on April 27, 2012. The premise of these recommendations provided insights on FMCSA's purpose to adopt a more concrete guideline to the management of OSA in CMV drivers. The released recommendations included standards that require drivers with BMI greater than 35 kg/m to have a mandatory sleep study within 60 days of conditional certification. If OSA is diagnosed and the driver is compliant with treatment, the conditional certification can be extended for another 90 days. Minimally acceptable compliance is defined here as CPAP treatment greater than 4 hours nightly for more than 70% of days and is based on the current standard of practice. The extension cannot be for more than 1 year without verification of continual compliance with treatment. Drivers with sleep apnea who fall asleep at the wheel, or are found not to be compliant with treatment, will have their certification disqualified.[47] It could be requested of the driver to produce data printed from CPAP machines to verify compliance before certification renewal.

The Federal Aviation Administration (FAA)

To educate pilots about fatigue, the Congress mandated a Fatigue Risk Management Plan (FRMP) for all airlines in 2010. In December 2011, new rules were incorporated by the FAA to set standards for fatigue management.[48] The new rules set requirements for pilot flight time, duty period, and rest; the rules include limitations on the number of flight segments and flight zone crossings.[48] With these rules, the FAA limits daily flight time to 9 hours and requires a 10-hour minimum rest period before the next flight duty period.[49] Pilots must have the opportunity for at least 8 hours of uninterrupted sleep during their 10-h rest period and on a weekly basis must have at least 30 consecutive hours free from duty.[49] In addition, the FAA has prescribed a fitness-for-duty expectation that pilots and airlines report fatigue and take a joint responsibility to be relieved of duty.[49]

Pilots with sleep apnea are not immediately disqualified from flying. The Assisted Special Issuance (AASI) now provides FAA physicians the ability to reissue an airman medical certificate under the provisions of an authorization for 14 CFR 67.401.[48] An FAA physician not only provides the initial certification decision but also grants the authorization. According to the FAA, a first-time issuance of such an authorization for sleep apnea requires that all requisite medical information be submitted and deferred to either the Aerospace Medical Certification Division (AMCD) or Regional Flight Surgeon (RFS).[48]

Examiners may reissue an airman medical certificate if the applicant provides evidence of previous authorization granted by the FAA and an optimal or no concerns report (within last 90 days) regarding the status of the treatment, compliance of the treatment, and whether the treatment is efficacious.[50] Specifically, a comment on daytime sleepiness that references the current treatment modality is required.[50] Examiners must defer to AMCD or RFS if there is a question regarding treatment adequacy, noncompliance, or other associated illnesses (eg, heart failure) or if the maintenance of wakefulness test (MWT) demonstrates sleep deficiency.[50]

An MWT will be requested for most pilots after treatment of sleep apnea. The MWT requires that patients be monitored in 40-minute intervals for their ability to stay awake sitting comfortably in bed.[51] Although many sleep specialists agree that the MWT may not adequately demonstrate sleep apnea control, as of yet no other objective testing has been validated for this purpose, or has been shown superior to the MWT.[50] As a result, it continues to be used as a certifying test for issuance of authorization.[52]

SCREENING AND DIAGNOSIS

The FMCSA does not require any standard protocol for OSA screening. Their guidelines do suggest that individuals scoring high risk on the Berlin questionnaire, or with specific findings and comorbities ascertained by history and physical examination such as snoring, sleepiness, witnessed apneas, advanced age, obesity, small upper airway, family history of OSA, or comorbid hypertension, diabetes type 2, or untreated hypothyroidism, should be considered high risk for OSA. Unfortunately, many of these measures are self-reported and there is strong incentive for drivers to deny a history or symptoms of a sleep disorder. Parks and colleagues[53] found that drivers who were subsequently found to have OSA on polysomnograph (PSG) denied related symptoms on their Commercial Driver Medical Examination. The Epworth Sleepiness Scale (ESS) is a common tool among sleep specialists to assess subjective daytime sleepiness. Unfortunately, ESS has not been shown to reliably predict OSA or automobile crashes.[54] In fact, Talmage and colleagues[51] found that subjective sleepiness as measured by the ESS was inversely related to the severity of sleep apnea as defined by the AHI on PSG in truck drivers undergoing required Department of Transportation (DOT) physicals. However, drivers were more willing to divulge symptoms related to sleep apnea when reporting anonymously. Smith and Phillips[55] found that among 595 truck drivers completing an anonymous online survey, an alarming 56% were positive on the Berlin questionnaire and 21% reported falling asleep at stoplights. Therefore, health care providers must maintain a high level of awareness for risk of OSA in commercial drivers and screen vigilantly regardless of self-reported symptoms.

The role of portable monitoring in screening and diagnosis of OSA in drivers remains undefined.

Portable monitoring when used as a screening tool for OSA in unselected commercial drivers has shown to have a positive predictive value of 64% and a negative predictive value of 87% for moderate-to-severe OSA in comparison to the in-laboratory PSG.[56] Therefore, portable monitoring for screening may be most useful in those highly suspected for OSA based on symptoms or clinical findings, and those who despite high clinical suspicion screen negative for OSA by portable monitoring should have a follow-up in-laboratory sleep test to confirm the negative findings. Despite limited data, portable monitoring remains an attractive screening mechanism for drivers because of its objectivity. As mentioned before, there is powerful incentive for many drivers to deny symptoms of sleep apnea. Sharwood and colleagues[57] found in a study of 517 drivers that at-home diagnostic testing found 41% of drivers to be positive for OSA, whereas only 4.4% of them reported a previous diagnosis of sleep apnea and only 12% of drivers reported daytime sleepiness (ESS score >10). Furthermore, a multivariable apnea prediction index based on numerous self-report measures showed poor agreement with the portable monitoring results. There is also a real concern for data manipulation of unattended sleep studies for similar reasons leading to inaccuracy of self-reported measures. However, portable monitoring will likely play a significant role in screening and diagnosing OSA in commercial drivers because of its primary advantage over in-laboratory PSGs of convenience and greater accessibility and potential for wider dissemination. As of now, the FMCSA recommends portable devices for screening only when they include all 3 measurements, namely, oxygen saturation, nasal pressure, and sleep/wake time.

TREATMENT

CPAP is the first-line treatment of OSA. A meta-analysis of 9 observational studies found a large risk reduction across all studies in crash risk of drivers with moderate-to-severe OSA (AHI ≥15) before and after CPAP treatment.[58] While the data was determined to be limited by study design, the consistent findings across all studies makes the conclusion that CPAP reduces crash risk a real likelihood. In another meta-analysis by Antonopoulos and colleagues,[59] CPAP treatment was associated with nearly 55% reduction in real crashes and near-miss crashes. Based on their analysis, treating 5 patients with OSA with CPAP is expected to prevent 1 real crash and treating 2 patients with OSA with CPAP is expected to prevent 1 near-miss crash.

Although oral appliances and surgery are considered second-line therapy for OSA in those who fail CPAP, there are no studies addressing these treatment options in drivers. Furthermore, unlike with current CPAP devices, there is no objective means of monitoring adherence with an oral appliance. The FMCSA currently recommends that these alternative therapies achieve an AHI less than or equal to 10 and result in improvement in daytime sleepiness in order for the driver to return to driving.

Some driving companies may request objective evidence of improvement in sleepiness with a Multiple Sleep Latency Test (MSLT) or MWT. In one study by Pizza and colleagues,[60] sleep latencies on the MSLT and more so on the MWT did in fact correlate with driving performance during a simulated driving test. However, whether the MSLT or MWT predict reduced crash risk in patients with OSA who have been treated have not been assessed. Despite limited evidence, however, the FAA, as mentioned earlier, requires MWT studies on most pilots with OSA on CPAP. Currently, an MLST or MWT is not recommended by the Joint Task Force for drivers diagnosed and treated for OSA to return to driving.[20]

The FMCSA Medical Expert Panel currently recommends immediate removal from active duty those with AHI greater than 20 who are not currently receiving treatment or are noncompliant with treatment or those who experience sleepiness with driving or have had a crash because of falling asleep while driving. However, more data are required to understand driving risks with abnormal sleep study findings and to make further recommendations for removing a driver from active duty.

IMPAIRMENT AND DISABILITY

The definition of disability varies based on the context of reference. The WHO international classification of functioning, disability, and health (IFC) defines an umbrella term disabilities that covers impairments, activity limitations, and participation restrictions. Although impairment is associated with disability, the 2 are not identical. Impairment is defined as loss or deviation in physiologic function, psychological function, or anatomic structure of the body.[61] Unlike disability, impairment does not incorporate a person's interaction with the environment. In addition, depending on the treatment or severity, impairment may be permanent, change over time, or completely resolve. Disability is recognized as a complex phenomenon, reflecting an interaction between features of an impaired body function and structure and the society in which affected people live.[62] It has also often been described as any restriction or lack of ability to perform an activity in the manner or within the range considered normal for a human being.[61]

Specifically, OSA has been found to contribute to work disability. It often arises as the interplay between disease, work, and personal factors. For example, based on the expectation of occupation, a bus driver who falls asleep or has trouble staying awake while driving would have a higher claim to disability than a clerical worker who dozes off at the desk. From the case of the clerical worker, he or she may have impairments from sleep apnea, but not be disabled. In actuality, receiving disability benefits for OSA would require implication that no gainful work could be obtained. Significant documentation of treatment course, impairments, and justification under the preface of documented cor pulmonale or mental cognitive decline would need to be obtained for consideration for disability.[63] Even with this documentation, there is no absolute threshold of function or specific cause that marks whether a person is disabled or not.[64]

OSA can contribute to increased sick days and absenteeism.[6] It has been shown that even before obtaining a diagnosis of sleep apnea this affected population demonstrated excessive lost work days, calculated for females to be 1.8 times that of the control subjects and for males to be 1.6 times that of controls.[65] Even after adjusting for comorbid conditions, a large case-control study in Finland ($n = 4785$) revealed a statistically significant increased risk of absenteeism in those diagnosed with OSA as compared with controls.[65] EDS was found to be more strongly correlated to sick leave and disability than to snoring or breathing cessations.[66] The impact of OSA may not be apparent for years: excess risk of lost workdays was seen up to 5 years before diagnosis for women and up to 1 year before diagnosis for men.[65]

Consequently, self-reported symptoms of sleep apnea syndrome have been found to be independent risk factors for permanent disability.[15] Accordingly, patients with the combination of OSA and EDS (also referred to as OSAS), were at higher risk of both recent work disability (OR 13.7; 95% CI, 3.9–48) and longer term work duty modification (OR, 3.6; CI, 1.1–12).[67] In a Finnish study, both men and women with OSAS were found to have an approximately 2.5-fold increase in the risk of disability pensions 6 years after diagnosis of sleep apnea compared with their controls.[65] Employees diagnosed with OSAS had an increased risk of work disability in all diagnostic categories (mental and behavioral, musculoskeletal and connective tissue, circulatory system, injury, poisoning, and other external causes) and

were at particularly high risk for work disability caused by injuries and mental disorders.[66]

Finally, since consequences of sleep apnea may include physiologic conditions such as cognitive deficits, psychomotor coordination, fatigue, and cardiovascular comorbidities, it is not uncommon for patients with sleep apnea to have multiple comorbidities contributing to absenteeism.[6]

ECONOMIC IMPACT

In an effort to decrease the risk of crashes, focus has been directed at minimizing factors such as fatigue and sleepiness as well as their interplay with OSA.[68] Data provided by the National Highway Traffic Administration estimate that at least 1 million police-reported crashes were caused by driver fatigue each year, resulting in 1550 deaths, 71,000 injuries, and $12.5 billion in losses.[69] The combined direct and indirect costs of CMV crashes were estimated at US $7.2 million for a fatal crash and $331,000 for a nonfatal crash resulting in injury.[68] It has been projected that that if all US drivers having OSAS were treated with CPAP at a cost of $3.18 billion, every year $11.1 billion dollars in collision costs would be avoided and 980 lives would be saved.[18]

Patients with OSA also use more health care dollars and have more medical visits than the general population. Because OSA often coexists or interferes with other chronic diseases, data have suggested that undiagnosed sleep apnea may cost up to $3.4 billion in medical costs in the United States.[6] OSA is estimated to directly contribute $11 million because of hospitalization alone.[6] While the indirect costs of disability, absenteeism, decreased productivity, and modified work duties were not explicitly calculated, these certainly also have a large economic impact.[67]

COMORBID SLEEP DISORDERS

Patients with OSA not infrequently have other comorbid sleep disorders, all of which should be addressed in the assessment of job performance and safety. For this reason, a thorough evaluation by a sleep specialist is helpful to decipher the contribution of OSA compared with other sleep disorders on patients' sleepiness and daytime function. Most often, patients are treated aggressively for their OSA whether it be borderline/mild or severe. A minority of patients do not derive symptomatic improvements despite effective CPAP therapy. These patients are candidates for wake-promoting medications. Alternatively, their comorbid sleep disorders will require addressing and therapy as well.

Shift Work

Shift work is an essential component of the industrialized US economy. An estimated 21 million workers (17.7% of the American workforce) work alternate shifts that fall at least partially outside the range of daytime shifts.[70] According to a poll from 2010, 25% of working individuals claim that their current work schedule does not permit sufficient sleep.[71] This sort of long-term shift work increases the risk of obesity and hypertension, and it has also demonstrated changes in heart rate, hormone secretion, and metabolism.[72] Because obesity is frequently observed among patients with OSA, it has been postulated that shift workers are at a heightened vulnerability to development of OSA.[37]

Studies of shift work in patients with OSA show an increase in AHI per hour and greater oxygen desaturation on diurnal PSG after shift work compared with nocturnal PSG.[25] It has also been observed that AHI is greater during diurnal sleep after nighttime shifts. This result may suggest that there is a risk of underdiagnosing the severity of the disease in nocturnal PSG in shift workers.[25] Health care providers must consider the possibility that shift workers presenting with the typical history of somnolence and negative nighttime PSG may still have elevated AHI during diurnal PSG after a nighttime shift. In addition, CPAP titrated during nighttime sleep may be suboptimal for daytime sleep.[25]

COMORBID MEDICAL CONDITIONS
Cardiovascular Outcomes

OSA has been implicated in various worsening cardiovascular conditions. Chronic hypoxemia in patients with OSA is associated with neural, humoral, thrombotic, metabolic, and inflammatory disease mechanisms, each of which has also been implicated in the pathophysiology of cardiac and vascular disease.[72] The hypoxia found in OSA also contributes to lung diseases such as pulmonary hypertension and cor pulmonale, further compromising the cardiopulmonary system.[73] Compared with controls, patients with OSA have been found to have increased heart rates, decreased heart rate variability, and increased blood pressure variability.[74]

With respect to cardiovascular risk, studies have shown that decreased heart rate variability may lead to an increased risk of hypertension and increased mortality in patients with heart failure. Increased blood pressure variability has been correlated with an increased risk for target organ damage, and surges in blood pressure may result in myocardial ischemia.[72] Furthermore, vasoactive and trophic substances (eg, endothelin), coupled with the activation of inflammatory and procoagulative mechanisms, are thought to contribute to progression of coronary artery disease.[74]

Diabetes

OSA and insulin resistance often occur concomitantly, a correlation noted in both obese and nonobese individuals.[75] Recent studies suggest that OSA itself is an independent risk factor for insulin resistance and diabetes mellitus.[75] Population studies suggest that up to 40% of patients with OSA will also have diabetes.[75] There is strong evidence to indicate an association between OSA and the risk for type 2 diabetes, but whether a causal relationship exists is yet to be determined.[76] Some evidence suggests that cortisol may trigger mechanisms that cause accumulation of abdominal fat and ultimately lead to insulin resistance.[75]

Stroke

Determining which is the cause and which the effect with respect to OSA and stroke has proved to be a challenge. Numerous studies use snoring as an indicator of OSA, but this does not directly support OSA as a causal agent.[77] In correlation studies dealing with stroke and OSA, many subjects had a prior history of strokes, which confounds any possible conclusions of causality.[77] Despite this fact, many studies have supported the association between OSA and stroke. Various mechanisms have been postulated, including abnormal cerebral hemodynamics, increased platelet aggregation, increased fibrinogen concentration, increased blood viscosity, and abnormal vascular endothelial function.[77] Furthermore, it has been shown that the presence of sleep apnea in patients undergoing rehabilitation after stroke is associated with a more profound functional impairment and a longer period of hospitalization and rehabilitation.[75]

Obesity

Weight changes have been shown to be significantly correlated with OSA. One study by the Wisconsin Sleep Cohort found that a 10% weight increase was associated with a 32% increase in AHI and a 10% weight decrease was associated with 26% decrease in AHI.[78] Additionally, a 10% weight increase has been linked to a 6-fold increase in the odds of developing moderate-to-severe OSA.[78] Studies have suggested that comorbid conditions related to obesity may be better managed if patients are evaluated and treated for previously undiagnosed OSA.[79] Weight loss has

a large positive impact on OSA and CPAP requirements. Weight itself may be a risk factor for workplace injuries.

SUMMARY/RECOMMENDATIONS

Given the effectiveness of available treatments,
early intervention should be implemented to mini-
mize the decline of health and cognition associated with untreated OSA. Consequences of OSA
such as sleepiness and fatigue have major
impacts on both economics and public health.
For example, commercial vehicle drivers having
OSA-related sleepiness clearly affects the safety
of the roads; even police relations with the public
may be strained by OSA. OSA contributes to workplace disability and is also associated with other
chronic medical conditions that themselves lead
to disability. Furthermore, the association with
cardiovascular diseases, diabetes, stroke, and
obesity should prompt physicians to suspect,
evaluate, and treat OSA in an efficient manner.
Treating the effects of OSA reduces absenteeism,
length of modified work days, reaction time, and
production. Ultimately, effective treatment of
OSA results in improved quality of life for workers
and financial savings for employers. Although
recommendations for OSA screening and treatment exist for several specific work populations,
a large population of patients with OSA unfortunately remain undiagnosed. Continued collaborative effort between people with OSA, their
employers, and their physicians must exist to
ensure that provisions for educating, screening,
evaluating, and treating OSA in the workplace
are established.

REFERENCES

1. Young T, Palta M, Dempsey J, et al. The occurrence
   of sleep-disordered breathing among middle-aged
   adults. N Engl J Med 1993;328(17):1230.
2. Lurie A. Obstructive sleep apnea in adults: epidemiology, clinical presentation, and treatment options.
   Adv Cardiol 2011;46:1–42.
3. Finkelstein EA, DiBonaventura MC, Burgess SM,
   et al. The costs of obesity in the workplace.
   J Occup Environ Med 2010;52(10):971.
4. Wang Y, Beydoun MA, Liang L, et al. Will all Americans become overweight or obese? Estimating the
   progression and cost of the US obesity epidemic.
   Obesity (Silver Spring) 2008;16(10):2323.
5. Hymel PA, Loeppke R, Baase C, et al. Workplace
   health protection and promotion: a new pathway
   for a Healthier—and Safer—Workforce. J Occup
   Environ Med 2011;53(6):695.
6. Leger D, Bayon V, Laaban J, et al. Impact of sleep
   apnea on economics. Sleep Med Rev 2012;16(5):
   455–62.
7. Naëgelé B, Thouvard V, Pepin JL, et al. Deficits of
   cognitive executive functions in patients with sleep
   apnea syndrome. Sleep 1995;18(1):43–52.
8. Quan SF, Wright R, Baldwin CM, et al. Obstructive
   sleep apnea-hypopnea and neurocognitive functioning in the sleep heart health study. Sleep Med
   2006;7(6):498.
9. Smith IE, Shneerson JM. Is the SF 36 sensitive to
   sleep disruption? A study in subjects with sleep
   apnoea. J Sleep Res 1995;4(3):183.
10. Lee IS, Bardwell W, Ancoli-Israel S, et al. The rela-
    tionship between psychomotor vigilance perfor-
    mance and quality of life in obstructive sleep
    apnea. J Clin Sleep Med 2011;7(3):254–60.
11. Jackson M, Howard M, Barnes M. Cognition and
    daytime functioning in sleep-related breathing disor-
    ders. Prog Brain Res 2011;190:53–68.
12. Ayalon L, Peterson S. Functional central nervous
    system imaging in the investigation of obstructive
    sleep apnea. Curr Opin Pulm Med 2007;13(6):479.
13. Desai A, Marks G, Jankelson D, et al. Do sleep depri-
    vation and time of day interact with mild obstructive
    sleep apnea to worsen performance and neurobeha-
    vioral function? J Clin Sleep Med 2006;2(1):63–70.
14. Mulgrew AT, Ryan CF, Fleetham JA, et al. The impact
    of obstructive sleep apnea and daytime sleepiness
    on work limitation. Sleep Med 2007;9(1):42–53.
15. Nena E, Steiropoulos P, Constantinidis T, et al. Work
    productivity in obstructive sleep apnea patients.
    J Occup Environ Med 2010;52(6):622–5.
16. Viegas CA, de Oliveira H. Prevalence of risk factors
    for obstructive sleep apnea syndrome in interstate
    bus drivers. J Bras Pneumol 2006;32(2):144–9 [in
    English, Portuguese].
17. Heaton K, Rayens M. Feedback actigraphy and
    sleep among long-haul truck drivers. AAOHN J
    2010;58(4):137–45.
18. Philip P. Sleepiness of occupational drivers. Ind
    Health 2005;43(1):30–3.
19. Vakulin A, Balk SD, Catcheside PG, et al. Effects of
    alcohol and sleep restriction on simulated driving
    performance in untreated patients with obstructive
    sleep apnea. Ann Intern Med 2009;151(7):447.
20. Hartenbaum N, Callop N, Rosen IM, et al. Sleep
    apnea and commercial motor vehicle operators.
    Chest 2006;130(3):902.
21. Moreno CR, Carvelho FA, Lorenzi C, et al. High risk for
    obstructive sleep apnea in truck drivers estimated by
    the Berlin questionnaire: prevalence and associated
    factors. Chronobiol Int 2004;21(6):871.
22. Braeckman L, Verpraet R, Van Risseghem M, et al.
    Prevalence and correlates of poor sleep quality
    and daytime sleepiness in Belgian truck drivers.
    Chronobiol Int 2011;28(2):126–34.

23. Hoffman B, Wingenbach DD, Kagey AN, et al. The long-term health plan and disability cost benefit of obstructive sleep apnea treatment in a commercial motor vehicle driver population. J Occup Environ Med 2010;52(5):473–7.

24. Brown JR. Obstructive sleep apnea. In: federal aviation administration. 2012. Available at: www.faa.gov/pilots/safety/pilotsafetybrochures/media/Sleep_Apnea.pdf. Accessed April 2, 2012.

25. Rosekind MR. Sleep: a critical factor to enhance transportation safety in national transportation safety board. 2011. Available at: http://www.ntsb.gov/doclib/speeches/rosekind/Rosekind_031811.pdf. Accessed April 2, 2012.

26. Evans D. Pilot fatigue: unresponsive federal aviation. J Air Law Commerce 2000;65(3):567–604.

27. Price WJ, Holley DC. Shiftwork and safety in aviation. Occup Med 1990;5(2):343–77.

28. Rajaratnam SM, Barger L, Lockley S, et al. Sleep disorders, health, and safety in police officers. JAMA 2011;306(23):2567–78.

29. Klawe JJ, Laudencka A, Miskowiec I, et al. Occurrence of obstructive sleep apnea in a group of shift worked police officers. J Physiol Pharmacol 2005;56:115.

30. Sunderram J, Udasin I, Kelly-McNeil K, et al. Unique features of obstructive sleep apnea in World Trade Center responders with aerodigestive disorders. J Occup Environ Med 2011;53(9):975.

31. Webber MP, Lee R, Soo J, et al. Prevalence and incidence of high risk for obstructive sleep apnea in World Trade Center-exposed rescue/recovery workers. Sleep Breath 2011;15(3):283–94.

32. Spengler S, Browning S, Reed D. Sleep deprivation and injuries in part-time Kentucky farmers: impact of self reported sleep habits and sleep problems on injury risk. AAOHN J 2004;52(9):373–82.

33. Heaton K, Azuero A, Reed D. Obstructive sleep apnea indicators and injury in older farmers. J Agromedicine 2010;15(2):148.

34. Young A. VA sees sharp rise in apnea cases. In: USA Today. 2010. Available at: http://www.usatoday.com/news/health/2010-06-07-apnea_N.htm. Accessed March 29, 2012.

35. Sharafkhaneh A, Giray N, Richardson P, et al. Association of psychiatric disorders and sleep apnea in a large cohort. Sleep 2005;28(11):1405.

36. Yesavage JA, Kinoshita LM, Kimball T, et al. Sleep-disordered breathing in Vietnam veterans with post-traumatic stress disorder. Am J Geriatr Psychiatry 2012;20(3):199.

37. Asaoka S, Namba K, Tsuiki S, et al. Excessive daytime sleepiness among Japanese public transportation drivers engaged in shiftwork. J Occup Environ Med 2010;52(8):813–8.

38. Findley LJ, Smith C, Hooper J, et al. Automobile accidents involving patients with obstructive sleep apnea. Am J Respir Crit Care Med 1988;138(2):337.

39. Ferini Strambi L, Baietto C, Di Gioia MR, et al. Cognitive dysfunction in patients with obstructive sleep apnea (OSA): partial reversibility after continuous positive airway pressure (CPAP). Brain Res Bull 2003;61(1):87.

40. Lau EY, Eskes GA, Morrison DL, et al. Executive function in patients with obstructive sleep apnea treated with continuous positive airway pressure. J Int Neuropsychol Soc 2010;16(6):1077.

41. National Sleep Foundation. Sleep apnea and commercial drivers. In: National Transportation Safety Board. Available at: http://www.fmcsa.dot.gov/safety-security/sleepapnea/industry/commercial-drivers.aspx. Accessed March 27, 2012.

42. US GAO. Commercial drivers certification process for drivers with serious medical condition. 2008. Available at: http://www.gao.gov/new.items/d08826.pdf. Accessed April 4, 2012.

43. Federal Motor Carrier Safety Association. Physical qualifications for drivers. In: US Department of Transportation. 2011. Available at: http://www.fmcsa.dot.gov/rules-regulations/administration/fmcsr/fmcsrruletext.aspx?reg=391.41. Accessed April 4, 2012.

44. Federal Motor Carrier Safety Association. Frequently asked questions, medical. In: US Department of Transportation. 2011. Available at: http://www.fmcsa.dot.gov/rules-regulations/topics/medical/faqs.aspx#question61. Accessed July 6, 2012.

45. Federal Motor Carrier Safety Association. Summary of hours-of-services (HOS) regulation. In: US Department of Transportation. 2011. Available at: http://www.fmcsa.dot.gov/rules-regulations/topics/hos/index.htm. Accessed April 4, 2012.

46. Federal Motor Carrier Safety Association. News release, U.S. Department of Transportation takes action to ensure truck driver rest time and improve safety behind the wheel. In: US Department of Transportation. 2011. Available at: http://www.fmcsa.dot.gov/rules-regulations/topics/hos/statement.aspx. Accessed April 4, 2012.

47. Federal Motor Carrier Safety Administration. Proposed recommendations on sleep apnea. In: Federal Register. 2012. Available at: https://www.federalregister.gov/articles/search?conditions[term]=sleep+apnea+fmcsa&commit=Go. Accessed April 4, 2012.

48. Federal Aviation Administration. Flight crew member duty and rest requirements. In: US Department of Transportation. 2011. Available at: http://www.faa.gov/regulations_policies/rulemaking/recently_published/media/2120-AJ58-FinalRule.pdf. Accessed March 28, 2012.

49. Federal Aviation Administration. New rule seeks to prevent pilot fatigue. In: US Department of Transportation. 2011. Available at: http://fastlane.dot.gov/2011/12/flight-time-duty-time.html. Accessed April 3, 1012.

50. Federal Aviation Administration. Guide for aviation medical examiners. In: US Department of Transportation. 2011. Available at: http://www.faa.gov/about/office_org/headquarters_offices/avs/offices/aam/ame/guide/special_iss/all_classes/sleep_apnea/. Accessed March 28, 2012.

51. Talmage JB, Hudson TB, Hegmann KT, et al. Consensus criteria for screening commercial drivers for obstructive sleep apnea: evidence of efficacy. J Occup Environ Med 2008;50(3):324.

52. Crump G. FAA position on sleep apnea. In: Aircraft Owners and Pilots Association. 2011. Available at: http://www.aopa.org/membership/articles/2011/201101sleep.html. Accessed March 28, 2012.

53. Parks P, Durand G, Tsismenakis AJ, et al. Screening for obstructive sleep apnea during commercial driver medical examinations. J Occup Environ Med 2009;51(3):275.

54. Drake C, Nickel C, Burduvali E, et al. The 10-year risk of verified motor vehicle crashes in relation to physiologic sleepiness. Sleep 2010;33(6):745.

55. Smith B, Phillips B. Truckers drive their own assessment for obstructive sleep apnea: a collaborative approach to online self-assessment for obstructive sleep apnea. J Clin Sleep Med 2011;7(3):241–5.

56. Watkins MR, Talmage JB, Thiese MS, et al. Correlation between screening for obstructive sleep apnea using a portable device versus polysomnography testing in a commercial driving population. J Occup Environ Med 2009;51(10):1145.

57. Sharwood L, Elkington J, Stevenson M, et al. Assessing sleepiness and sleep disorders in Australian long-distance commercial vehicle drivers: self-report versus an "at home" monitoring device. Sleep 2012;35(4):469–75.

58. Tregear S, Reston J, Schoelles K, et al. Continuous positive airway pressure reduces risk of motor vehicle crash among drivers with obstructive sleep apnea: systematic review and meta-analysis. Sleep 2010;33(10):1373.

59. Antonopoulos CN, Sergentanis TS. Nasal continuous positive airway pressure (nCPAP) treatment for obstructive sleep apnea, road traffic accidents and driving simulator performance: a meta-analysis. Sleep Med Rev 2010;15(5):301–10.

60. Pizza F, Contardi S, Mondini S, et al. Daytime sleepiness and driving performance in patients with obstructive sleep apnea: comparison of the MSLT, the MWT, and a simulated driving task. Sleep 2009;32(3):382.

61. Taiwo O, Cantley L. Impairment and disability evaluation: the role of the family physician. Am Fam Physician 2008;77(12):1689–94.

62. WHO. Disability and health. In: World Health Organization. 2011. Available at: http://www.who.int/topics/disabilities/en/. Accessed April 1, 2012.

63. Social Security Online. Disability evaluation under social security (Blue Book- September 2008). In: social security disability programs medical/professional relations 2008. Available at: http://www.ssa.gov/disability/professionals/bluebook/3.00-Respiratory-Adult.htm. Accessed July 6, 2012.

64. Leonardi M, Bickebbach J, Ustun TB, et al. The definition of disability: what is in a name? Lancet 2006; 368(9543):1219.

65. Sjsten N, Vahtera J, Salo P, et al. Increased risk of lost workdays prior to the diagnosis of sleep apnea. Chest 2009;136(1):130–6.

66. Sivertsen B, Overland S, Glozier N, et al. The effect of OSAS on sick leave and work disability. Eur Respir J 2008;32(6):1497–503.

67. Omachi T, Claman D, Blanc P, et al. Obstructive sleep apnea: a risk factor for work disability. Sleep 2009;32(6):791–8.

68. Hiestand D, Phillips B. Obstructive sleep apnea syndrome: assessing and managing risk in the motor vehicle operator. Curr Opin Pulm Med 2011; 17(6):1.

69. NCSDR/NHTSA Expert Panel on Driver Fatigue and Sleepiness. Drowsy driving and automobile crashes. DOT HS 808 707. Washington, DC: USA Author; 1998.

70. McMenamin TM. Time to work: recent trends in shift work and flexible schedules. Mon Labor Rev 2007; 130:3.

71. Drexel C, Merlo K. Shift work and sleep optimizing health, safety, and performance. J Occup Environ Med 2011;53:S1.

72. Shamsuzzaman AS, Bernard JG, Virend KS, et al. Obstructive sleep apnea. JAMA 2003;290(14):1906.

73. Fletcher EC, Schaaf JW, Miller J, et al. Long-term cardiopulmonary sequelae in patients with sleep apnea and chronic lung disease. Am Rev Respir Dis 1987;135(3):525–33.

74. Ip MS, Lam B, Matthew M, et al. Obstructive sleep apnea is independently associated with insulin resistance. Am J Respir Crit Care Med 2002;165(5):670.

75. Shaw JE, Punjabi NM, Wilding JP, et al. Sleep-disordered breathing and type 2 diabetes: a report from the international diabetes federation taskforce on epidemiology and prevention. Diabetes Res Clin Pract 2008;81(1):2.

76. Tasali E, Mokhlesi B, Van Cauter E. Obstructive sleep apnea and type 2 diabetes. Chest 2008;133(2):496.

77. Gibson GJ. Sleep disordered breathing and the outcome of stroke. Thorax 2004;59(5):361.

78. Punjabi NM. The epidemiology of adult obstructive sleep apnea. Proc Am Thorac Soc 2008;5(2):136.

79. Gami AS, Capples SM, Somers VK, et al. Obesity and obstructive sleep apnea. Endocrinol Metab Clin North Am 2003;32(4):869.

The Classic Pneumoconioses
New Epidemiological and Laboratory Observations

A. Scott Laney, PhD, David N. Weissman, MD*

KEYWORDS

- Coal • Coal workers' pneumoconiosis • Silica • Silicosis • Asbestos • Asbestosis

KEY POINTS

- Digital chest imaging can now be used in the International Labor Office's classification system for the presence and severity of changes of pneumoconiosis with equivalent results to classification of analog film-screen radiographs.
- The role of lung cancer screening of asbestos-exposed individuals with low-dose chest computed tomography scanning is still evolving.
- Coal workers' pneumoconiosis, including severe forms, such as progressive massive fibrosis, is still occurring in the United States and has been seen in relatively young miners.
- Emerging exposure situations include longer work hours, work in small mines, and silica exposure from thin-seam coal mining in Appalachia, construction work, and natural gas extraction by hydraulic fracturing and environmental exposures to asbestos associated with human contamination of the environment or the presence of natural deposits.
- Newly or poorly recognized adverse health effects of exposures include lower-zone, irregular opacities in coal miners; antibodies against citrullinated peptide antigens–positive rheumatoid arthritis and antineutrophil cytoplasmic antibody-positive vasculitis in silicotics; and laryngeal and ovarian cancer in asbestos-exposed individuals.
- Soluble mesothelin-related peptides can be measured in serum to monitor the course of malignant mesothelioma with epithelioid features. The test is not approved in the United States for diagnostic purposes and its diagnostic potential is limited by low sensitivity for malignant mesothelioma at threshold serum values providing good specificity.

INTRODUCTION

The pneumoconioses are a group of lung diseases caused by the inhalation of mineral dust. They have long histories. Classic authorities, such as Agricola and Ramazzini, described silicosis and coal workers' pneumoconiosis (CWP) centuries ago.[1,2] Although eliminating causative inhalation exposures can prevent pneumoconioses, they continue to occur. This brief review addresses selected issues of current interest and recent developments related to 3 types of inorganic mineral dust exposures that cause classic forms of pneumoconiosis: coal mine dust, crystalline

Funding sources: Dr Laney, Dr Weissman: US Government (CDC-NIOSH).
Conflict of interest: Dr Laney, Dr Weissman: Nil.
Disclaimer: The findings and conclusions in this report are those of the authors and do not necessarily represent the views of the National Institute for Occupational Safety and Health.
Division of Respiratory Disease Studies, National Institute for Occupational Safety and Health, Centers for Disease Control and Prevention, 1095 Willowdale Road, Morgantown, WV 26505, USA
* Corresponding author.
E-mail address: DWeissman@cdc.gov

Clin Chest Med 33 (2012) 745–758
http://dx.doi.org/10.1016/j.ccm.2012.08.005
0272-5231/12/$ – see front matter Published by Elsevier Inc.

chestmed.theclinics.com

silica, and asbestos. More comprehensive reviews are also available.[3–6] Although this review has a US perspective, mineral dust exposures and the pneumoconioses they cause are an important global issue.[7]

CHEST IMAGING IN PNEUMOCONIOSIS

Recent advances in chest imaging are relevant to all types of pneumoconiosis because imaging technology is critical to identifying these conditions in medical screening and surveillance and in epidemiologic research. Issues discussed in this section include use of digital chest imaging to classify the presence and severity of changes of pneumoconiosis using the International Labor Organization's (ILO) classification system and use of chest computed tomography (CT) for early detection of dust-induced disease.

Use of Digital Chest Imaging for ILO Classification

The ILO classification system is used worldwide to assess the presence and severity of chest radiographic changes of pneumoconiosis.[8] Before 2011, the classification system could only be applied to film-based chest radiographs. However, access to film-based radiography has markedly declined in the United States in recent years because of replacement by modern digital radiographic imaging systems. This replacement has hindered access to ILO classification when it was needed in research and other settings.

To address this issue, in 2009, the National Institute for Occupational Safety and Health (NIOSH), together with partners, including the ILO, established a plan to develop the ILO classification of digital chest images.[9] Since then, several studies have been conducted with the goal of establishing whether and how contemporary digital chest images could be used to perform ILO classifications and yield results equivalent to classifications using film-based images.[10–14] Together, these studies indicate that with appropriate attention to image acquisition and when images are displayed on medical-grade monitors, direct readout digital systems and computed radiography systems provide comparable classification results to traditional film-based radiographs. In addition, a consistent finding across studies is that digital image quality is significantly better than film-screen image quality. The equivalence between digital and film radiography for the classification of pneumoconiosis has also been demonstrated using the Chinese classification system (GBZ 70–2002).[15,16]

Reader variability is an important source of variability in the classification of chest images. Although a variety of measures can be used to reduce within and between reader variation, human subjectivity continues to be an important issue. To address this, efforts have been made to develop computer-assisted classification of chest radiographs for findings of pneumoconiosis. Studies were initially published in the 1970s.[17,18] Although much remains to be done, computer-aided ILO classification of digital chest images may someday be achievable.[19,20]

Medical Screening with Chest CT

High-resolution CT is more sensitive for detecting the earliest stages of pneumoconiosis than conventional chest radiography.[21–26] However, the potential benefits to patients of very early detection of pneumoconiosis, which generally progresses slowly and lacks specific curative treatment, are limited in comparison with the early detection of lung cancer, which can be life saving. A recently published, large, randomized controlled trial, the National Lung Screening Trial (NLST), has documented the effectiveness of early detection of lung cancer in older heavy smokers undergoing annual screening with low-dose chest CT scans (LDCT) as compared with annual screening with plain chest imaging. Its finding of reduced mortality in the group randomized to LDCT has been of great interest to those caring for individuals previously exposed to other carcinogens, including asbestos.[27] LDCT was used for screening instead of conventional CT to limit the potential harmful consequences of radiation exposure.

In the wake of the NLST, 4 medical societies collaborated to conduct a systematic review of the evidence of benefits and harms of lung cancer screening with LDCT.[28] The review found NLST to be the most informative study. Patients included in the NLST were smokers and former smokers aged 55 to 74 years who had smoked for 30 pack-years or more and either continued to smoke or had quit within the past 15 years. After 3 rounds of annual LDCT imaging and appropriate follow-up care for those with abnormal findings, the relative risk of lung cancer mortality was decreased by 20% and absolute risk by 0.33%. Unfortunately, screening does result in false positives. Across studies, nearly 20% of individuals had positive results requiring follow-up, whereas approximately 1% had lung cancer. The review concluded: "For smokers and former smokers aged 55 to 74 years who have smoked for 30 pack-years or more and either continue to smoke or have quit within the past 15 years, we suggest that annual screening with...LDCT... should be offered over both annual screening with chest radiograph or no screening..."[28] The review categorized this as a weak recommendation based on moderate-quality evidence.

It is unclear how these general screening recommendations for lung cancer might apply to workers at an increased risk from lung cancer caused by exposures, such as asbestos. The American Association for Thoracic Surgery suggested the following group be screened in addition to the one already noted: "Screening may begin at age 50 years with a 20 pack-year history of smoking and additional comorbidity that produces a cumulative risk of developing lung cancer of 5% or greater over the following 5 years."[29] Thus, LDCT screening under this recommendation might target LDCT screening to those with sufficient risk from past asbestos exposure and cigarette smoking.[30]

COAL MINE DUST

Despite marked improvements in the United States relative to several decades ago, several recent studies have documented that CWP, including advanced forms, such as progressive massive fibrosis (PMF), continues to be an important problem. Issues discussed in this section include the persistence of CWP in the United States, underlying factors associated with persistence, respiratory health outcomes among coal dust–exposed workers other than classic CWP, and new technology for personal dust monitoring.

Persistence of CWP in the United States

As a result of the 1969 Federal Coal Mine Health and Safety Act (Coal Act),[31] the United States established and has subsequently maintained an ongoing medical monitoring program for CWP. This monitoring program, called the Coal Workers' X-ray Surveillance Program (CWXSP), provides chest radiographs at about 5-year intervals to underground coal miners at no cost to them. It documented that interventions specified in the Coal Act to track and reduce dust exposures were highly successful. The impact can be seen most markedly in miners of long tenure because CWP typically takes one or more decades to develop after the first exposure. For example, the prevalence of CWP among underground miners with greater than 25 years' tenure who participated in the program in 1970 was 44%. This decreased markedly through the 1990s, reaching a nadir of 2.4% in 1997 (**Fig. 1**).[32–37]

In 1999, NIOSH collaborated with the Mine Safety and Health Administration (MSHA) to

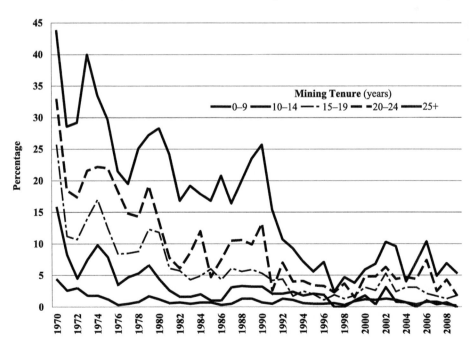

Fig. 1. Percentage of examined underground miners with coal workers' pneumoconiosis (ILO category 1/0+) by tenure in mining, 1970–2009. (*From* CDC/NIOSH. Work-Related Lung Disease Surveillance System (eWoRLD) Coal Workers' Pneumoconiosis and Related Exposures. Available at: http://www2a.cdc.gov/drds/WorldReportData/FigureTableDetails.asp?FigureTableID=2549&GroupRefNumber=F02-05. Accessed August 14, 2012.)

provide chest radiographs to both underground and surface miners through the CWXSP and a supplemental program called Miners' Choice. The effort lasted from October 1, 1999 to September 30, 2002. A total of 35 983 chest films were analyzed. CWP prevalence was 3.2% for underground miners and 1.9% for surface miners.[34] Of concern, advanced CWP, including PMF, was still occurring. Because of concerns about continued occurrence of CWP, including PMF among relatively young coal miners, Antao and colleagues[38] conducted a study that focused on rapidly progressive disease among underground miners from 1996 to 2002. Among the 29 521 miners examined, 886 cases of CWP were identified. Among the miners with CWP who contributed serial radiographs, 35.4% had evidence of rapidly progressive CWP, defined as the development of PMF or an increase in one or more small opacity profusion subcategories within 5 years. The cases of rapidly progressive CWP were clustered in Eastern Kentucky and Western Virginia, with more than 60% of evaluated miners in this region with CWP showing advanced and rapidly progressive CWP. A total of 41 cases of PMF (0.14%) were identified.

In 2005, NIOSH established the Enhanced Coal Workers' Health Surveillance Program (ECWHSP). This program used a mobile examination unit to conduct surveillance outreach. The goals of ECWHSP were to better define the scope and magnitude of the problem of lung disease in coal miners and to identify potentially remediable causes. The mobile unit conducted surveys in March and May of 2006 in the Lee and Wise counties of Virginia.[39] Among the miners surveyed, the prevalence of CWP was 9.0% and the prevalence of PMF was 1.5% (greater than the 1.3% observed in US miners for the period 1968–1972). A subsequent report in 2007 included information from surveys in Southwest Virginia and Eastern Kentucky and found a prevalence of PMF of 1.8%.[40]

Overall national trends of PMF prevalence in underground coal miners with 15 or more years of tenure showed marked decreases from the 1970s to the 1990s. Although prevalence remains far less than in the 1970s, it has trended upward since then.[41] At the state level, West Virginia has reported a similar experience. A large case series of 138 miners with PMF was reported for the 2000–2009 period using data from the West Virginia State Occupational Pneumoconiosis Board (WVSOPB).[42] The average age in this group was 52.6 years (range 40–77 years). The study noted that PMF was more frequent, more aggressive, and occurring at an earlier age among West Virginian miners compensated by the WVSOPB in this period compared with previous years. The rate of premature mortality was significantly elevated in this group.

Years of potential life lost (YPLL) is an important metric for the burden of premature mortality. It is particularly affected by deaths at an early age. At the national level, Mazurek and colleagues[43] reported in 2009 that YPLL before 65 years of age and, to a greater extent, mean YPLL per decedent increased from 2002 to 2006. Recent reports of lung transplantation for severe CWP also document a continued burden of severe cases.[44–46]

Underlying Factors Associated with the Persistence of CWP

A consistent finding among the studies conducted since 2000, which have assessed the effect of mine size (number of employees), is a significant correlation between small mine size and greater levels of CWP.[37,38,47,48] In a large study of US underground miners, miners from small mines (less than 50 employees) had a 3.5-fold greater prevalence of CWP and a 5-fold greater prevalence of PMF compared with miners from larger mines (50 or more employees).[47] The reason CWP risk and severity are highly correlated with mine size is not fully known. However, this finding is similar to injury fatality rates; miner fatalities are highest in the smallest mines.[49–52] It has been observed that smaller mines tend to use younger miners,[47,49] and it is hypothesized that this average inexperience leads to higher rates of injuries. How this would impact respiratory illness is unclear. It is likely that larger mines are more likely to have the resources required to effectively monitor and control dust exposures, whereas smaller mines may lack the capital to upgrade ventilation systems or purchase advanced dust control technologies. In addition, dedicated health and safety officers are less likely to be available in a small workforce.[53]

Another hypothesis for the new epidemiologic observations in CWP is that exposure to crystalline silica has increased in recent years.[47,54,55] Although the available quartz exposure data in coal mining do not provide evidence for an appreciable upward trend, the validity and representativeness of these measures has been questioned.[56–58] One piece of evidence that supports a role for silica exposure as causing pneumoconiosis in at least some miners is that a radiographic abnormality suggestive of silicosis (rounded pneumoconiotic opacities exceeding 3 mm in diameter [designated r-type under the ILO classification system]) has increased among underground coal miners since

2000.[59] Among miners in Kentucky, Virginia, and West Virginia, r-type opacities were 7.6 times more common in the 2000–2008 period compared with the 1980s. However, r-type opacities were found in only a small minority of these Appalachian miners, increasing from approximately 0.2% to about 1.4%. This increase was noted only in Appalachia. Silica exposure in Appalachia might be the result of thin-seam mining (defined as a coal seam less than 43 in). Crystalline silica is most often found in a higher concentration in the rock strata outside of the coal seam than within the coal seam itself, and the practice of breaching the coal/rock interface is more common in thin-seam mines.[60] Often rock is intentionally mined from the floor and roof to provide greater clearance for mining equipment.[37,60] Ninety-six percent of US underground thin-seam mines are located in Kentucky, Virginia, and West Virginia.[61]

Range of Respiratory Outcomes Associated with Coal Mine Dust Exposure

Exposure to coal mine dust can result in pulmonary diseases other than pneumoconiosis with the classical nodular interstitial appearance and upper zone predominance. Several studies have evaluated the zonal distribution of pneumoconiotic small opacities on radiographs of US coal miners.[62–64] Each of these found that the distribution of small opacities was not predominantly in the upper lung zones, despite what is commonly found in textbooks and review articles. In general, the distribution of small pneumoconiotic opacities is associated with the primary shape observed on the radiograph. Irregularly shaped opacities tend to be more common in the lower lung zones, whereas nodular opacities are more presently observed in the upper lung zones. This finding has also been observed among Canadian hard rock miners.[65] Another important adverse health effect of coal mine dust exposure is chronic obstructive pulmonary disease (COPD), including chronic bronchitis and emphysema.[41,66–68]

Real-time Monitors for Exposure Assessment

An important recent advance has been the development of an essentially real-time personal respirable dust monitor (PDM) that can be worn by coal miners at risk for excessive coal mine dust exposures.[69,70] The PDM uses a tapered-element oscillating microbalance to measure the mass of dust deposited on a filter. It provides continuous measurement of the concentration of respirable coal mine dust in a wearer's breathing zone. Validation testing showed 95% confidence that the individual PDM measurements were within ±25% of the reference measurements obtained using conventional gravimetric samplers. Having immediate information about excessive exposures has great advantages over conventional methods, which do not provide this feedback. If aware of situations causing exposures, coal miners can immediately take steps to correct them. The potential benefits have led to regulatory efforts by MSHA to enable the use of PDM in its proposed rule, "Lowering Miners' Exposure to Respirable Coal Mine Dust Including Continuous Personal Dust Monitors."[71]

CRYSTALLINE SILICA

Exposure to respirable crystalline silica has been associated with several health effects, including silicosis, increased susceptibility to tuberculosis, lung cancer, COPD, autoimmune diseases, and chronic renal disease.[4,72] Issues discussed in this section include the current burden of silica exposure and silicosis in the United States; new occupational settings for respirable crystalline silica exposure and silicosis; and brief updates on selected silica-related health effects, including lymph node involvement and silica-related immune dysfunction and immunologic disease.

Current Burden of Silica Exposure and Silicosis in the United States

Inhalation exposure to crystalline silica is a potential hazard across many occupations and industries. One type of crystalline silica, quartz, is a major component of soil and rocks. Many occupations and industries involve activities that aerosolize quartz-containing dust from soil and/or rocks. Examples include drilling, tunneling, and quarrying or cutting, breaking, or crushing materials, such as stone that contains quartz. Cristobalite and tridymite are types of crystalline silica that can be produced by industrial processes that involve heating quartz or amorphous silica. Examples of such processes include foundry work whereby clay molds are heated by molten metal or in manufacturing brick or ceramics.

Yassin and colleagues[73] analyzed inspection data from the Occupational Safety and Health Administration (OSHA) collected between 1988 and 2003 to assess the level of occupational exposure to respirable crystalline silica in the United States. Although exposures had declined in some industries and occupations, others were still overexposed. It was estimated that about 119 000 employees were potentially exposed in the United States. The industries with the greatest numbers of potentially exposed individuals were automotive repair paint shop; masonry, stonework; testing laboratories services; and repair shops, not classified elsewhere.

There is no ongoing, organized national surveillance specifically targeted to silicosis in the United States. An especially important gap is information at the national level about silicosis morbidity. A major source of such information in the United States is the Bureau of Labor Statistics' (BLS) *Survey of Occupational Injuries and Illnesses.*[74] It contains information about work-related illnesses provided by employers. However, diseases with long latencies, like silicosis, are undercounted.[75] Silicosis can take decades since first exposure to develop and often manifests long after a worker has left a causative job. Thus, employers will be unaware and not able to enter such cases into BLS' reporting system.

Much of what is known about the burden of silicosis in the United States is gleaned from mortality data. The number of silicosis-related deaths has declined markedly over the past several decades (**Fig. 2**). In the late 1960s, death certificates indicated that in excess of 1000 people died of or with silicosis annually. By 2007, silicosis mortality had declined markedly. In that year, 123 people had death certificates indicating death from or with silicosis, an approximately 10-fold reduction. Rosenman and colleagues[76] have proposed that silicosis mortality can be used to estimate how many of those still living in the population have silicosis. They reported a capture-recapture analysis performed in Michigan that found a ratio of the number of living silicosis cases to deceased confirmed silicosis cases of 6.44. An important metric related to mortality is YPLL. Mazurek and Wood[77] reported that deaths in individuals aged 15 to 44 years accounted for 37% of silicosis-related YPLL in the United States before 65 years of age over the 2000–2005 period.

Emerging Settings of Exposure to Crystalline Silica

Because crystalline silica is present in so many materials, or can be created by heating amorphous silica in a range of industrial processes, new settings for exposure continue to emerge. An important development over the past decade has been increasing recognition of exposures in the construction industry.[78–80] The burden of silicosis in construction (and perhaps other industries) is underestimated when screening is performed using plain chest films, which are less sensitive to early disease than chest CT scans.[81] Another emerging source of exposure is natural gas extraction by hydraulic fracturing.[82] The process involves use of air pumps to transport and drive dry, fine sand into fracture sites to keep them open for gas extraction. Leaks in systems for transporting the sand used in this process can result in substantial overexposures to respirable crystalline silica. Another industry whereby exposures may occur is agriculture, particularly when farming dry, sandy soil.[83] Sand blasting is a well-known source of overexposure and is illegal in many countries. Akgun and colleagues[84] recently reported an outbreak of silicosis among denim sandblasters. This outbreak highlights the

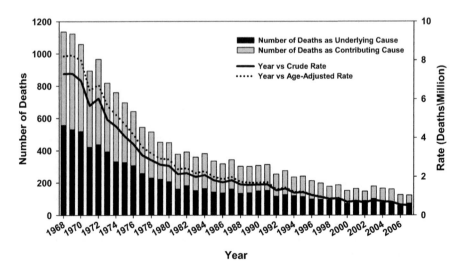

Fig. 2. Silicosis: number of deaths, crude and age-adjusted death rates, US residents aged 15 years and older, 1968–2007. (*From* CDC/NIOSH. Work-Related Lung Disease Surveillance System (eWoRLD) Silicosis and Related Exposures. Available at: http://www2a.cdc.gov/drds/WorldReportData/FigureTableDetails.asp?FigureTableID=2595&Group RefNumber=F03-01. Accessed August 14. 2012.)

risk when an industry that is unfamiliar with the hazard associated with inhaling crystalline silica, such as the textile industry, implements new processes that create such exposures.

Silica-Related Health Effects

As already described, exposure to respirable crystalline silica can result in a range of adverse health effects. Recent developments in the area of silica-induced adverse health effects described in this section include intrathoracic lymph node involvement, the association between silica exposure and lung cancer, immune dysfunction, and immunologically mediated disease.

Two recent publications have evaluated lung and lymph node histopathology in specimens obtained from an autopsy archive of German uranium miners.[85,86] Occupational history and exposure information were also available to the investigators. Both studies found that lymph node–only silicosis was associated with lower exposures than lung silicosis. In one of the studies, as cumulative exposure to silica increased, lung silicosis increased at the expense of lymph node–only silicosis and no silicosis.[86] Although cross-sectional, these studies' findings suggest that, in at least some individuals, lymph node silicosis precedes lung silicosis.

The International Agency for Research on Cancer (IARC) has classified crystalline silica in group 1, carcinogenic to humans, since 1997. An IARC working group reconfirmed IARC's classification in 2010.[87] The 2010 working group found sufficient evidence in humans for the carcinogenicity of crystalline silica in the form of quartz or cristobalite and remarked that crystalline silica in the form of quartz or cristobalite dust causes lung cancer in humans. It found sufficient evidence in experimental animals for the carcinogenicity of quartz.

An area of controversy has been whether crystalline silica exposure without silicosis is associated with increased risk for lung cancer. Erren and colleagues[88] reported a meta-analysis of epidemiologic studies published from 1979 to 2006. The investigators noted that, in patients with silicosis, lung cancer risks were about double in 38 studies. In 8 studies of patients without silicosis without smoking adjustment, relative risk for lung cancer was smaller at 1.2; this increase was marginal from the standpoint of statistical significance. In 3 studies of patients without silicosis with smoking adjustment, no increased risk was observed. Guha and colleagues[87] discussed the issue of cancer risk in silica-exposed patients without silicosis in their discussion of the IARC

classification of crystalline silica as a human carcinogen:

The analyses including only patients without silicosis showed no statistically significant association between crystalline silica exposure and lung cancer risk. However, the IARC Working Group noted that studies that restrict their analysis to individuals without silicosis potentially limit their range of silica exposure which would result in reduced power to detect associations and tend to omit individuals with the highest exposures.[87]

It is likely that this issue will continue to be controversial, especially in view of its important social and economic implications. In 2011, the Italian Society of Occupational Medicine and Industrial Hygiene sought to address issues of liability and compensation. It recommended that, for legal purposes, only lung cancer cases associated with silicosis should be recognized as occupational.[89]

It has long been known that silica exposure, with or without silicosis, is associated with an increased risk for tuberculous and nontuberculous mycobacterial-related diseases.[90] A recent publication documented similarly impaired pulmonary host defense for fungal infections. It showed that patients with silicosis were more likely to die with pulmonary mycosis than those without pneumoconiosis or those with more common pneumoconioses.[91]

The association between silicosis and various connective tissue disorders is well recognized. Makol and colleagues[92] recently published an evaluation of connective tissue disease among 790 patients with silicosis with available medical records identified between 1985 and 2006 by a statewide surveillance system in Michigan. They found that rheumatoid arthritis was the most common classic connective tissue disease in this population of patients with silicosis (33 cases out of 790 patients with silicosis, 4.2%). Scleroderma occurred in 2 of the patients with silicosis (0.3%). A surprising finding was the prevalence of antineutrophilic cytoplasmic antibody (ANCA)–positive vasculitis (6 cases out of 790 patients with silicosis, 0.8%). Prevalence ratios were significantly increased relative to the general population for all of these conditions (rheumatoid arthritis 2.26–6.96, depending on the reference rate used; scleroderma 28.3; ANCA-vasculitis 25.3).

To further characterize rheumatoid arthritis in silica-exposed individuals, Stolt and colleagues[93] evaluated the prevalence of antibodies against citrullinated peptide antigens (ACPA) in rheumatoid arthritis cases and controls with and without histories of silica exposure. It had previously been demonstrated that increased risk for rheumatoid arthritis associated with cigarette smoking was limited to the ACPA-positive subset of rheumatoid arthritis. There was about a 1.5-fold increased risk for ACPA-positive rheumatoid arthritis among patients exposed to silica. There was no increase in the risk of developing ACPA-negative rheumatoid arthritis, as compared with patients unexposed to silica. There was a strong interaction between silica exposure and smoking, with silica-exposed current smokers having a more than 7-fold increase in the risk of having ACPA-positive rheumatoid arthritis. Thus, ACPA may have some potential as biomarkers for silica-induced rheumatoid arthritis.

ASBESTOS

Asbestos is a commercial name, not a mineralogical definition. It is applied to a group of fibrous minerals with properties such as strength, flexibility, resistance to thermal and chemical degradation, and electrical resistance. These properties resulted in widespread use of asbestos in the last century for a range of purposes, including insulation, construction materials, brake pads, and fireproof woven textiles. Unfortunately, because of long latency, it took decades after the use of asbestos became common for the inhalation of asbestos-containing dust to be recognized as a serious health risk.[5]

There are currently 6 regulated types of asbestos fibers: a serpentine mineral (chrysotile asbestos) and 5 amphibole minerals, including cummingtonite-grunerite asbestos (amosite), riebeckite asbestos (crocidolite), actinolite asbestos, anthophyllite asbestos, and tremolite asbestos. The distinctive constellation of pleural and pulmonary health effects resulting from inhalation of these materials is well recognized, as is the need for preventing exposures. Pleural effects include pleural effusion, parietal pleural plaque, visceral diffuse pleural disease, rounded atelectasis, and mesothelioma. Pulmonary parenchymal effects include asbestosis and lung cancer.[3,5]

This section describes several areas that are controversial or where there have been important new developments. These areas include how asbestos should be defined; recent developments in documenting the nonpleuropulmonary malignancies associated with asbestos; hazards associated with environmental exposures to asbestos, whether from human contamination of the environment or natural deposits; and recent developments in mesothelioma biomarkers.

Definition of Asbestos

Regulated forms of asbestos in the United States are the 6 previously noted asbestos minerals in an asbestiform crystalline morphology or habit. The term *asbestiform* is generally used to describe populations of single-crystal fibrils (the smallest structural unit of a fiber), which occur in bundles and possess certain characteristics, including high aspect ratio, high tensile strength, and flexibility (**Fig. 3**).[94] Several authorities have commented on problems and controversies in how asbestos is defined.[5,94–97] For example, some mineral types other than those named in regulations can occur in asbestiform habit and cause the same diseases. One such mineral is erionite, which is responsible for outbreaks of mesothelioma in residents of some Turkish villages where erionite-containing rock was used to construct homes.[98] Two other such minerals are winchite and richterite. These minerals constitute a major portion of the asbestiform amphibole fibers contaminating vermiculite from Libby, Montana. They also exemplify problems with terminology related to asbestos because winchite and richterite were once included within the definition of tremolite asbestos but have more recently been redefined as separate minerals based on elemental content.[94]

More controversial is whether fibers of asbestos minerals in habits other than asbestiform should be counted as asbestos. Examples include cleavage fragments created by the breakage of mineral in massive crystalline habit or needlelike acicular fibers that grow as single crystals instead of

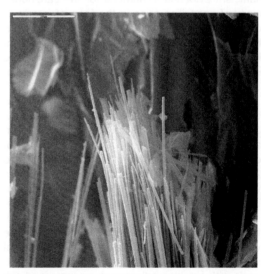

Fig. 3. Winchite-richterite asbestos, Libby, Montana. (*Courtesy of* the U.S. Geological Survey. Available at: http://usgsprobe.cr.usgs.gov/picts2.html.   Accessed August 14, 2012.)

asbestiform bundles. This controversy is a source of a long-standing difference between NIOSH, OSHA, and MSHA, with NIOSH recommending that cleavage fragments of the asbestos minerals be counted as asbestos if they meet the dimensional criteria of a fiber and the permissible exposure limits of OSHA and MSHA not including such elongate mineral particles within their definitions of asbestos. An important source of these differences is imperfect information about the toxicology of such particles.[5]

Certain counting methods are specified in regulatory definitions of asbestos fibers. The most commonly used analytical method to count asbestos fibers in air samples or bulk materials is phase-contrast light microscopy (PCM). The dimensions of asbestos fibers counted using this method are generally defined as a length/width (aspect) ratio of 3:1 and a length of at least 5 μm. Some methods also specify a width no more than 3 μm. An important limitation of PCM is that it does not count thin fibers of less than about 0.25 μm. These fibers can be visualized and counted by electron microscopy, which is used far less frequently than PCM in asbestos exposure assessment. A recent reevaluation of a cohort of chrysotile textile workers documented the important role of thin fibers not visualized by PCM in causing respiratory disease.[99] Fiber dimensions were evaluated in archived samples by transmission electron microscopy. Both lung cancer and asbestosis were most strongly associated with exposure to thin fibers less than 0.25 μm. Long fibers greater than 10 μm were the strongest predictors of lung cancer, but there was not a clear relationship between fiber length and asbestosis.

Nonpleuropulmonary Malignancies Associated with Asbestos

In 2006, the Institute of Medicine (IOM) released the report *Asbestos: Selected Cancers*.[100] The IOM committee writing the report was charged to evaluate evidence for causation of cancers of the pharynx, larynx, esophagus, stomach, and colon and rectum by asbestos. It found sufficient evidence for a causal relationship only for laryngeal cancer. There was suggestive evidence for all the others except esophageal cancer for which there was inadequate evidence. Another extrathoracic malignancy recently recognized as related to asbestos exposure is ovarian cancer. Based on a meta-analysis of available studies, IARC recently concluded that there was sufficient evidence for a causal relationship.[101] The overall pooled standardized mortality ratio estimate for ovarian cancer was 1.77.

Environmental Exposures to Asbestos

Many recent reports have highlighted the potential importance of environmental exposure to asbestos. Human contamination has been an important factor in several outbreaks of asbestos-associated disease. Widespread contamination of Libby, Montana occurred when asbestos-contaminated material from the vermiculite mine there was used across the community as gravel on roads, driveways, playgrounds, and so forth. Even tree bark has been suggested as a contaminated reservoir of asbestos fibers that, if disturbed, could result in exposure.[102] Excess morbidity and mortality has been documented even in those with nonoccupational sources of exposure.[103] A similar environmental disaster with widespread contamination and asbestos-related disease even among those not engaged in mining occurred in the Australian town of Witenoom where riebeckite asbestos (crocidolite) was mined.[104]

Use of asbestos-containing materials to gravel roads is another type of human activity that can result in environmental contamination and disease. Exposure can occur when these materials are disturbed by driving or by road work. Baumann and colleagues[105] investigated malignant mesothelioma in New Caledonia and found that presence of serpentinite on roads was a major environmental risk factor for the disease. Several recent investigations resulted from the realization that roads in Southwestern North Dakota had been graveled with materials contaminated with asbestiform fibrous erionite.[98,106] Two people with histories of road maintenance work were identified with asbestos-related pleuropulmonary disease visualized by chest CT.

Exposure can also occur through disturbance of natural deposits. In 2005, Pan and colleagues[107] reported residential proximity to naturally occurring asbestos in California as an independent risk factor for mesothelioma. Exposure from naturally occurring asbestos has been recognized in California for several years. In 1979, Cooper and colleagues[108] noted that dust fall along roads and trails used recreationally in the Clear Creek area of San Benito County, California was 90% or more chrysotile asbestos. Riding motorcycles on trails was associated with exposures well in excess of occupational exposure limits. A series of studies done since then have confirmed the presence of asbestos and the potential for exposures.[109] Another example of human exposure from natural deposits was in El Dorado Hills, California where the Environmental Protection Agency was petitioned to assess asbestos exposure after asbestos was found in the soil at a high school.[109] Asbestos was subsequently found in many air and soil samples from across the community. Highest exposures occur when people are engaged in activities that disturb contaminated soil. Both of these situations have been challenging to manage. In such situations, it is often hard to balance desires to preserve land access and property values versus minimizing health risks.

Mesothelioma Biomarkers

An important recent advance has been the development of blood biomarkers for malignant mesothelioma.[110,111] One of these, Mesomark, measures soluble mesothelin-related peptides (SMRP). The US Food and Drug Administration approved it in 2007 for monitoring the course of mesothelioma with epithelioid features. Although not approved for diagnosis of malignant mesothelioma, there has been great interest in this potential application of serum SMRP levels. A recent meta-analysis of available studies found that at a threshold level with 95% specificity, serum mesothelin had a sensitivity of 32%. It was suggested that low sensitivity limited the value of the test for early diagnosis.[112] Osteopontin is another potential blood marker for malignant mesothelioma that has received much attention. A recent study suggests that plasma osteopontin has better performance characteristics for diagnosis than serum osteopontin, but neither performed as well as serum mesothelin. Combining serum mesothelin and plasma osteopontin results did not improve diagnostic performance.[113]

SUMMARY

There is a long history of recognition that coal mine dust, respirable crystalline silica, and asbestos are hazards that can be controlled. However, new settings for exposure continue to emerge and dust-related disease persists. Examples of emerging settings for exposure include thin-seam coal mining in Appalachia, construction work, and natural gas extraction by hydraulic fracturing (all of which can result in exposure to crystalline silica) and environmental exposures to asbestos associated with human contamination of the environment or the presence of natural deposits. New adverse health effects also continue to be recognized, such as ACPA-positive rheumatoid arthritis and ANCA-positive vasculitis in silicotics and laryngeal and ovarian cancer in asbestos-exposed individuals. Important advances continue to be made. Examples include advancements in the application

of modern chest imaging and the development of blood markers for malignant mesothelioma. Until they are eliminated, pneumoconioses and related conditions will continue to be an important and dynamic aspect of chest medicine.

REFERENCES

1. Agricola G, De Re Metallica. (Translated from the first Latin edition of 1556. Translated by Hoover HC, Henry LH). New York: Dover; 1950. Available at: http://www.gutenberg.org/files/38015/38015-h/38015-h.htm. Accessed September 25, 2012.
2. Ramazzini B. De Morbis Artificum Diatriba [Diseases of Workers] (The Latin text of 1713 revised, with translation and notes by Wilmer Cave Wright). Chicago, IL: University of Chicago Press; 1940. Am J Public Health 2001;91(9):1380–2 [reprint].
3. American Thoracic Society. Diagnosis and initial management of nonmalignant diseases related to asbestos. Am J Respir Crit Care Med 2004; 170(6):691–715.
4. NIOSH. Health effects of occupational exposure to respirable crystalline silica. Publication No. 2002-129. Cincinnati (OH): DHHS (NIOSH); 2002.
5. NIOSH. Current intelligence bulletin 62. Asbestos fibers and other elongate mineral particles: state of the science and roadmap for research. DHHS (NIOSH) Publication No. 2011–159. Cincinnati (OH): DHHS (NIOSH); 2011.
6. NIOSH. Coal mine dust exposures and associated health outcomes. A review of information published since 1995. DHHS (NIOSH) Publication No. 2011–172. Cincinnati (OH): DHHS (NIOSH); 2011.
7. Driscoll T, Nelson DI, Steenland K, et al. The global burden of non-malignant respiratory disease due to occupational airborne exposures. Am J Ind Med 2005;48(6):432–45.
8. International Labour Office. Guidelines for the use of the ILO international classification of radiographs of pneumoconioses. Geneva (Switzerland): International Labour Office; 2011.
9. Levine BA, Ingeholm ML, Prior F, et al. Conversion to use of digital chest images for surveillance of coal workers' pneumoconiosis (black lung). Conf Proc IEEE Eng Med Biol Soc 2009;2009: 2161–3.
10. Franzblau A, Kazerooni EA, Sen A, et al. Comparison of digital radiographs with film radiographs for the classification of pneumoconiosis. Acad Radiol 2009;16(6):669–77.
11. Laney AS, Petsonk EL, Attfield MD. Intramodality and intermodality comparisons of storage phosphor computed radiography and conventional film-screen radiography in the recognition of small pneumoconiotic opacities. Chest 2011;140(6): 1574–80.

12. Laney AS, Petsonk EL, Wolfe AL, et al. Comparison of storage phosphor computed radiography with conventional film-screen radiography in the recognition of pneumoconiosis. Eur Respir J 2010;36(1):122–7.

13. Larson TC, Holiday DB, Antao VC, et al. Comparison of digital with film radiographs for the classification of pneumoconiotic pleural abnormalities. Acad Radiol 2012;19(2):131–40.

14. Sen A, Lee SY, Gillespie BW, et al. Comparing film and digital radiographs for reliability of pneumoconiosis classifications: a modeling approach. Acad Radiol 2010;17(4):511–9.

15. Mao L, Huang J, Zhou S, et al. Feasibility study of direct readout radiography in pneumoconiosis diagnosis. J Environ Occup Med (Chinese) 2011;28(3):1212–6.

16. Mao L, Laney AS, Wang ML, et al. Comparison of digital direct readout radiography with conventional film-screen radiography for the recognition of pneumoconiosis in dust-exposed Chinese workers. J Occup Health 2011;53(5):320–6.

17. Jagoe JR, Paton KA. Reading chest radiographs for pneumoconiosis by computer. Br J Ind Med 1975;32(4):267–72.

18. Turner AF, Kruger RP, Thompson WB. Automated computer screening of chest radiographs for pneumoconiosis. Invest Radiol 1976;11(4):258–66.

19. Okumura E, Kawashita I, Ishida T. Computerized analysis of pneumoconiosis in digital chest radiography: effect of artificial neural network trained with power spectra. J Digit Imaging 2011;24(6):1126–32.

20. Yu P, Xu H, Zhu Y, et al. An automatic computer-aided detection scheme for pneumoconiosis on digital chest radiographs. J Digit Imaging 2011;24(3):382–93.

21. Gevenois PA, Pichot E, Dargent F, et al. Low grade coal worker's pneumoconiosis. Comparison of CT and chest radiography. Acta Radiol 1994;35(4):351–6.

22. Lamers RJ, Schins RP, Wouters EF, et al. High-resolution computed tomography of the lungs in coal miners with a normal chest radiograph. Exp Lung Res 1994;20(5):411–9.

23. Remy-Jardin M, Degreef JM, Beuscart R, et al. Coal worker's pneumoconiosis: CT assessment in exposed workers and correlation with radiographic findings. Radiology 1990;177(2):363–71.

24. Remy-Jardin M, Remy J, Farre I, et al. Computed tomographic evaluation of silicosis and coal workers' pneumoconiosis. Radiol Clin North Am 1992;30(6):1155–76.

25. Rose C, Lynch D. The role of CT scanning in pneumoconiosis. DHHS (NIOSH) Publication No. 2009-140. In: The NIOSH B reader certification program: looking to the future. Cincinnati, OH: DHHS (NIOSH); 2009. p. 28–56. Available at: http://www.cdc.gov/niosh/docs/2009-140/. Accessed August 14, 2012.

26. Savranlar A, Altin R, Mahmutyazicioglu K, et al. Comparison of chest radiography and high-resolution computed tomography findings in early and low-grade coal worker's pneumoconiosis. Eur J Radiol 2004;51(2):175–80.

27. National Lung Screening Trial Research Team, Aberle DR, Adams AM, et al. Reduced lung-cancer mortality with low-dose computed tomographic screening. N Engl J Med 2011;365(5):395–409.

28. Bach PB, Mirkin JN, Oliver TK, et al. Benefits and harms of CT screening for lung cancer: a systematic review. JAMA 2012;307(22):2418–29.

29. Jacobson FL, Austin JH, Field JK, et al. Development of the American Association for Thoracic Surgery guidelines for low-dose computed tomography scans to screen for lung cancer in North America: recommendations of the American Association for Thoracic Surgery Task Force for Lung Cancer Screening and Surveillance. J Thorac Cardiovasc Surg 2012;144(1):25–32.

30. Hodgson JT, Darnton A. The quantitative risks of mesothelioma and lung cancer in relation to asbestos exposure. Ann Occup Hyg 2000;44(8):565–601.

31. Federal Coal Mine Health and Safety Act of 1969. Pub. L. No. 91–173, S. 29171969.

32. Attfield MD, Althouse RB. Surveillance data on US coal miners' pneumoconiosis, 1970 to 1986. Am J Public Health 1992;82(7):971–7.

33. Attfield MD, Castellan RM. Epidemiological data on US coal miners' pneumoconiosis, 1960 to 1988. Am J Public Health 1992;82(7):964–70.

34. Pon MR, Roper RA, Petsonk EL, et al. Pneumoconiosis prevalence among working coal miners examined in federal chest radiograph surveillance programs–United States, 1996-2002. MMWR Morb Mortal Wkly Rep 2003;52(15):336–40.

35. National Institute for Occupational Safety and Health. Coal workers' pneumoconiosis and related conditions. DHHS (NIOSH) Publication No. 2008-143a. In: Work-related lung disease surveillance report 2007. Cincinnati, OH: DHHS (NIOSH); 2008. p. 27–52. Available at: http://www.cdc.gov/niosh/docs/2008-143/. Accessed August 14, 2012

36. National Institute for Occupational Safety and Health. Coal Workers' Health Surveillance Program (CWHSP) data query system. 2011. Available at: http://webappa.cdc.gov/ords/cwhsp-database.html. Accessed August 15, 2012.

37. Suarthana E, Laney AS, Storey E, et al. Coal workers' pneumoconiosis in the United States: regional differences 40 years after implementation of the 1969 Federal Coal Mine Health and Safety Act. Occup Environ Med 2011;68(12):908–13.

38. Antao VC, Petsonk EL, Sokolow LZ, et al. Rapidly progressive coal workers' pneumoconiosis in the

United States: geographic clustering and other factors. Occup Environ Med 2005;62(10):670–4.

39. Antao VC, Petsonk EL, Attfield MD. Advanced cases of coal workers' pneumoconiosis–two counties, Virginia, 2006. MMWR Morb Mortal Wkly Rep 2006;55(33):909–13.

40. Attfield MD, Petsonk EL. Advanced pneumoconiosis among working underground coal miners–Eastern Kentucky and Southwestern Virginia, 2006. MMWR Morb Mortal Wkly Rep 2007;56(26):652–5.

41. National Institute for Occupational Safety and Health. Coal mine dust exposures and associated health outcomes: a review of information published since 1995. Current intelligence bulletin 64. DHHS (NIOSH) Publication No. 2011-172. Washington, DC: DHHS (NIOSH); 2011.

42. Wade WA, Petsonk EL, Young B, et al. Severe occupational pneumoconiosis among West Virginian coal miners: one hundred thirty-eight cases of progressive massive fibrosis compensated between 2000 and 2009. Chest 2011;139(6):1458–62.

43. Mazurek JM, Laney AS, Wood JM, et al. Coal workers' pneumoconiosis-related years of potential life lost before age 65 years - United States, 1968-2006. MMWR Morb Mortal Wkly Rep 2009;58(50):1412–6.

44. Diaz-Guzman E, Zwischenberger JB, Hoopes CW. Lung transplantation in coal workers pneumoconiosis. Chest 2011;140(5):1387–8 [author reply: 1388–9].

45. Enfield KB, Floyd S, Peach P, et al. Transplant outcome for coal workers pneumoconiosis. Paper presented at: American Transplant Congress, May 2–5, 2010, San Diego.

46. Hayes D Jr, Diaz-Guzman E, Davenport DL, et al. Lung transplantation in patients with coal workers' pneumoconiosis. Clin Transplant 2012;26(4):629–34.

47. Laney AS, Attfield MD. Coal workers' pneumoconiosis and progressive massive fibrosis are increasingly more prevalent among workers in small underground coal mines in the United States. Occup Environ Med 2010;67(6):428–31.

48. Laney AS, Petsonk EL, Hale JM, et al. Potential determinants of coal workers' pneumoconiosis, advanced pneumoconiosis, and progressive massive fibrosis among underground coal miners in the United States, 2005-2009. Am J Public Health 2012;102(Suppl 2):S279–83.

49. Hunting KL, Weeks JL. Transport injuries in small coal mines: an exploratory analysis. Am J Ind Med 1993;23(3):391–406.

50. National Academy of Sciences. Toward safer underground coal mines. Washington, DC: National Academy Press; 1982.

51. Fotta B, Mallett LG. Effects of mining height on injury rates in U.S. underground nonlongwall bituminous coal mines. DHHS (NIOSH) Information Circular 9447. Pittsburgh: DHHS (NIOSH); 1997.

52. Randolph RF. Injury analysis of Pennsylvania small surface coal mines. Proc third health and safety seminar for small mines (Somerset, PA). University Park (PA): The Pennsylvania State University; 1998. p. 83–92.

53. Seaton A. Coal workers' pneumoconiosis in small underground coal mines in the United States. Occup Environ Med 2010;67(6):364.

54. Cohen RA. Is the increasing prevalence and severity of coal workers' pneumoconiosis in the United States due to increasing silica exposure? Occup Environ Med 2010;67(10):649–50.

55. Laney AS, Attfield MD. Quartz exposure can cause pneumoconiosis in coal workers. J Occup Environ Med 2009;51(8):867 [author reply: 868].

56. Tomb TF, Gero AJ, Kogut J. Analysis of quartz exposure data obtained from underground and surface coal mining operations. Appl Occup Environ Hyg 1995;10(12):1019–26.

57. Weeks JL. Tampering with dust samples in coal mines (again). Am J Ind Med 1991;20(2):141–4.

58. Weeks JL. The fox guarding the chicken coop: monitoring exposure to respirable coal mine dust, 1969-2000. Am J Public Health 2003;93(8):1236–44.

59. Laney AS, Petsonk EL, Attfield MD. Pneumoconiosis among underground bituminous coal miners in the United States: is silicosis becoming more frequent? Occup Environ Med 2010;67(10):652–6.

60. Pollock DE, Potts JD, Joy GJ. Investigation into dust exposures and mining practices in the southern Appalachian region. Min Eng 2010;62(2):44–9.

61. Peters RH, Fotta B, Mallett LG. The influence of seam height on lost-time injury and fatality rates at small underground bituminous coal mines. Appl Occup Environ Hyg 2001;16(11):1028–34.

62. Amandus HE, Lapp NL, Morgan WK, et al. Pulmonary zonal involvement in coal workers' pneumoconiosis. J Occup Med 1974;16(4):245–7.

63. Laney AS, Petsonk EL. Small pneumoconiotic opacities on U.S. coal worker surveillance chest radiographs are not predominantly in the upper lung zones. Am J Ind Med 2012;55(9):793–8.

64. Young RC Jr, Rachal RE, Carr PG, et al. Patterns of coal workers' pneumoconiosis in Appalachian former coal miners. J Natl Med Assoc 1992;84(1):41–8.

65. Liddell FD. Radiological assessment of small pneumoconiotic opacities. Br J Ind Med 1977;34(2):85–94.

66. Coggon D, Newman Taylor A. Coal mining and chronic obstructive pulmonary disease: a review of the evidence. Thorax 1998;53(5):398–407.

67. Cohen RA, Patel A, Green FH. Lung disease caused by exposure to coal mine and silica dust. Semin Respir Crit Care Med 2008;29(6):651–61.
68. Kuempel ED, Stayner LT, Attfield MD, et al. Exposure-response analysis of mortality among coal miners in the United States. Am J Ind Med 1995; 28(2):167–84.
69. Page SJ, Volkwein JC, Vinson RP, et al. Equivalency of a personal dust monitor to the current United States coal mine respirable dust sampler. J Environ Monit 2008;10(1):96–101.
70. Volkwein JC, Vinson RP, McWilliams LJ, et al. Performance of a new personal respirable dust monitor for mine use. DHHS (NIOSH) Publication No. 2004-151. Pittsburgh: DHHS (NIOSH); 2004.
71. US Department of Labor, Mine Safety and Health Administration. Lowering miners' exposure to respirable coal mine dust including continuous personal dust monitors. 75 FR 64411. 2010:64411–506.
72. American Thoracic Society. Adverse effects of crystalline silica exposure. Am J Respir Crit Care Med 1997;155(2):761–8.
73. Yassin A, Yebesi F, Tingle R. Occupational exposure to crystalline silica dust in the United States, 1988-2003. Environ Health Perspect 2005;113(3):255–60.
74. Bureau of Labor Statistics. Injuries, illnesses, and fatalities. 2012.Available at: http://www.bls.gov/iif/. Accessed August 15, 2012.
75. Bureau of Labor Statistics. Frequently asked questions (FAQs). 2. Does the BLS "undercount" workplace injuries and illnesses? 2012. Available at: http://www.bls.gov/iif/oshfaq1.htm#q02. Accessed August 15, 2012.
76. Rosenman KD, Reilly MJ, Henneberger PK. Estimating the total number of newly-recognized silicosis cases in the United States. Am J Ind Med 2003;44(2):141–7.
77. Mazurek JM, Wood JM. Silicosis-related years of potential life lost before age 65 years - United States, 1968-2005. MMWR Morb Mortal Wkly Rep 2008;57(28):771–5.
78. Meeker JD, Cooper MR, Lefkowitz D, et al. Engineering control technologies to reduce occupational silica exposures in masonry cutting and tuckpointing. Public Health Rep 2009;124(Suppl 1): 101–11.
79. Suarthana E, Moons KG, Heederik D, et al. A simple diagnostic model for ruling out pneumoconiosis among construction workers. Occup Environ Med 2007;64(9):595–601.
80. Valiante DJ, Schill DP, Rosenman KD, et al. Highway repair: a new silicosis threat. Am J Public Health 2004;94(5):876–80.
81. Meijer E, Tjoe Nij E, Kraus T, et al. Pneumoconiosis and emphysema in construction workers: results of HRCT and lung function findings. Occup Environ Med 2011;68(7):542–6.
82. Occupational Safety and Health Administration and National Institute for Occupational Safety and Health. OSHA-NIOSH hazard alert. Worker exposure to silica during hydraulic fracturing. 2012. Available at: http://www.osha.gov/dts/hazardalerts/hydraulic_frac_hazard_alert.html. Accessed August 15, 2012.
83. Swanepoel AJ, Rees D, Renton K, et al. Quartz exposure in agriculture: literature review and South African survey. Ann Occup Hyg 2010;54(3):281–92.
84. Akgun M, Araz O, Akkurt I, et al. An epidemic of silicosis among former denim sandblasters. Eur Respir J 2008;32(5):1295–303.
85. Cox-Ganser JM, Burchfiel CM, Fekedulegn D, et al. Silicosis in lymph nodes: the canary in the miner? J Occup Environ Med 2009;51(2):164–9.
86. Taeger D, Bruning T, Pesch B, et al. Association between lymph node silicosis and lung silicosis in 4,384 German uranium miners with lung cancer. Arch Environ Occup Health 2011;66(1):34–42.
87. Guha N, Straif K, Benbrahim-Tallaa L. The IARC monographs on the carcinogenicity of crystalline silica. Med Lav 2011;102(4):310–20.
88. Erren TC, Morfeld P, Glende CB, et al. Meta-analyses of published epidemiological studies, 1979-2006, point to open causal questions in silica-silicosis-lung cancer research. Med Lav 2011;102(4):321–35.
89. Piolatto G, Pira E. The opinion of the Italian Society of Occupational Medicine and Industrial Hygiene (SIMLII) on silica-exposure and lung cancer risk. Med Lav 2011;102(4):336–42.
90. Barboza CE, Winter DH, Seiscento M, et al. Tuberculosis and silicosis: epidemiology, diagnosis and chemoprophylaxis. J Bras Pneumol 2008;34(11): 959–66.
91. Iossifova Y, Bailey R, Wood J, et al. Concurrent silicosis and pulmonary mycosis at death. Emerg Infect Dis 2010;16(2):318–20.
92. Makol A, Reilly MJ, Rosenman KD. Prevalence of connective tissue disease in silicosis (1985-2006)- a report from the state of Michigan surveillance system for silicosis. Am J Ind Med 2011;54(4):255–62.
93. Stolt P, Yahya A, Bengtsson C, et al. Silica exposure among male current smokers is associated with a high risk of developing ACPA-positive rheumatoid arthritis. Ann Rheum Dis 2010;69(6): 1072–6.
94. Meeker GP, Bern AM, Brownfield IK, et al. The composition and morphology of amphiboles from the Rainy Creek complex, near Libby, Montana. Am Mineral 2003;88(11–12):1955–69.
95. Case BW, Abraham JL, Meeker G, et al. Applying definitions of "asbestos" to environmental and "low-dose" exposure levels and health effects, particularly malignant mesothelioma. J Toxicol Environ Health B Crit Rev 2011;14(1–4):3–39.

96. Gunter ME. Defining asbestos: differences between the built and natural environments. Chimia 2010;64(10):747–52.

97. Lee RJ, Strohmeier BR, Bunker KL, et al. Naturally occurring asbestos: a recurring public policy challenge. J Hazard Mater 2008;153(1–2):1–21.

98. Carbone M, Baris YI, Bertino P, et al. Erionite exposure in North Dakota and Turkish villages with mesothelioma. Proc Natl Acad Sci U S A 2011; 108(33):13618–23.

99. Stayner L, Kuempel E, Gilbert S, et al. An epidemiological study of the role of chrysotile asbestos fibre dimensions in determining respiratory disease risk in exposed workers. Occup Environ Med 2008; 65(9):613–9.

100. Institute of Medicine. Asbestos: selected cancers. Washington, DC: National Academies Press; 2006.

101. Camargo MC, Stayner LT, Straif K, et al. Occupational exposure to asbestos and ovarian cancer: a meta-analysis. Environ Health Perspect 2011; 119(9):1211–7.

102. Ward TJ, Spear TM, Hart JF, et al. Amphibole asbestos in tree bark–a review of findings for this inhalational exposure source in Libby, Montana. J Occup Environ Hyg 2012;9(6):387–97.

103. Antao VC, Larson TC, Horton DK. Libby vermiculite exposure and risk of developing asbestos-related lung and pleural diseases. Curr Opin Pulm Med 2012;18(2):161–7.

104. Reid A, Heyworth J, de Klerk N, et al. The mortality of women exposed environmentally and domestically to blue asbestos at Wittenoom, Western Australia. Occup Environ Med 2008;65(11):743–9.

105. Baumann F, Maurizot P, Mangeas M, et al. Pleural mesothelioma in New Caledonia: associations with environmental risk factors. Environ Health Perspect 2011;119(5):695–700.

106. Ryan PH, Dihle M, Griffin S, et al. Erionite in road gravel associated with interstitial and pleural changes–an occupational hazard in Western United States. J Occup Environ Med 2011;53(8):892–8.

107. Pan XL, Day HW, Wang W, et al. Residential proximity to naturally occurring asbestos and mesothelioma risk in California. Am J Respir Crit Care Med 2005;172(8):1019–25.

108. Cooper WC, Murchio J, Popendorf W, et al. Chrysotile asbestos in a California recreational area. Science 1979;206(4419):685–8.

109. Environmental Protection Agency, Region 9. Naturally occurring asbestos. 2012. Available at: http://www.epa.gov/region9/toxic/noa/. Accessed August 15, 2012.

110. Creaney J, Robinson BW. Serum and pleural fluid biomarkers for mesothelioma. Curr Opin Pulm Med 2009;15(4):366–70.

111. Cristaudo A, Bonotti A, Simonini S, et al. Soluble markers for diagnosis of malignant pleural mesothelioma. Biomark Med 2011;5(2):261–73.

112. Hollevoet K, Reitsma JB, Creaney J, et al. Serum mesothelin for diagnosing malignant pleural mesothelioma: an individual patient data meta-analysis. J Clin Oncol 2012;30(13):1541–9.

113. Creaney J, Yeoman D, Musk AW, et al. Plasma versus serum levels of osteopontin and mesothelin in patients with malignant mesothelioma–which is best? Lung Cancer 2011;74(1):55–60.

Respiratory Health Effects of Ambient Air Pollution: An Update

Francesco Sava, MD, MSc, FRCPC[a,b],
Chris Carlsten, MD, MPH[a,b],*

KEYWORDS

- Air pollution • Gene • Environment • Respiratory health • Asthma • COPD • Lung cancer

KEY POINTS

- The last decade of research on ambient air pollution (AAP) has confirmed its adverse impact on respiratory morbidity and mortality, quality of life, and economic burden on health care systems.
- Efforts to reduce AAP have been fruitful, in terms of reduced mortality, but the concentration-effect relationship seems steepest at the lower end of the concentration range, suggesting that further reductions in AAP may confer marked additional benefit.
- Evidence for incident asthma caused by AAP has proliferated, strengthening the claim of a cause-effect relationship, particularly in children.
- This finding is of critical importance because such insight may support additional efforts to prevent new lung disease, and prevention of new disease generally has a larger impact than does preventing exacerbations of existing disease.
- Research has demonstrated that co-exposures have the potential to dramatically augment the effects of AAP and, thus, lower the threshold of effect of a given pollutant.

INTRODUCTION

A lot has happened since the topic of the health effects of ambient air pollution (AAP) was last reviewed in the *Clinics in Chest Medicine* 10 years ago,[1] with major contributions from epidemiology, toxicology, and particularly genetics and epigenetics. With this review, the authors do not aim to be comprehensive regarding the effect of AAP on human respiratory health because the topic has been covered from several perspectives in recent years.[2–5] Instead, the purpose of the current review is to reflect on specific areas where progress has been most significant in the last decade. For each such topic, the authors include the most up-to-date evidence and explain how it has advanced our understanding of long-standing concerns. The authors' approach is to integrate findings from epidemiology, controlled human experimental exposures, and toxicology, highlighting key areas of novel insight and describing prominent gaps in the evidence to motivate future research. AAP generally refers to particulate matter, as well as ozone and other gasses, largely generated by the combustion of fossil fuels by vehicles or power plants, outdoor biomass burning, and a variety of industrial processes and then dispersed within the commonly inhabited airspace. Therefore, the authors are not covering indoor air, including indoor biomass burning, cardiovascular disease (the subject of much attention, appropriately, elsewhere[6]), or disorders outside the lung.

The authors have no disclosures.
[a] Air Pollution Exposure Laboratory (APEL), Vancouver Coastal Health Research Institute, University of British Columbia, Vancouver General Hospital (VGH)-Research Pavilion, 828 West 10th Avenue, Vancouver, British Columbia V5Z 1L8, Canada; [b] The Lung Centre, Department of Medicine, Vancouver General Hospital, 7th Floor, 2775 Laurel Street, Vancouver, British Columbia V5Z 1M9, Canada
* Corresponding author.
E-mail address: Carlsten@mail.ubc.ca

Clin Chest Med 33 (2012) 759–769
http://dx.doi.org/10.1016/j.ccm.2012.07.003
0272-5231/12/$ – see front matter

The authors divide the material into (1) epidemiologic findings, (2) experimental results (especially as they are oriented to mechanistic support for observational population-based findings), and (3) genetic and epigenetic insights, given the particularly prominent role of these disciplines in recent literature and their potential to identify at-risk populations and novel mechanisms that might guide upcoming policy decisions and further research.

EPIDEMIOLOGIC STUDIES
Particulate Matter: Acute Effects

The most powerful epidemiologic evidence of the effects of short-term exposure to air pollution has typically come from large cooperative efforts that allow the standardization of analytic methods and reporting across a broad range of international jurisdictions. One of the biggest such collaborative studies, Air Pollution and Health: A Combined European and North American Approach (APHENA), includes studies from the Air Pollution and Health: A European Approach (APHEA) study in Europe; the National Morbidity, Mortality, and Air Pollution Study (NMMAPS) in the United States; and others from Canada.[7,8] The effect of particulate matter with a diameter less than 10 μm (PM10) on increased daily death rates ranged from 0.2% to 0.6% for each 10 μg/m^3 increase in ambient PM10 concentration. The main objective of APHENA was to assess the coherence of the findings of the multicity studies carried out on different continents; APHENA found similar effects when comparing Europe and the United States, showing the robustness of the data and the different modeling approaches. Across regions, effects were stronger for people older than 75 years. Most of the effect was driven by cardiovascular mortality, but a significant increase in respiratory mortality was also noted.

The daily variation in disease burden caused by urban air pollution was further assessed by measuring the number of emergency visits and hospital admissions caused by respiratory diseases. In the APHEA cohorts, a 10 μg/m^3 increase in PM10 was associated with increases of 1.2% in children asthma admissions, 1.1% in adult asthma admissions, and 0.9% in respiratory diseases as a combined end point (chronic obstructive pulmonary disease [COPD], asthma, and other respiratory diseases). Effects were stronger in children with asthma without antiinflammatory medication; notably, the association between PM10 and respiratory hospital admissions was significant on the same day of the PM10 assessment (zero day lag) and also over lags of several subsequent days. The principle novelty in APHENA is its assessment of the acute effects of AAP across such diverse geographic regions with such different modeling approaches, and the coherence of its findings adds substantial confidence in the collective evidence of prior decades connecting AAP to the exacerbation of respiratory disease.

Progress has also been made regarding the acute impact of PM on patients with established respiratory conditions, such as asthma and COPD. Such individuals are considered vulnerable because of their compromised respiratory reserve. In a national database comprising daily measurements of PM2.5, Dominici and colleagues[9] showed an association between acute changes in the PM2.5 concentration and hospitalizations for heart failure and COPD. Halonen and colleagues[10] showed, similarly, that acute changes in levels of PM2.5 were associated with hospital admissions for asthma and COPD with a lag of 4 days in children but additionally demonstrated an immediate effect in the elderly. Children may be another vulnerable group and one whose vulnerability to traffic-related air pollution (TRAP) may not always be apparent. Rabinovitch and colleagues[11] found that environmental tobacco smoke (ETS) obscured the relationship between morning maximum ambient PM2.5 levels and urinary leukotriene E4 (LTE4) in a group of asthmatic children; notably, only in the absence of elevated ETS exposure was PM2.5 significantly associated with significant increases in LTE4.

Although fine PM has become a dominant focus of concern over the past decades, there remains interest in toxicity attributable to the coarse fraction of PM (between 2.5 and 10 μm in diameter). A Danish study by Iskandar and colleagues[12] studied the association between pediatric hospital admissions for asthma and daily PM measurements, stratifying by particle size within a case-crossover design. There was a significant association of admissions with PM10 and PM2.5 but not ultrafine particles, suggesting a prominent role for coarse PM. Another study in patients with asthma noted a significant positive correlation between daily coarse particle exposure and peripheral blood eosinophils but not pulmonary function.[13]

Particulate Matter: Chronic Effects

Teasing out the contribution of each component of TRAP, inherently a mixture of PM and gases, is difficult because of the substantial correlation between TRAP components within epidemiologic studies. With that caveat, the association of particulate matter with mortality has been most extensively documented. Studies from 4 landmark cohorts, the Harvard Six Cities Study,[14] NMMAPS,[15–17] the American Cancer Society's Cancer Prevention Study II (CPS-II),[18] and APHEA,[19] have demonstrated a strong correlation between levels of PM in different cities in the United States and Europe and all-cause mortality. Much of the harm was attributed to fine particles with a diameter less than 2.5 μm (PM2.5).[20,21] A more recent study showed that residential PM2.5, but not PM10, was associated with respiratory mortality regardless of occupational exposure.[22]

Collectively, these observational data have been extremely influential in the creation, updating, and enforcement of international law and regulations, such as the Clean Air Act and the National Ambient Air Quality Standards (NAAQS).[23,24] The benefit of these statutory requirements seems apparent from an 8-year follow-up analysis of the Six Cities Study, which reaffirmed the impact of PM on mortality but also demonstrated the significant mortality reduction associated with a reduction in PM.[25] The average annual concentration of PM2.5 in the original 6 cities was reduced by between 1 and 7 μg/m^3, with the largest decreases in Steubenville and St Louis (which, notably, had the higher concentrations at the beginning of the study); they observed a relative risk for mortality of 0.77 associated with a 10 μg/m^3 decrease of PM2.5. Similar results were observed in a reanalysis of 1.2 million patients from the CPS-II cohort. Comparing mortality between 2 time periods, the late 1970s to the early 1980s and the late 1990s to the early 2000s, and carefully adjusting for key socioeconomic and demographic variables as well as cigarette smoking, a decrease of 10 μg/m^3 PM2.5 was associated with an estimated increase in mean life expectancy of 0.61 years.[26]

These decreasing trends in PM2.5 concentration and their associated mortality reductions are encouraging because they suggest a substantial benefit caused by decades of hard-fought PM reductions, but other novel findings temper this optimism. In the CPS II cohort, the concentration-effect relationship between PM and cardiovascular, cardiopulmonary, or all-cause mortality was exponential, with the steepest portion of the curve apparent at lower concentrations. The regression is almost linear at more than 50 μg/m^3 PM2.5, with a relatively modest additional increase in relative risk.[27] This observation suggests that ongoing reduction in PM2.5 levels, even well below the NAAQS for PM, may yield dramatic further reductions in mortality despite the additional cost.

The effect of long-term PM exposure on lung function has been a major area of research insight in the past decade, with 2 cohorts having made particular contributions. In the Children's Health Study (CHS), lung function in more than 1700 southern California children was observed prospectively from 10 to 18 years of age.[28,29]

PM2.5 and elemental carbon were each associated with reduced growth of forced expiratory volume in 1 second (FEV$_1$).[30] In the Swiss Cohort Study on Air Pollution and Lung Diseases in Adults (SAPALDIA),[31] lung function was assessed prospectively over 11 years in 9000 patients from 18 to 60 years of age. The annual exposure to PM10 for individual patients was estimated with a dispersion model, and multiple regression analyses (adjusting for cigarette smoking and other potential confounders) showed an inverse relationship between PM10 exposure and both the ratio of FEV$_1$ over forced vital capacity (FVC) as well as the forced expiratory flow (FEF) between 25% and 75% of the FVC.[32] Taken together, these observations from CHS and SAPALDIA were groundbreaking in connecting PM concentrations to physiologic end points of clear clinical significance in such large and well-characterized cohorts with prospective data.

The past decade has also been remarkable in advancing the evidence that PM is associated with incident asthma, particularly in children. A prospective cohort from the Netherlands, the Prevention and Incidence of Asthma and Mite Allergy (PIAMA) study,[33] demonstrated that PM2.5 levels were independently associated with significant increases in incidence and prevalence of asthma, as well as asthma symptoms[34] in a multi-pollutant model, including nitrogen dioxide (NO$_2$), soot, and PM2.5. Similar results were found in the CHS whereby there was an association between new onset asthma and levels of TRAP exposure.[35] PIAMA and several other birth cohorts have associated in utero and early life exposure to PM2.5, black carbon, and soot with incidence of asthma, wheeze, and atopy to common allergens later in life.[36–38] A case-control study from British Columbia looking at infants in the Georgia Air Basin showed an association of lifetime exposure to air pollutants from several sources, including wood smoke and TRAP, with an increased risk of consultation for bronchiolitis,[39] which could conceivably be interpreted as asthma in some settings.

Although the evidence for the causative role of PM exposure for an increased incidence of asthma in *adults* is not as well developed, several recent studies have substantially strengthened the rationale therein. A case-control study from Sweden suggested that living close to roads with high traffic volumes increases asthma incidence in people 20 to 60 years of age,[40] and another report showed similar findings in a broader age range (18–80 years of age).[41] In SAPALDIA, PM10 was significantly associated with adult-onset asthma in never-smokers, with a hazard ratio of 1.30 for each μg/m^3 increase in PM10 over the study period of 11 years.[42] Collectively, these observations strongly suggest that TRAP, even at concentrations typically considered acceptable by current regulatory standards, can cause asthma.

Chronic exposure to particulate matter is also associated with adverse outcomes in patients with preexisting asthma. Andersen and colleagues[43] found an association between long-term exposure to TRAP and the risk of asthma hospitalizations in the elderly within the Diet, Cancer, and Health study.

TRAP has also been associated with an increased incidence of COPD. In the Danish prospective cohort study, Diet, Cancer, and Health, which included 57 000 adult participants,[44] there was a positive association between COPD incidence and long-term exposure to TRAP[45]; the hazard ratio for COPD incidence was 1.08 for a 5.8 $\mu g/m^3$ increase in the 35-year mean NOx (used as a surrogate marker for TRAP). Again, it is difficult to tease out the specific contribution of PM among all the components of TRAP because of colinearity. In a recent policy statement by the American Thoracic Society on novel risk factors for COPD, the evidence supporting traffic and other outdoor air pollution as causal was deemed insufficient.[46]

Another area that has attracted a lot of interest in the last decade is the association between PM and lung cancer. In the CPS-II, the incidence of lung cancer increased by 8% per 10 $\mu g/m^3$ increase in PM2.5.[47] A subanalysis of the nearly 190 000 never-smokers in this cohort showed an even more dramatic effect of long-term exposure to PM, with a 15% to 27% increase in cancer mortality per 10 $\mu g/m^3$ increase in PM2.5.[48] With the same confounding caveats, the Danish Diet, Cancer, and Health study showed that the lung cancer incidence increased by 3.7% per 10 $\mu g/m^3$ increase in NOx (again used as a surrogate for TRAP).[49]

The tragic collapse of the World Trade Center (WTC) in New York City led to very high levels of airborne PM and served, sadly, as a fertile ground for novel insight into the subacute effects of such exposure. Banauch and colleagues[50] assessed pulmonary function of 12 000 rescue workers of the New York City Fire Department and showed an average decrease in FEV_1 of 372 mL 1 year after the tragedy; exposure intensity, estimated by the initial arrival time at the disaster site, correlated linearly with FEV_1 reduction. Related findings were reported by Herbert and colleagues[51] who showed novel respiratory symptoms in 61% of workers and abnormal spirometry in 28%. These abnormalities persisted for up to 2.5 years. Although the particulate matter released during the collapse of the WTC (mainly comprised of coarse [>53 μm in diameter] cement and fiberglass particles and less than 2% PM10 and PM2.5)[52] is substantially different than traditional AAP, the findings are generally consistent with the literature, summarized earlier in this review, regarding changes in lung function caused by longer-term but less intensive PM exposure.

Ozone

Although particulate matter has dominated the literature on AAP and respiratory health over the past decade, there is also remarkable new evidence regarding the impact of ozone on respiratory health. The most compelling epidemiologic data comes again from the CPS-II. As already mentioned, there was a significant correlation with long-term PM2.5 exposure and mortality. Long-term exposure to ozone was also associated with decreased life expectancy. Notably, when combining the two pollutants in the same model, PM2.5 was associated with mortality from cardiovascular causes and ozone with mortality from respiratory causes.[53]

To assess the impact of long-term ozone exposure on lung function, Tager and colleagues[54] investigated 255 students from the University of California in Berkley who were lifelong residents of Los Angeles or the San Francisco Bay Area and who were never-smokers. Lifetime exposure to ozone, PM10, and NO_2 was estimated based on spatial interpolation to all residences where the students had lived. There was a significant association between ozone exposure and small airway disease as measured by the ratio of FEF between 25% and 75% of FVC to FVC (FEF25–75/FVC), even after controlling for atopy, environmental tobacco smoke exposure, and other ambient pollutants. These results are consistent with the known deposition pattern of ozone in smaller airway.

Acute effects of ozone were studied by Luginaah and colleagues[55] in Ontario, who looked at the association between ambient air quality indicators, including NO_2, sulfur dioxide (SO_2), carbon monoxide, ozone, and PM10, and respiratory hospitalizations. Acute changes in PM had a significant effect on hospital admissions with a 1-day lag, but there was no such association with ozone.

Other Gases

Although recent years have shown less focus on components of AAP other than ozone and PM, an analysis of the APHEA-2 study found significant associations between NO_2 and respiratory mortality. Each increase of 10 $\mu g/m^3$ in peak daily levels of hourly measured NO_2 was associated with a 0.34% increase in respiratory mortality, even after correction for other pollutants (PM10, SO_2, and ozone).[56] O'Connor and colleagues[57] studied 861 children with asthma living in 7 US inner cities. Daily pollution measurements were correlated with asthma symptoms and lung function measured over a period of 2 months. Notably, almost all pollutant concentrations were within the NAAQS levels. Higher concentrations of NO_2, SO_2, and PM2.5 were independently associated with more symptoms and lower pulmonary function. Rosenlund and colleagues[58] studied an Italian cohort of more than 2000 children aged 9 to 14 years. Long-term exposure to NO_2 was estimated with a land-use regression model. Although the levels of NO_2 were not corrected for any other air pollutant in this study, there was a strong association between estimated long-term NO_2 exposure and lung function, with a larger effect in atopic children. The association with NO_2 in these studies is interesting, but firm conclusions are difficult to make because it is difficult to tease out its effect from that of TRAP in general. In some European studies mentioned earlier, NO_2 is the only pollutant measured as a surrogate for TRAP. For this reason, epidemiologic studies are not likely to be very informative about the independent respiratory effects of NO_2.

Co-exposures

There have been few studies looking at the impact of co-exposures on the respiratory health effects of AAP. An interesting finding by McConnell and colleagues[59] showed stronger associations between various air pollutants and asthma symptoms among children owning a dog compared with those who did not. They concluded that this observation suggests that a source of endotoxin, like dog ownership, may worsen the impact of AAP on children with asthma. This epidemiologic association, however, needs further confirmation in experimental studies.

EXPERIMENTAL STUDIES

Epidemiologic approaches are adept at identifying associations between AAP and clinical or biologic outcomes. In general, however, they alone cannot fully establish causality because key criteria for causality, such as biologic plausibility and dose response, typically require supplementary data from experimental models. The aim of experimental studies on air pollution is often to provide a mechanistic explanation to corroborate the epidemiologic observations; in the following sections, the authors describe some of the experimental data that have helped construct such plausibility.

Diesel Exhaust

The experimental literature on diesel exhaust's respiratory health effects has focused mainly on airway inflammation and hyperresponsiveness. A landmark study by McCreanor and colleagues[60] in London, England included 60 patients with mild or moderate asthma in a crossover design. Each individual walked for 2 hours on Oxford Street and, on a separate occasion, in Hyde Park. Oxford Street is notable because its vehicular traffic is almost exclusively diesel-powered buses and taxicabs, whereas Hyde Park is a large urban park in central London where no vehicular traffic is allowed. Pulmonary function, in terms of FEV_1, was significantly lower after the walk on Oxford Street compared with the walk in Hyde Park, and this effect was largest in patients with mild asthma. The exhaled breath condensate acidity and sputum neutrophil count was also measured as markers of airway inflammation, and both were increased by the Oxford Street exposure relative to the exposure in Hyde Park.[60]

The long-standing group from Umea, Sweden has also used a crossover design, but the exposures take place in a chamber where the level of particulate matter generated by a diesel engine can be tightly controlled. They have demonstrated that diesel exhaust induces bronchial hyperresponsiveness[61] in patients with moderate asthma (despite their taking inhaled corticosteroids), whereas it induces airway inflammation in healthy patients but not in patients with asthma.[62,63]

Ozone

Early, controlled, human exposure studies of healthy adults were critical in establishing that ozone reduces lung function, increases respiratory symptoms and airway responsiveness, and increases airway inflammation,[64,65] even at concentrations as low as 60 ppb.[66] In a more recent meta-analysis, Mudway and Kelly[67] revealed a dose-response relation between ozone and neutrophil concentrations in bronchoalveolar lavage (BAL). Arjomandi and colleagues[68] found increases in BAL macrophages after short-term repeated exposures to a low ozone concentration (20 ppb) in patients with asthma. Other recent studies have identified genetic risk factors of susceptibility to ozone and are discussed later.

Co-exposure Studies

Experimental co-exposure studies are important because they attempt to capture the complexity of real-world exposure to AAP within a tightly controlled model. A general summary of these studies is that co-exposures typically worsen the respiratory effects of AAP. In an animal model of asthma, Jaspers and colleagues[69] showed that the presence of diesel exhaust particles is able to markedly increase the inflammatory response to influenza virus. McDonald and colleagues[70] stressed the importance of particle composition to explain the impact of diesel exhaust particles on the susceptibility of viral infection in a mouse model. Recent in vitro experiments have shown that diesel exhaust particles are able to promote dendritic cell maturation, thus, suggesting that particulate pollutants act as adjuvants during allergic sensitization.[71,72] Others have suggested a role of diesel exhaust on T helper cells type 2 (TH2) polarization,[73] or a role of polycyclic hydrocarbon on smooth muscle beta-adrenergic receptor function.[74] These studies are only a few examples to show the relevance of these co-exposure studies and how they can allow a better understanding of the mechanisms that take place in real-world exposure.

GENETICS AND EPIGENETICS
Interindividual Variability in the Respiratory Effects of Air Pollutants

The studies mentioned earlier describe the effect of AAP on respiratory health and try to provide mechanistic explanations to its effects. However, it is clear that there is marked interindividual variability in the physiologic response to AAP. For example, a small proportion of ozone-exposed patients have relatively large airway responses.[75–77] Understanding this observation is one of the motivations for the study of genetic predispositions and epigenetic changes associated with AAP.

Antioxidant Gene Polymorphism

Much attention has been given to polymorphisms in genes related to oxidative stress because of the evidence that effects of AAP are often mediated by reactive oxidative species.[78,79] Notably, Gilliland and colleagues[80] used a co-exposure model of diesel exhaust and intranasal ragweed exposure in sensitized patients. Patients were divided into 3 subgroups according to single-nucleotide polymorphisms in genes coding for glutathione-S-transferases (GSTs), which are enzymes responsible for the metabolism of reactive oxygen species. The specific polymorphisms of interest were null genotypes for GSTM1 and GSTT1 and the GSTP1 codon 105 variant, all of which effectively confer loss of function. Patients with GSTM1 null or the GSTP1 codon 105 variant showed a significantly larger increase in immunoglobulin E production and histamine release following ragweed exposure in the presence of

diesel exhaust. This finding suggests that diesel adjuvancy of allergic responses is particularly potent in people with these genotypes.

Curjuric and colleagues[81] showed, using the SAPALDIA study, a significant interaction between PM10-associated decline in FEF25-75 and polymorphisms in GSTP1 and heme oxygenase-1 genes. Similar results were found by Schroer and colleagues[82] in the Cincinnati Childhood Allergy and Air Pollution Study, in which high Diesel exhaust particles (DEP) exposure conferred an increased risk for wheezing phenotypes but only among those with the GSTP1 codon 105 variant.

Another gene implicated in the oxidative stress pathway, NAD(P)H:quinine oxidoreductase (NQO1) gene, was identified by Castro-Giner and colleagues[83] as modifying the impact of AAP on asthma prevalence. Close to 3000 adults from the European Community Respiratory Health Survey were stratified by genotype and a significant interaction was found between NQO1 rs2917666 genotype and NO_2 for both asthma prevalence and new-onset asthma. Romieu and colleagues[84] found similar interactions with ozone and GSTs in children living in Mexico City. In a birth cohort from British Columbia, Carlsten and colleagues[85] also found an interaction between GSTP1 single-nucleotide polymorphisms and AAP in the risk for incident asthma in children.

Other Genes

The toll-like receptors (TLR) are implicated in innate immune response and have been suggested to participate in the response to different air pollutants.[86,87] Kerkhof and colleagues,[88] in the PIAMA birth cohort, identified single-nucleotide polymorphisms in TLR2 and TLR4 genes as significantly modifying the effect of PM2.5 on the prevalence of doctor-diagnosed asthma from birth up to 8 years of age.

Transforming growth factor (TGF)-b1 is involved in airway inflammation and remodeling, which are 2 key processes in asthma pathogenesis. Salam and colleagues,[89] using the CHS, showed that those with the TGF-b1 2509TT genotype are at an increased risk of asthma when exposed to maternal smoking in utero or to traffic-related emissions.

Epigenetics of Air Pollution

Efforts to understand mechanisms by which AAP can affect respiratory health increasingly include investigation of how AAP may directly alter DNA or genomic expression. Baccarelli and colleagues[90] showed that traffic-related particles could decrease global levels of DNA methylation in an older adult cohort as measured by 2 repeated elements: the long interspersed elements and the Alu elements. Interestingly, this group also demonstrated a significant interaction between GSTM1 single-nucleotide polymorphisms and PM on DNA methylation, suggesting a role for oxidative stress on the mechanism by which AAP can induce epigenetic changes.[91] Some have proposed a biochemical explanation for this observation in which particulate matter could induce the production of reactive oxygen species (ROS), which would then consume S-adenosylmethionine, the substrate used by DNA methyltransferases.[92] The same group also showed that the promoter region of the gene coding for the enzyme-inducible nitric oxide synthase was hypomethylated in peripheral blood leukocytes following exposure to particulate matter.[93] Soberanes and colleagues[94] showed hypermethylation of the p16 promoter region in alveolar epithelial cells in relation to particulate matter, suggesting precarcinogenic changes. Reflecting interest in AAP-related changes in gene expression in the lung, Jardim and colleagues[95] demonstrated changes in micro-RNA profiles in airway epithelial cells.

Overall, exploration of gene-environment interactions shows promise in terms of understanding mechanisms of respiratory disease related to AAP, but the full potential of genetics in this context may best lie in supporting lower exposure limits to protect vulnerable populations.[96] There is further promise for genome-wide interaction studies (GWIS) to elucidate new pathways of vulnerability, although GWIS has not been successfully applied to AAP.

SUMMARY AND FUTURE RESEARCH

In summary, the last decade of research on AAP has confirmed its adverse impact on respiratory morbidity and mortality, quality of life, and economic burden on health care systems. Efforts to reduce AAP have been fruitful in terms of reduced mortality, but the concentration-effect relationship seems steepest at the lower end of the concentration range, suggesting that further reductions in AAP may confer marked additional benefit.

Evidence for incident asthma caused by AAP has proliferated, strengthening the claim of a cause-effect relationship, particularly in children. Moreover, there is new evidence for AAP leading to the increased incidence of respiratory diseases in adults, including asthma, COPD, and lung cancer, which collectively may contribute substantially to global respiratory health and, thus, should motivate corresponding regulations. This point is of critical importance because such insight may support additional efforts to prevent new lung

disease, and the prevention of new disease generally has a larger impact than does preventing exacerbations of existing disease.

Research has demonstrated that co-exposures have the potential to dramatically augment the effects of AAP and, thus, lower the threshold of effect of a given pollutant. Interactions between genes related to oxidative stress and AAP seem to significantly alter the effect of AAP on an individual and population basis. Better definition of vulnerable populations, those particularly susceptible to AAP, may bolster local or regional efforts to remediate AAP. Advances in genetic research tools, including GWIS, have the potential to identify candidate genes that can guide further research.

More work on potential therapeutics and interventions needs be done. For example, despite considerable efforts to implicate oxidative stress as a major mechanism for AAP-related lung disease, there is currently insufficient evidence to recommend antioxidants routinely therein.[97] Further reductions of PM seem well motivated,[26] but further such reductions will require innovation, integrating land-use and urban planning decisions,[98] to optimize the health impacts of AAP at the individual and community levels. The use of air filters has also been suggested as being part of the solution,[99] perhaps even as applied to reducing acute exposures to high levels of TRAP in road congestions during rush hour commutes,[100] but more research in this field is needed.[101,102]

REFERENCES

1. Vedal S. Update on the health effects of outdoor air pollution. Clin Chest Med 2002;23:763–75, vi.
2. Laumbach RJ. Outdoor air pollutants and patient health. Am Fam Physician 2010;81:175–80.
3. Laumbach RJ, Kipen HM. Respiratory health effects of air pollution: update on biomass smoke and traffic pollution. J Allergy Clin Immunol 2012;129:3–11 [Quiz: 2–3].
4. Ruckerl R, Schneider A, Breitner S, et al. Health effects of particulate air pollution: a review of epidemiological evidence. Inhal Toxicol 2011;23:555–92.
5. Braback L, Forsberg B. Does traffic exhaust contribute to the development of asthma and allergic sensitization in children: findings from recent cohort studies. Environ Health 2009;8:17.
6. Brook RD, Rajagopalan S, Pope CA 3rd, et al. Particulate matter air pollution and cardiovascular disease: an update to the scientific statement from the American Heart Association. Circulation 2010;121:2331–78.
7. Katsouyanni K, Samet JM, Anderson HR, et al. Air pollution and health: a European and North

American approach (APHENA). Res Rep Health Eff Inst 2009;5–90.

8. Samoli E, Peng R, Ramsay T, et al. Acute effects of ambient particulate matter on mortality in Europe and North America: results from the APHENA study. Environ Health Perspect 2008;116:1480–6.

9. Dominici F, Peng RD, Bell ML, et al. Fine particulate air pollution and hospital admission for cardiovascular and respiratory diseases. JAMA 2006;295: 1127–34.

10. Halonen JI, Lanki T, Yli-Tuomi T, et al. Urban air pollution, and asthma and COPD hospital emergency room visits. Thorax 2008;63:635–41.

11. Rabinovitch N, Silveira L, Gelfand EW, et al. The response of children with asthma to ambient particulate is modified by tobacco smoke exposure. Am J Respir Crit Care Med 2011;184:1350–7.

12. Iskandar A, Andersen ZJ, Bonnelykke K, et al. Coarse and fine particles but not ultrafine particles in urban air trigger hospital admission for asthma in children. Thorax 2012;67:252–7.

13. Yeatts K, Svendsen E, Creason J, et al. Coarse particulate matter (PM2.5–10) affects heart rate variability, blood lipids, and circulating eosinophils in adults with asthma. Environ Health Perspect 2007;115:709–14.

14. Dockery DW, Pope CA 3rd, Xu X, et al. An association between air pollution and mortality in six U.S. cities. N Engl J Med 1993;329:1753–9.

15. Samet JM, Dominici F, Zeger SL, et al. The National Morbidity, Mortality, and Air Pollution Study. Part I: methods and methodologic issues. Res Rep Health Eff Inst 2000;5–14 [discussion: 75–84].

16. Samet JM, Zeger SL, Dominici F, et al. The National Morbidity, Mortality, and Air Pollution Study. Part II: morbidity and mortality from air pollution in the United States. Res Rep Health Eff Inst 2000;94: 5–70 [discussion: 1–9].

17. Daniels MJ, Dominici F, Zeger SL, et al. The National Morbidity, Mortality, and Air Pollution Study. Part III: PM10 concentration-response curves and thresholds for the 20 largest US cities. Res Rep Health Eff Inst 2004;1–21 [discussion: 3–30].

18. Cancer Prevention Study II. The American Cancer Society Prospective Study. Stat Bull Metrop Insur Co 1992;73:21–9.

19. Katsouyanni K, Zmirou D, Spix C, et al. Short-term effects of air pollution on health: a European approach using epidemiological time-series data. The APHEA project: background, objectives, design. Eur Respir J 1995;8:1030–8.

20. Krewski D, Burnett RT, Goldberg M, et al. Reanalysis of the Harvard Six Cities Study, part I: validation and replication. Inhal Toxicol 2005;17:335–42.

21. Krewski D, Burnett RT, Goldberg M, et al. Reanalysis of the Harvard Six Cities Study, part II: sensitivity analysis. Inhal Toxicol 2005;17:343–53.

22. Hart JE, Garshick E, Dockery DW, et al. Long-term ambient multipollutant exposures and mortality. Am J Respir Crit Care Med 2011;183:73–8.

23. Samet JM. The Clean Air Act and health–a clearer view from 2011. N Engl J Med 2011;365:198–201.

24. Huang YC, Brook RD. The Clean Air Act: science, policy, and politics. Chest 2011;140:1–2.

25. Laden F, Schwartz J, Speizer FE, et al. Reduction in fine particulate air pollution and mortality: extended follow-up of the Harvard Six Cities study. Am J Respir Crit Care Med 2006;173:667–72.

26. Pope CA 3rd, Ezzati M, Dockery DW. Fine-particulate air pollution and life expectancy in the United States. N Engl J Med 2009;360:376–86.

27. Pope CA 3rd, Burnett RT, Turner MC, et al. Lung cancer and cardiovascular disease mortality associated with ambient air pollution and cigarette smoke: shape of the exposure-response relationships. Environ Health Perspect 2011;119:1616–21.

28. Peters JM, Avol E, Navidi W, et al. A study of twelve Southern California communities with differing levels and types of air pollution. I. Prevalence of respiratory morbidity. Am J Respir Crit Care Med 1999;159:760–7.

29. Peters JM, Avol E, Gauderman WJ, et al. A study of twelve Southern California communities with differing levels and types of air pollution. II. Effects on pulmonary function. Am J Respir Crit Care Med 1999;159:768–75.

30. Gauderman WJ, Avol E, Gilliland F, et al. The effect of air pollution on lung development from 10 to 18 years of age. N Engl J Med 2004;351:1057–67.

31. Ackermann-Liebrich U, Leuenberger P, Schwartz J, et al. Lung function and long term exposure to air pollutants in Switzerland. Study on Air Pollution and Lung Diseases in Adults (SAPALDIA) team. Am J Respir Crit Care Med 1997;155:122–9.

32. Downs SH, Schindler C, Liu LJ, et al. Reduced exposure to PM10 and attenuated age-related decline in lung function. N Engl J Med 2007;357: 2338–47.

33. Brunekreef B, Smit J, de Jongste J, et al. The prevention and incidence of asthma and mite allergy (PIAMA) birth cohort study: design and first results. Pediatr Allergy Immunol 2002;15(Suppl 13): 55–60.

34. Gehring U, Wijga AH, Brauer M, et al. Traffic-related air pollution and the development of asthma and allergies during the first 8 years of life. Am J Respir Crit Care Med 2010;181:596–603.

35. Jerrett M, Shankardass K, Berhane K, et al. Traffic-related air pollution and asthma onset in children: a prospective cohort study with individual exposure measurement. Environ Health Perspect 2008;116:1433–8.

36. Carlsten C, Dybuncio A, Becker A, et al. Traffic-related air pollution and incident asthma in

a high-risk birth cohort. Occup Environ Med 2011; 68:291–5.

37. Brauer M, Hoek G, Smit HA, et al. Air pollution and development of asthma, allergy and infections in a birth cohort. Eur Respir J 2007;29:879–88.

38. Clark NA, Demers PA, Karr CJ, et al. Effect of early life exposure to air pollution on development of childhood asthma. Environ Health Perspect 2010; 118:284–90.

39. Karr CJ, Demers PA, Koehoorn MW, et al. Influence of ambient air pollutant sources on clinical encounters for infant bronchiolitis. Am J Respir Crit Care Med 2009;180:995–1001.

40. Modig L, Jarvholm B, Ronnmark E, et al. Vehicle exhaust exposure in an incident case-control study of adult asthma. Eur Respir J 2006;28:75–81.

41. Lindgren A, Bjork J, Stroh E, et al. Adult asthma and traffic exposure at residential address, workplace address, and self-reported daily time outdoor in traffic: a two-stage case-control study. BMC Public Health 2010;10:716.

42. Kunzli N, Bridevaux PO, Liu LJ, et al. Traffic-related air pollution correlates with adult-onset asthma among never-smokers. Thorax 2009;64:664–70.

43. Andersen ZJ, Bonnelykke K, Hvidberg M, et al. Long-term exposure to air pollution and asthma hospitalisations in older adults: a cohort study. Thorax 2012;67:6–11.

44. Tjonneland A, Olsen A, Boll K, et al. Study design, exposure variables, and socioeconomic determinants of participation in Diet, Cancer and Health: a population-based prospective cohort study of 57,053 men and women in Denmark. Scand J Public Health 2007;35:432–41.

45. Andersen ZJ, Hvidberg M, Jensen SS, et al. Chronic obstructive pulmonary disease and long-term exposure to traffic-related air pollution: a cohort study. Am J Respir Crit Care Med 2011; 183:455–61.

46. Eisner MD, Anthonisen N, Coultas D, et al. An official American Thoracic Society public policy statement: novel risk factors and the global burden of chronic obstructive pulmonary disease. Am J Respir Crit Care Med 2010;182:693–718.

47. Pope CA 3rd, Burnett RT, Thun MJ, et al. Lung cancer, cardiopulmonary mortality, and long-term exposure to fine particulate air pollution. JAMA 2002;287:1132–41.

48. Turner MC, Krewski D, Pope CA 3rd, et al. Long-term ambient fine particulate matter air pollution and lung cancer in a large cohort of never-smokers. Am J Respir Crit Care Med 2011;184: 1374–81.

49. Raaschou-Nielsen O, Andersen ZJ, Hvidberg M, et al. Lung cancer incidence and long-term exposure to air pollution from traffic. Environ Health Perspect 2011;119:860–5.

50. Banauch GI, Hall C, Weiden M, et al. Pulmonary function after exposure to the World Trade Center collapse in the New York City Fire Department. Am J Respir Crit Care Med 2006;174:312–9.

51. Herbert R, Moline J, Skloot G, et al. The World Trade Center disaster and the health of workers: five-year assessment of a unique medical screening program. Environ Health Perspect 2006;114:1853–8.

52. Lioy PJ, Weisel CP, Millette JR, et al. Characterization of the dust/smoke aerosol that settled east of the World Trade Center (WTC) in lower Manhattan after the collapse of the WTC 11 September 2001. Environ Health Perspect 2002;110:703–14.

53. Jerrett M, Burnett RT, Pope CA 3rd, et al. Long-term ozone exposure and mortality. N Engl J Med 2009;360:1085–95.

54. Tager IB, Balmes J, Lurmann F, et al. Chronic exposure to ambient ozone and lung function in young adults. Epidemiology 2005;16:751–9.

55. Luginaah IN, Fung KY, Gorey KM, et al. Association of ambient air pollution with respiratory hospitalization in a government-designated "area of concern": the case of Windsor, Ontario. Environ Health Perspect 2005;113:290–6.

56. Samoli E, Aga E, Touloumi G, et al. Short-term effects of nitrogen dioxide on mortality: an analysis within the APHEA project. Eur Respir J 2006;27: 1129–38.

57. O'Connor GT, Neas L, Vaughn B, et al. Acute respiratory health effects of air pollution on children with asthma in US inner cities. J Allergy Clin Immunol 2008;121:1133–1139.e1.

58. Rosenlund M, Forastiere F, Porta D, et al. Traffic-related air pollution in relation to respiratory symptoms, allergic sensitisation and lung function in schoolchildren. Thorax 2009;64:573–80.

59. McConnell R, Berhane K, Molitor J, et al. Dog ownership enhances symptomatic responses to air pollution in children with asthma. Environ Health Perspect 2006;114:1910–5.

60. McCreanor J, Cullinan P, Nieuwenhuijsen MJ, et al. Respiratory effects of exposure to diesel traffic in persons with asthma. N Engl J Med 2007;357: 2348–58.

61. Nordenhall C, Pourazar J, Ledin MC, et al. Diesel exhaust enhances airway responsiveness in asthmatic subjects. Eur Respir J 2001;17:909–15.

62. Behndig AF, Larsson N, Brown JL, et al. Proinflammatory doses of diesel exhaust in healthy subjects fail to elicit equivalent or augmented airway inflammation in subjects with asthma. Thorax 2011;66: 12–9.

63. Stenfors N, Nordenhall C, Salvi SS, et al. Different airway inflammatory responses in asthmatic and healthy humans exposed to diesel. Eur Respir J 2004;23:82–6.

64. Devlin RB, McDonnell WF, Mann R, et al. Exposure of humans to ambient levels of ozone for 6.6 hours causes cellular and biochemical changes in the lung. Am J Respir Cell Mol Biol 1991;4:72–81.

65. Horstman DH, Folinsbee LJ, Ives PJ, et al. Ozone concentration and pulmonary response relationships for 6.6-hour exposures with five hours of moderate exercise to 0.08, 0.10, and 0.12 ppm. Am Rev Respir Dis 1990;142:1158–63.

66. Kinney PL, Nilsen DM, Lippmann M, et al. Biomarkers of lung inflammation in recreational joggers exposed to ozone. Am J Respir Crit Care Med 1996;154:1430–5.

67. Mudway IS, Kelly FJ. An investigation of inhaled ozone dose and the magnitude of airway inflammation in healthy adults. Am J Respir Crit Care Med 2004;169:1089–95.

68. Arjomandi M, Witten A, Abbritti E, et al. Repeated exposure to ozone increases alveolar macrophage recruitment into asthmatic airways. Am J Respir Crit Care Med 2005;172:427–32.

69. Jaspers I, Sheridan PA, Zhang W, et al. Exacerbation of allergic inflammation in mice exposed to diesel exhaust particles prior to viral infection. Part Fibre Toxicol 2009;6:22.

70. McDonald JD, Campen MJ, Harrod KS, et al. Engine-operating load influences diesel exhaust composition and cardiopulmonary and immune responses. Environ Health Perspect 2011;119:1136–41.

71. Bleck B, Tse DB, Curotto de Lafaille MA, et al. Diesel exhaust particle-exposed human bronchial epithelial cells induce dendritic cell maturation and polarization via thymic stromal lymphopoietin. J Clin Immunol 2008;28:147–56.

72. Bleck B, Tse DB, Jaspers I, et al. Diesel exhaust particle-exposed human bronchial epithelial cells induce dendritic cell maturation. J Immunol 2006; 176:7431–7.

73. Finkelman FD, Yang M, Orekhova T, et al. Diesel exhaust particles suppress in vivo IFN-gamma production by inhibiting cytokine effects on NK and NKT cells. J Immunol 2004;172:3808–13.

74. Factor P, Akhmedov AT, McDonald JD, et al. Polycyclic aromatic hydrocarbons impair function of beta2-adrenergic receptors in airway epithelial and smooth muscle cells. Am J Respir Cell Mol Biol 2011;45:1045–9.

75. McDonnell WF 3rd, Horstman DH, Abdul-Salaam S, et al. Reproducibility of individual responses to ozone exposure. Am Rev Respir Dis 1985;131:36–40.

76. Holz O, Jorres RA, Timm P, et al. Ozone-induced airway inflammatory changes differ between individuals and are reproducible. Am J Respir Crit Care Med 1999;159:776–84.

77. McDonnell WF. Individual variability in human lung function responses to ozone exposure. Environ Toxicol Pharmacol 1996;2:171–5.

78. Minelli C, Wei I, Sagoo G, et al. Interactive effects of antioxidant genes and air pollution on respiratory function and airway disease: a HuGE review. Am J Epidemiol 2011;173:603–20.

79. Li N, Hao M, Phalen RF, et al. Particulate air pollutants and asthma. A paradigm for the role of oxidative stress in PM-induced adverse health effects. Clin Immunol 2003;109:250–65.

80. Gilliland FD, Li YF, Saxon A, et al. Effect of glutathione-S-transferase M1 and P1 genotypes on xenobiotic enhancement of allergic responses: randomised, placebo-controlled crossover study. Lancet 2004;363:119–25.

81. Curjuric I, Imboden M, Schindler C, et al. HMOX1 and GST variants modify attenuation of FEF25-75% decline due to PM10 reduction. Eur Respir J 2010;35:505–14.

82. Schroer KT, Biagini Myers JM, Ryan PH, et al. Associations between multiple environmental exposures and Glutathione S-Transferase P1 on persistent wheezing in a birth cohort. J Pediatr 2009;154:401–8, 408.e1.

83. Castro-Giner F, Kunzli N, Jacquemin B, et al. Traffic-related air pollution, oxidative stress genes, and asthma (ECHRS). Environ Health Perspect 2009;117:1919–24.

84. Romieu I, Ramirez-Aguilar M, Sienra-Monge JJ, et al. GSTM1 and GSTP1 and respiratory health in asthmatic children exposed to ozone. Eur Respir J 2006;28:953–9.

85. Carlsten C, Dybuncio A, Becker A, et al. GSTP1 polymorphism modifies risk for incident asthma associated with nitrogen dioxide in a high-risk birth cohort. Occup Environ Med 2011;68:308.

86. Becker S, Mundandhara S, Devlin RB, et al. Regulation of cytokine production in human alveolar macrophages and airway epithelial cells in response to ambient air pollution particles: further mechanistic studies. Toxicol Appl Pharmacol 2005;207:269–75.

87. Becker S, Fenton MJ, Soukup JM. Involvement of microbial components and toll-like receptors 2 and 4 in cytokine responses to air pollution particles. Am J Respir Cell Mol Biol 2002;27:611–8.

88. Kerkhof M, Postma DS, Brunekreef B, et al. Toll-like receptor 2 and 4 genes influence susceptibility to adverse effects of traffic-related air pollution on childhood asthma. Thorax 2010;65:690–7.

89. Salam MT, Gauderman WJ, McConnell R, et al. Transforming growth factor- 1 C-509T polymorphism, oxidant stress, and early-onset childhood asthma. Am J Respir Crit Care Med 2007;176:1192–9.

90. Baccarelli A, Wright RO, Bollati V, et al. Rapid DNA methylation changes after exposure to traffic particles. Am J Respir Crit Care Med 2009;179:572–8.

91. Madrigano J, Baccarelli A, Mittleman MA, et al. Prolonged exposure to particulate pollution, genes

associated with glutathione pathways, and DNA methylation in a cohort of older men. Environ Health Perspect 2011;119:977–82.

92. Ji H, Khurana Hershey GK. Genetic and epigenetic influence on the response to environmental particulate matter. J Allergy Clin Immunol 2012;129:33–41.

93. Tarantini L, Bonzini M, Apostoli P, et al. Effects of particulate matter on genomic DNA methylation content and iNOS promoter methylation. Environ Health Perspect 2009;117:217–22.

94. Soberanes S, Gonzalez A, Urich D, et al. Particulate matter air pollution induces hypermethylation of the p16 promoter via a mitochondrial ROS-JNK-DNMT1 pathway. Sci Rep 2012;2:275.

95. Jardim MJ, Fry RC, Jaspers I, et al. Disruption of microRNA expression in human airway cells by diesel exhaust particles is linked to tumorigenesis-associated pathways. Environ Health Perspect 2009;117:1745–51.

96. Gilliland FD. Outdoor air pollution, genetic susceptibility, and asthma management: opportunities for intervention to reduce the burden of asthma. Pediatrics 2009;123(Suppl 3):S168–73.

97. Tashakkor AY, Chow KS, Carlsten C. Modification by antioxidant supplementation of changes in human lung function associated with air pollutant exposure: a systematic review. BMC Public Health 2011;11:532.

98. Giles LV, Barn P, Kunzli N, et al. From good intentions to proven interventions: effectiveness of actions to reduce the health impacts of air pollution. Environ Health Perspect 2011;119:29–36.

99. Sublett JL. Effectiveness of air filters and air cleaners in allergic respiratory diseases: a review of the recent literature. Curr Allergy Asthma Rep 2011;11:395–402.

100. Zuurbier M, Hoek G, Oldenwening M, et al. In-traffic air pollution exposure and CC16, blood coagulation, and inflammation markers in healthy adults. Environ Health Perspect 2011; 119:1384–9.

101. Balmes J, Pinkerton K. Clearing the air. Am J Respir Crit Care Med 2012;185:1–2.

102. Brunekreef B, Annesi-Maesano I, Ayres JG, et al. Ten principles for clean air. Eur Respir J 2012;39: 525–8.

Induced Sputum, Exhaled Nitric Oxide, and Particles in Exhaled Air in Assessing Airways Inflammation in Occupational Exposures

Anna-Carin Olin, PhD, MD

KEYWORDS

- Exhaled nitric oxide • Induced sputum • Exhaled particles • Occupational exposure

KEY POINTS

- Sensitive methods to detect airways inflammation caused by exposures associated with adverse respiratory effects are crucial, as is the identification of individuals with early-stage disease.
- In this review, the use of induced sputum and sampling of the fraction of nitric oxide methods to identify airways inflammation associated with occupational exposures is discussed.

INTRODUCTION

Several new, noninvasive methods have been developed in the last decade to study inflammation in the airways. These methods address, in part, the need for objective and easy methods to characterize such inflammatory processes. The key methods are quantifying the fraction of exhaled nitric oxide (FENO), characterizing induced sputum (IS), and sampling exhaled breath condensate (EBC) and particles in exhaled air (PEx). In the clinical context of occupational health, identification of exposures associated with adverse respiratory effects is a priority, and, in particular, there is a pressing need for sensitive methods to identify individuals with disease in the early stages of airway inflammation.

Over the last decade, IS has emerged as a well-recognized method in occupational medicine research, enabling characterization of inflammatory patterns associated with work-related exposures. The use of IS has informed several studies addressing inflammatory mechanisms and pathways in work-related airway disease. Despite its research applications, IS can be cumbersome and time-consuming. This characteristic limits its suitability for screening applications or its adoption in clinical occupational health services.

For these reasons, FENO measurement, an easier method to perform, can be a compelling alternative to IS analysis. However, a central question is whether or not FENO can be used to substitute for the assessment of eosinophilic airways inflammation as directly quantified by IS. Studies have shown that FENO is associated with eosinophils in sputum or in bronchoalveolar lavage, yet that association, as shown by Berry and colleagues in one of the largest studies of adults thus far,[1] is only modest, and in children, as reported by Manso and colleagues,[2] it is poor. This variability may reflect the reality that the use of FENO to study inflammation is not straightforward. For example, both cigarette smoking and airway

Occupational and Environmental Medicine, Sahlgrenska Academy, Gothenburg University, Box 414 S- 405 30 Göteborg, Sweden
E-mail address: anna-carin.olin@amm.gu.se

Clin Chest Med 33 (2012) 771–782
http://dx.doi.org/10.1016/j.ccm.2012.08.002
0272-5231/12/$ – see front matter © 2012 Elsevier Inc. All rights reserved.

obstruction may confound the results of FENO, a set of problems that are discussed further later.

This review focuses on the recent biomedical literature reporting on the use of noninvasive methods to assess airways inflammation in association with occupational exposures, emphasizing studies using IS or FENO methods. The studies reviewed were identified via an on-line search of PubMed using the mesh-terms occupation* AND exposure AND nitric oxide/induced sputum. There have been several excellent recent reviews of IS.[3–5] For that reason, results presented here for IS emphasize new findings and approaches in the application of this method, as well as studies comparing IS and FENO. Furthermore, case reports using FENO have been omitted. An alternative novel, noninvasive method to assess airways inflammation in small airways is reviewed, the sampling of PEx. This method is juxtaposed with sampling EBC, addressing several serious methodologic challenges with the EBC approach.

New methods to assess airways inflammation need to be compared with a reference method. The gold standard to define airways inflammation is by bronchial biopsy (eg, via bronchoscopy). In practice, this method is relatively invasive, expensive, and rarely applicable in the study of large cohorts. Moreover, bronchial biopsies are limited to the central airways, limiting their generalizability to more distal inflammation. Hence newer methods of measuring airway inflammation are often compared with each other rather than with biopsy data. In addition, correlation with one or more indirect measures of airways inflammation, such as bronchial hyperresponsiveness (BHR) or respiratory symptoms, may be reported.

Another central problem to the validation of newer methods is that there are many subtypes of airways inflammation. There have been attempts to phenotype inflammation, but, so far, the most pragmatic approach has been to subdivide it into eosinophilic (allergic) versus neutrophilic airways inflammation, because this has proved helpful, for example, in guiding the treatment.[6] In generic asthma, Wentzel and colleagues[7] have suggested delineation of a paucigranular phenotype as well, but this has not yet been applied in occupational asthma (OA). Transcriptional analysis of IS has been used to phenotype 59 patients with asthma by Baines and colleagues.[8] Cluster analysis of the gene expression profiles supported the presence of 3 distinct asthma phenotypes: (1) an eosinophilic phenotype, with higher FENO and lower FEV_1 (forced expiratory volume in first second of expiration) predicted; (2) a neutrophilic phenotype, with decrements of both FEV_1 and FVC (forced vital capacity); and (3) a third phenotype, with increased number of macrophages and with almost normal lung function. Haldar and colleagues[9] presented a more clinically oriented approach, based on level of eosinophils in IS and symptoms from 371 patients with asthma, resulting in 3 major groups of asthma: concordant disease (symptoms are associated with levels of eosinophils); discordant symptoms (more symptoms and fewer eosinophils); and discordant inflammation (few or no symptoms, but with eosinophilia).

IS IN OCCUPATIONAL RESPIRATORY DISEASE

Analysis of IS promises to be a valuable tool in identifying inflammatory patterns and recognizing disease phenotypes in OA as well, although data are limited.[4,10] Studies have used IS to classify the subtype of inflammation after various exposures. However, the same exposure does not seem to elicit the same pattern of inflammation in all individuals. Moreover, both low-molecular-weight (LMW) and high-molecular-weight (HMW) agents, despite their presumed differences in immunologic pathways, seem to be able to induce eosinophilic inflammation.[11] Further, Prince and colleagues[3] observed that both LMW and HMW agents induced eosinophils or neutrophils, but these agents were also associated with an increase in macrophages and lymphocytes as measured by IS.

The mechanisms underlying this heterogeneity are unclear and may depend on individual host factors as well as other exposures. For example, smoking has been shown to enhance the neutrophilic response seen in IS.[3,12] These results may also reflect the time at which the response is measured, because neutrophils and eosinophils may have different kinetics within the natural history of the inflammatory process. This question is particularly challenging because methodologic aspects of IS (eg, its proinflammatory effect) make it difficult to repeat this test to follow the short-term time course of shifting populations of effector cells. Specifically, the method gives rise to neutrophilic influx, limiting short-term, repeated sampling within the same patient, although it seems safe to repeat the test within 24 hours.[4,13]

Methodologic Aspects

A major limitation of the IS method is that it is more or less laboratory-based. Samples have to be prepared within short after sampling and their handling is not straightforward. For this reason, IS is most often used in controlled-exposure challenge studies, in which the complexity of real-world exposures can be lost. This disadvantage is shown by a study by Sundblad and colleagues[12] in which patients were exposed to endotoxins (either 3 hours in real life in a barn or by lipopolysaccharide [LPS] inhalation in the laboratory); the former exposure induced a profoundly stronger inflammatory reaction, despite the fact that the LPS concentration in the field was 200 times lower than that administered in the laboratory. Another limitation of IS is that around 20% of patients cannot produce a sputum sample adequate for analysis.

IS and Specific Inhalation Challenge Testing

In the diagnosis of OA, specific inhalation challenge (SIC) is the reference test performed in many locations, for example, Quebec, Canada, and Finland. SIC can induce an immediate, late, or dual asthmatic reaction, defined by the pattern of FEV_1 after challenge, where a 20% drop in FEV_1 is defined as a positive test. SIC is often used in combination with IS, a valuable adjunct to spirometry that can give better insights into the airway inflammatory aspect of the disease. In parallel with spirometric changes that can vary over time, the influx of inflammatory cells into the airways also have certain time-dependent patterns of response. However, as noted earlier, it is not possible to follow this pattern by serial same-day IS measurement.

In the context of SIC, IS has been used to classify effects of exposure to a wide variety of substances that have the potential to induce asthma, both LMW and HMW agents. Both LMW and HMW compounds seem to be able to induce both eosinophilic and neutrophilic inflammation, and there does not seem to be a clear association between type of exposure and inflammatory pattern. Again, the interpretation of the results is limited because IS gives only a snapshot of the induced inflammatory pattern. For example, a recent retrospective study by Malo and colleagues[10] analyzed data from 519 patients who underwent an SIC test for the suspected diagnosis of OA. On a control day without exposure, increased levels of sputum eosinophils were found in only half of the patients diagnosed with OA and 27% were found to have normal BHR in the control assessment. The positive predictive value (PPV) and the negative predictive value (NPV) for identifying OA among the entire pool of tested patients (some who did not have asthma of any kind) were similar for post-SIC sputum eosinophilia and PC_{20} (the provocative concentration causing a 20% decrease in FEV_1). Limiting the study pool to asthma alone, post-SIC increased levels of eosinophils by IS performed better than PC_{20} in predicting occupational disease (PPV 44% vs 35%; NPV 58% vs 30%).

Vandenplas and colleagues[14] also investigated whether IS after SIC improves the predictive value of the test, studying 68 consecutive patients examined for respiratory symptoms suggestive of OA. They were first challenged to a sham agent and then up to 3 times with the suspected agent (including both HMW and LMW agents). Of 68 patients, 39 had a positive SIC. Receiver-operator-curve (ROC) analysis found that an increase in sputum eosinophils after the first challenge had the highest discriminating power to predict OA defined by a positive SIC. An increase of at least 3% in sputum eosinophils achieved the best combination of specificity (97%) and sensitivity (67%).

IS and Pathophysiologic Processes in OA

Sputum induction has provided new insights into inflammatory pathways associated with various occupational exposures. Hur and colleagues[15] studied IS after challenge with methyl diphenyl diisocyanate (MDI) among 13 MDI-exposed workers with respiratory symptoms and 2 control individuals. Exposure was associated with mast-cell activation (indicated by an increase in tryptase), interleukin 8, and vascular endothelial growth factor in IS, and eosinophilic activation. It was suggested that these proinflammatory mediators were responsible for eosinophil recruitment and activation.

IS has also been used to examine the degree of vascular leakage in the respiratory tract, a measure that may show more general harmful effects to the airways. Moreira and colleagues[16] developed a vascular permeability index though measurements of albumin in IS and serum, examining 13 elite swimmers, 6 asthmatic swimmers, and 19 individuals with asthma using IS, FENO, and methacholine challenge testing. Each unit change in the vascular permeability index was associated with an increase of 1% in eosinophils and 2.6% in neutrophils in IS, whereas no association with FENO was observed nor was there any significant difference in the vascular permeability index among the groups.

IS and Prognosis in OA

In a study by Lemiere and colleagues,[17] 19 patients with diagnosis of OA by a SIC test were followed at 2 weeks, 6 months, and 1, 2, 3, and 4 years after removal from exposure with IS, spirometry, and metacholine-challenge test at each time point (13 patients had OA caused by HMW agents and 11 patients by LMW agents). There was no significant improvement in clinical parameters; those with a neutrophilic predominance in sputum after

SIC had a poorer prognosis and there was an inverse correlation between eosinophil counts and PC_{20} 3 years after removal from exposure. Those having less than a 2% increase in eosinophils after SIC but reacting with an increase in neutrophils also had significantly lower lung function (predicted FEV_1 81.3% vs 89.2%) after 4 years.

IS and Occupational Eosinophilic Bronchitis

Eosinophilic bronchitis is defined as chronic cough in patients with no symptoms of or objective evidence of variable airflow obstruction (normal BHR) and sputum eosinophilia.[18] The discriminative power of FENO for this IS-defined diagnosis has not yet been elucidated, and data on the prevalence of occupational eosinophilic bronchitis are scarce.[19] This diagnostic entity warrants additional study given that up to 8% of patients with OA can have a normal BHR test and thus could have findings consistent with this syndrome.[10]

EXHALED NITRIC OXIDE IN THE ASSESSMENT OF OCCUPATIONAL EXPOSURE EFFECTS

Since it first came to the fore two decades ago, FENO measurement has gained a great deal of interest as a biomarker of inflammation. Nonetheless, its usefulness in the assessment of occupational respiratory disease is far from clear. Eosinophilic airway inflammation measured by IS correlates with FENO, but the two approaches are not interchangeable. Rather, each approach seems to provide another piece that is a part of the puzzle of inflammation. Large comparative studies of eosinophils in IS and FENO have shown only a modest degree of correlation: $R^2 = 0.26$ (albeit statistically significant).[1] Although data are limited, the post-SIC challenge time course of an increase in FENO and an increase in eosinophils in sputum seems not to run in parallel (potentially because the increase of FENO may be a result of induced nitric oxide synthase [NOS] induction); FENO seem to peak later than eosinophils measured in sputum by IS.[20] Elucidating exposure-specific FENO effects (ie, HMW or LMW agents) is further complicated by the likelihood that individual factors, possibly linked to genetics[21] and present or previous exposures, are as important in driving the measured response to the specific agents studied.

Methodologic Aspects

Smoking is known to downregulate the NO synthases, resulting in substantially lower FENO values. Thus, the usefulness of FENO in assessing airways inflammation associated with occupational exposures in smokers is unclear. Previous studies have had varying success in showing increased NO production among smokers after exposures that are believed to induce airways inflammation.[22,23] Analyses of FENO outcomes do benefit from smoking stratification.[24,25]

FENO measurement also seems to be confounded by airway narrowing, that is, manifesting lower levels in the presence of bronchial obstruction.[20,26,27] Thus, if possible, FENO should be measured after bronchodilation in persons with airway obstruction. Further, repeated spirometric maneuvers may also lower FENO, and should be avoided before measurement as well.[28]

Off-line FENO methods are attractive in occupational settings. Early attempts were associated with methodologic difficulties. However, considerable methodologic developments seem to have achieved good accuracy using such measurements, including constant and well-defined exhalation flow, inhalation of NO free air before measurement, and an increased mouth pressure to ensure closure of the velum, all of which are necessary for reliable measurement.

FENO and Exposure to HMW Allergens

Adisesh and colleagues[29] performed the first FENO study in an occupational setting in 1998, showing higher levels with increased symptoms of laboratory animal allergy: patients sensitized to animal dander with rhinoconjunctivitis had higher levels of FENO than nonsensitized workers, but lower levels than patients with asthma. More recently, Hewitt and colleagues[30] followed 50 laboratory animal workers and measured FENO at the end of a working week (Friday) and every morning and at the end of the work day the following weekend. Eleven patients had work-related symptoms and 2 were seropositive for laboratory animal antigens. In one of the seropositive individuals, but not the other, there was a progressive increase in FENO during the working week. Two other patients also had an increase of FENO of more than 25 ppb during the working week, but no symptoms and no changes in peak expiratory flow measurements. In all other patients, no significant changes in FENO occurred during the working week.

In 1999, Chan-Yeung and colleagues[31] found no relation between FENO and respiratory impairment (lung function, BHR, or response to bronchodilator and medication) among 71 workers with western red cedar asthma; sputum eosinophilia, on the other hand, significantly correlated with FENO ($r = 0.42$). Relevant to the same exposure,

17 patients with suspected western red cedar asthma were challenged with plicatic acid in a study by Obata and colleagues.[32] Nine of the patients were defined as responders from bronchoconstriction after the SIC. Levels of FENO increased 24 hours after the exposure, although only significantly among the nonresponders, and the changes were not related to changes in lung function.

Tan and colleagues[33] challenged 8 patients with self-reported latex sensitivity (3/8 positive for latex on the radioallergosorbent test, and 6/8 positive on the skin-prick test), and eye or nasal symptoms, with latex; no change in FENO was found after the challenge. In another study of the same exposure, Allmers and colleagues[34] challenged 12 patients with natural rubber latex allergy (positive skin-prick test) and 6 controls; 3 of the patients reacted with bronchoconstriction, of whom 1 also reacted with increased FENO. More recently, Shiryaeva and colleagues[35] examined 139 salmon workers, from fish slaughteries and fillet-processing factories, who were exposed to both fish proteins as well as endotoxins, along with 214 control individuals (administrative workers). The control individuals had higher FENO levels than the exposed group, but there seemed to be a large influence of healthy worker effect, because 27% of the control group and only 10% of the exposed group reported allergy. In a multivariable regression analysis, FENO was associated with work-related dry cough. Underscoring the variability in such observations, the same group went on to study 127 trawler fishermen (presumably with fish protein and endotoxin exposure) and 118 merchant seafarers without such exposures; there was a difference in measures of FENO between the 2 groups.[36]

Van der Walt and colleagues[37] examined FENO in 3 spice-mill workers reporting symptoms of asthma and allergy. The mill workers were examined 4 times daily over 2 working weeks and 2 weeks away from work, and 2 weeks back at work. In 1 of 3 workers, FENO was increased both before (84 ppb) and after the work shift (76 ppb); the other 2 patients had normal FENO without any changes during the work shifts. The patient with increased FENO had high levels of specific IgE against garlic (208 kU/L) (a workplace exposure); the other patients had lower levels (2.37 and 0.63, respectively).

One longitudinal study is particularly relevant to the question of FENO in HMW exposures. Tossa and colleagues[38] followed 351 apprentices of various types for 2 years; before being exposed and 3 times during the following 2-year period, examined serially with FENO, methacholine challenge test, and skin-prick test. The apprentices were working as bakers, pasta-makers, or hairdressers. In patients with new-onset BHR, or those who had an increase of BHR during the study period, the level of FENO increased: 20% in nonatopic and 16% in atopic patients. In a multiple regression model, the OR for developing BHR was doubled for each log-ppb increase of FENO. The sensitization rate was 11.8% among bakers, 8.1% in pasta-makers, and 4.1% in hairdressers.

FENO and Exposure to LMW Allergens and Irritants

There have also been several studies of FENO in relation to LMW agents and to irritant substances. Nonsmoking aluminum pot-room workers (n = 99), exposed to fluorides and dust, had 63% higher FENO compared with 40 nonsmoking controls; however, the increased FENO was not related to respiratory symptoms.[39] Ulvestad and colleagues[40] compared 29 nonsmoking underground tunnel workers who had been exposed to a variety of substances, including dust and nitrogen dioxide, with 26 controls; the tunnel workers had 50% higher FENO compared with nonsmoking controls, and those reporting wheeze had the highest levels of FENO.

We investigated bleachery workers in 3 pulp-mills repeatedly exposed to high levels of ozone in Swedish pulp-mills. In the first small study, the 29 highest-exposed workers had 63% higher FENO compared with 39 control workers.[41] These findings were confirmed in a larger study on 228 bleachery workers exposed to ozone and 63 controls; the highest-exposed workers had 23% higher FENO compared with control workers (19.2 vs 15.7 ppb).[42]

In the study of latex cited earlier, 9 patients with suspected MDI sensitivity were also challenged; 3 of them showed a significant bronchoconstriction (-20% of FEV_1) after exposure and 2 also had an increase in FENO 20 hours after the exposure.[34] Barbinova and colleagues[22] also challenged 55 workers with isocyanate-related respiratory symptoms (44 of whom were smokers). The 12 patients (22%) who had a positive test showed the highest changes of FENO 22 hours after challenge; 8 of them had a FENO increase of more than 50%. Yet, 12 patients of 43 with a negative challenge also had a similar increase. In a third study of isocyanates, Pronk and colleagues[43] examined 229 isocyanate exposed workers and did not find any association between FENO and exposure, even although the BHR was related to degree of exposure. Limiting the analysis to nonsmokers without atopy, FENO was related to asthmalike symptoms and rhinitis in exposed workers.

Sue-Chu and colleagues[44] examined professional skiers (n = 9) exposed to cold air with asthma and found FENO to be in the same range as in healthy controls. FENO has also been used to assess airways inflammation after exposure in swimming pools: among 39 lifeguards, those showing BHR (n = 15) had significantly higher FENO than those who did not have BHR (18.9 vs 12.5 ppb).[45] Potentially relevant to the chlorine exposure of swimming pools as well, Sastre and colleagues[46] examined 13 cleaning employees before and after challenge to 0.4 ppm chlorine. Three patients developed airway obstruction, but there was no change in FENO.

There have been several studies related to building material exposures. Fell and colleagues[47] examined FENO preshift and postshift FENO in 85 cement-exposed workers; FENO levels decreased after the shift, along with reductions in FEV_1 and peak expiratory flow. Carlsten and colleagues[48] examined cement-exposed apprentices (n = 11) and electrician (control) apprentices (n = 21); even although the cement-exposed apprentices had higher levels of proinflammatory mediators in serum, there was no difference in FENO between the groups. In another environment characterized in part by alkaline dust, Mauer and colleagues[49] examined first responders to the World Trade Center disaster 6 years later, finding no association between exposure and FENO.

FENO in SIC Diagnostic Testing for OA

In a study from Finland,[50] SIC tests were performed in 40 persons with suspected OA. In those challenges in which a bronchoconstriction occurred, a significant increase in FENO also occurred, but only in those patients with normal or slightly increased basal FENO levels. The increase in FENO occurred both after SIC to LMW and HMW agents. There was no increase among those with high basal FENO levels.

FENO and Endotoxin Exposure

Many studies have been performed exploring the effects of endotoxin on exhaled NO. Von Essen and colleagues[51] observed slightly increased FENO and an increased prevalence of respiratory symptoms among workers who had been exposed to swine dust. More recently, a large cohort (n = 425) of farmers and agriculture workers in Holland, thoroughly characterized in terms of endotoxin exposure, were tested for FENO (this study has already been cited in terms of confounding factors in FENO assessment).[23]

FENO was associated with endotoxin exposure, but only in nonatopic, nonsmoking individuals. Patients with wheezing and asthma symptoms had increased FENO, irrespective of atopy; the association between exposure and symptoms was marginally explained by FENO. The investigators conclude that FENO seems not to be an intermediate factor (mediator) between exposure and symptoms.

Kölbeck and colleagues[52] exposed 17 healthy individuals to swine dust, but found no significant changes of FENO; however, they measured FENO with an old method and after repeated spirometries (histamine challenges), which is known to decrease FENO. In a more recent study,[53] 33 healthy nonatopic individuals were exposed to a swine confinement environment; among the 22 individuals who were not wearing a breathing mask during the provocation, the FENO increased from 7.5 ppb to 13.4 ppb, whereas among those wearing a breathing mask the FENO was unaltered, from 8.3 ppb at baseline to 8.6 ppb after exposure. The same research group also examined whether the acute inflammatory reaction is related to previous exposure: swine farmers (n = 11), current smokers (n = 12), and controls (n = 11) underwent both endotoxin bronchial challenge and, on a separate occasion, spent 3 hours in a swine confinement environment.[12] The farmers, adapted to the exposure, reacted with fewer symptoms, less increase in hyperreactivity, a smaller decrease in lung function, and a smaller increase in inflammatory markers in nasal lavage and IS than controls. Spending 3 hours in the barn increased FENO, both in smokers and in controls, but not in farmers, possibly explained by higher preexposure FENO levels among the farmers; postexposure levels were similar in all groups. Smokers, on the other hand, appeared to have an enhanced response in terms of FENO and inflammation (total cell number and inflammatory cytokines) in both IS and nasal lavage. Experimental endotoxin challenge, on the other hand, did not change the FENO in any of the groups and elicited a smaller reaction in all of the tests, despite involving a higher endotoxin exposure than experienced in the field component of the study. This group has also performed an intervention study[54] to examine the effect of using robotic cleaning of the swine confinement environment to reduce exposure to endotoxins, which was also shown to reduce the increments of FENO. In another, related study, Heldal and colleagues[55] examined 44 sewage workers exposed to endotoxins and 36 controls (office workers); these investigators did not find any significant changes of FENO, despite high levels of endotoxin exposure.

FENO and Indoor Environments

FENO has also been used in a study of adverse health effects of indoor environment. The workers (n = 33) in a moisture-damaged school were compared with workers from a referent school (n = 23), with FENO measurements at the end of the spring term, at the end of summer vacation, and during the winter term.[56] No difference in FENO was found between the groups at any of the time points. Similar results were found in another Finnish study[57] in which working in a moisture-damaged school was not associated with any increase of FENO. Further, FENO was not associated with exposure in a large North American study comprising 207 nonsmoking individuals working in a water-damaged office building.[58] Studies of other indoor environment exposures have yielded more positive results. In an Australian study, 224 children were investigated with an extensive questionnaire, sampling of formaldehyde in the bedrooms and living rooms, skin-prick tests, and measurement of FENO.[59] Significantly higher FENO values were observed among children living in homes with average formaldehyde levels exceeding 50 ppb, with FENO levels of 15.5 ppb versus 8.7 ppb.

Exposure to indoor allergens in sensitized persons has also been associated with increased FENO. A study of 38 patients with mild asthma observed higher FENO values in patients sensitized to mite, cat, and dog and with current exposure to relevant allergen, compared with sensitized patients but without current exposure (17.7 ppb vs 9.1 ppb).[60] Similar results were found among 311 persons with asthma; those sensitized to mites and cat and with current exposure had significantly higher FENO.[61]

Phenotype of OA Based on FENO

Moore and colleagues,[62] testing FENO in 60 workers currently exposed to both HMW and LMW agents, concluded that there seem to be 2 variants of OA: 1 with increased FENO and lower PC_{20} and a second variant with normal FENO and less BHR, even although both groups may have similar peak expiratory flow rate changes in relation to work.

NO from Small Airways: Alveolar NO

In Finland, considerable research has been focusing on airways inflammation in small airways. Lehtimaki[63] was one of the first to report on increased alveolar NO levels in patients with alveolitis. The principle behind the alveolar NO value is mathematical modeling of measured NO concentrations using different exhalation flow rates; using high flow rates yields a sample with a higher contribution of NO from small airways, whereas low flow rates are more representative for central airways. Multiplying the NO concentration by the flow rate creates a value of the NO output at that flow rate. The NO outputs can then be plotted against the different flows; the slope represents an estimation of the alveolar NO concentration.[64] Several models have been created,[65] but none is perfect.[64] Preliminary reports of alveolar NO in relation to asbestos and silica from the Finnish group are intriguing.[66,67]

Comparison of IS and FENO

Lemiere and colleagues[68] analyzed SIC tests performed in Canada and Belgium using a similar protocol in both centers, yielding IS and FENO 7 and 24 hours after a positive SIC, and after 3 days of serial attempts in a negative SIC. In patients with a positive SIC test (n = 20), there was a significant increase in both sputum eosinophil count by IS and FENO, whereas no significant changes were found in the patients with negative SIC (n = 16). There was a moderate, statistically significant correlation between change in percent sputum eosinophilic counts and change in FENO (r = 0.4, p = 0.02). Analyzing ROC curves, a 2.2% change in sputum eosinophil counts provided the best sensitivity and specificity to identify a positive SIC, but no relevant cutoff value for FENO change could be detected (using a 10% increase in FENO as an arbitrary value achieved lower sensitivity and specificity than the IS-based criterion). The results of this study show one of the difficulties in comparing FENO at different time points with change in FEV_1, because, as noted earlier, the FENO may decrease in the presence of airflow obstruction. This possible confounding effect was also apparent in a study of 15 patients with isocyanate asthma, 3 patients with isocyanate-induced rhinitis, and 24 control individuals who were exposed to SIC with isocyanate by Ferrazzoni and colleagues,[20] in which IS was sampled before and 24 and 48 hours after SIC, whereas FENO and FEV_1 were examined daily for 5 days. There was a strong correlation between falling FEV_1 and decreasing in FENO; moreover the FENO levels were significantly increased only at 24 hours after SIC, at a time point when FEV_1 was on its way back to normal. The maximum FENO levels were reached between 24 and 48 hours after exposure, and changes in IS eosinophils and FENO were correlated at 24 hours and 48 hours, although the former returned to baseline only days later. Swiercybska-Machura and colleagues,[69] in another study comparing IS and FENO after SIC, showed that those with a positive SIC test (n = 19 of 42 challenged) had increased FENO and IS eosinophils 24 hours after exposure.

EXHALED BREATH CONDENSATE
Methodologic Problems with EBC

Exhaled breath condensate (EBC) is a technique based on the cooling of expired air, which thus condenses. The water vapor turns to water and simultaneously captures the nonvolatile and semivolatile substances in exhaled breath. It is likely that the nonvolatile matter contained in the EBC is transported from the respiratory tract lining fluid in the form of small particles in the aerosol that is exhaled.

Condensation is affected by temperature and the surface of the condenser, which can have different adhesive properties, potentially trapping proteins.[70] During condensation, the exhaled air is cooled and the water vapor is released in aqueous form, where particles (as droplets) are also trapped. However, condensation of the particles is random; many of the exhaled particles can bypass the condenser without being collected. This problem was clearly observed in an early study of EBC sampling, in which 2 condensers were serially connected and similar levels of analytes were identified in both.[71] Further, the extent to which dilution with water vapor varies between and within individuals is still uncertain. Attempts have been made to overcome this problem by measuring the so-called conductivity in the sample (sodium and potassium or conductivity), but this has not been shown to increase the reproducibility of results.[72] Because the substances in EBC are diluted with water and only present at extremely low concentrations, they are difficult to measure using existing enzyme-linked immunosorbent assays. Another problem is contamination of the EBC with substances present in the saliva.[73] These concerns with the EBC are particularly relevant when the method is used to study nonvolatile substances. For semivolatile substances, some of these issues may be less important, but contamination from the oral cavity is probably an even bigger problem in that case.

Condensate pH

EBC pH (ie, the presence of H+) is perhaps the biomarker most used in applying this method. pH in the EBC decreases with asthma exacerbation, a phenomenon that is believed to be caused by the respiratory tract lining fluid becoming more acidic, possibly because of an increase in the concentration of acetic acid. In studies of chronic obstructive pulmonary disease as opposed to asthma, conflicting results have been presented.[74,75] One of the concerns in the measurement of pH in the EBC is the presence of ammonium ions in the oral cavity that may affect the pH, although data on this are conflicting.[76,77] To achieve a stable pH of the collected condensate, the sample needs aerosation so that CO_2 absorbed from the ambient air disappears (ie, bubbling through an inert gas). Another way is to saturate the sample with CO_2, which requires about 40 minutes.[78] Even although the value of pH measurement in condensate is unclear, these studies have shown that the pH of the airways may be important in respiratory disease.

PARTICLES IN EXHALED AIR

Our research group has addressed the methodologic problems inherent in EBC by finding more efficient methods to sample nonvolatile components in exhaled breath (ie, exhaled particles in the exhaled aerosol [PEx]).[79] This is a noninvasive method, easy to perform, which may be repeated without affecting the airways. We have shown that this is a more efficient method than EBC. When comparing levels of surfactant protein A, the most abundant surfactant protein, the levels sampled by the PEx method are 10 to 50 times higher than in EBC using the same volume of exhaled air.[80] This method also avoids the problem of contamination from the oral cavity, because no particles can be formed from a liquid surface unless the flow is extremely high. Consistent with this finding, amylase (a saliva marker) is not found in PEx.[81] The same study identified 124 proteins, which is approximately 3 times more than previously detected in EBC. Nevertheless, 70% to 80% of the exhaled particles consist of lipids, mainly phospholipids from the surfactant. Further, the phospholipid composition was different in a small pilot study of 15 patients with asthma compared with healthy controls.[82]

These particles seem to be formed variously during different breathing maneuvers. Breathing that allows for airway closure and reopening causes a large increase in particle formation, indicating that the particles derive from the small airways, a part of the respiratory tract thus far difficult to assess by other noninvasive methods. During tidal breathing, particles are probably also formed by airway reopening, but the smallest fraction, particles less than 0.3 μm, seem to be formed by another, as yet unidentified, mechanism.[83]

SUMMARY

The use of IS to assess health effects after occupational exposure has led to a further understanding of inflammatory processes after exposure and represents an important step forward, even although the general picture is that the knowledge of the inflammatory pathways in OA is still limited. Moreover, the measurement of eosinophils in IS provides an objective measure of adverse respiratory effects that seems to be useful for early detection of disease and also may be related to prospective outcomes.[14,17,84] In light of the many contradictory results of using FENO after exposures known to induce inflammation in the airways, the picture is less clear. FENO can be correlated with eosinophilic airways inflammation, but both the increase in eosinophils and the increase of FENO may reflect separate underlying mechanisms. This situation may explain why FENO is also increased after exposures normally associated with a neutrophilic inflammation. The interpretation of FENO data is further hampered because it is profoundly influenced by smoking and many studies have not stratified their results by smoking status. In addition, FENO decreases with airway obstruction, which obscures the data from SIC studies, in which positive responders are defined by postexposure airway obstruction. Clearly, FENO data are not interchangeable with measurement of IS-defined eosinophilia. FENO seems not only to increase after exposure to high-molecular agents but also after exposures that are normally associated with a predominantly neutrophilic airways inflammation, such as endotoxins and isocyanates. However, our knowledge is limited in terms of time kinetics for the influx of inflammatory cells associated with airway inflammatory process in vivo. In atopic patients, FENO is strongly influenced by exposure to a sensitizing agent. In the subgroup of patients sensitized and exposed to common aeroallergens, this situation may limit the usefulness of FENO to assess effect of workplace exposures, because it may be difficult to discriminate the effect of possible occupational allergens or irritants.

If our knowledge of the longitudinal relevance of increased eosinophils is limited based on IS findings, the prospective data on FENO are even more sparse. There is an obvious need for longitudinal studies of exposed workers to further understand the value of both IS and FENO in relation to inflammatory pathways and the development of disease. Further examination of the alveolar fraction of NO in occupational lung disease may yield rich results. There are also interesting recent data using IS to study the particulate burden in cells as markers of occupational exposure.[85,86] The use of EBC is problem-ridden, and at present this method lags behind either IS or FENO. Attempts to circumvent some of the problems of EBC with PEx methods may prove worthwhile.

REFERENCES

1. Berry MA, Shaw DE, Green RH, et al. The use of exhaled nitric oxide concentration to identify eosinophilic airway inflammation: an observational study in adults with asthma. Clin Exp Allergy 2005;35(9):1175–9.
2. Manso L, Madero MF, Ruiz-Garcia M, et al. Comparison of bronchial hyperresponsiveness to methacholine and adenosine and airway inflammation markers in patients with suspected asthma. J Asthma 2011;48(4):335–40.
3. Prince P, Lemiere C, Dufour MH, et al. Airway inflammatory responses following exposure to occupational agents. Chest 2012;141(6):1522–7.
4. Quirce S, Lemiere C, de Blay F, et al. Noninvasive methods for assessment of airway inflammation in occupational settings. Allergy 2010;65(4):445–58.
5. Gautrin D, Malo JL. Risk factors, predictors, and markers for work-related asthma and rhinitis. Curr Allergy Asthma Rep 2010;10(5):365–72.
6. Green RH, Brightling CE, McKenna S, et al. Asthma exacerbations and sputum eosinophil counts: a randomised controlled trial. Lancet 2002;360(9347):1715–21.
7. Wenzel SE. Asthma: defining of the persistent adult phenotypes. Lancet 2006;368(9537):804–13.
8. Baines KJ, Simpson JL, Wood LG, et al. Transcriptional phenotypes of asthma defined by gene expression profiling of induced sputum samples. J Allergy Clin Immunol 2011;127(1):153–60.
9. Haldar P, Pavord ID, Shaw DE, et al. Cluster analysis and clinical asthma phenotypes. Am J Respir Crit Care Med 2008;178(3):218–24.
10. Malo JL, Cardinal S, Ghezzo H, et al. Association of bronchial reactivity to occupational agents with methacholine reactivity, sputum cells and immunoglobulin E-mediated reactivity. Clin Exp Allergy 2011;41(4):497–504.
11. Fernandez-Nieto M, Sastre B, Sastre J, et al. Changes in sputum eicosanoids and inflammatory markers after inhalation challenges with occupational agents. Chest 2009;136(5):1308–15.
12. Sundblad BM, von Scheele I, Palmberg L, et al. Repeated exposure to organic material alters inflammatory and physiological airway responses. Eur Respir J 2009;34(1):80–8.
13. Holz O, Richter K, Jorres RA, et al. Changes in sputum composition between two inductions performed on consecutive days. Thorax 1998;53(2):83–6.

14. Vandenplas O, D'Alpaos V, Heymans J, et al. Sputum eosinophilia: an early marker of bronchial response to occupational agents. Allergy 2009; 64(5):754–61.

15. Hur GY, Sheen SS, Kang YM, et al. Histamine release and inflammatory cell infiltration in airway mucosa in methylene diphenyl diisocyanate (MDI)-induced occupational asthma. J Clin Immunol 2008;28(5): 571–80.

16. Moreira A, Palmares C, Lopes C, et al. Airway vascular damage in elite swimmers. Respir Med 2011;105(11):1761–5.

17. Lemiere C, Chaboillez S, Welman M, et al. Outcome of occupational asthma after removal from exposure: a follow-up study. Can Respir J 2010;17(2):61–6.

18. Brightling CE. Cough due to asthma and nonasthmatic eosinophilic bronchitis. Lung 2010;188(Suppl 1): S13–7.

19. Pala G, Pignatti P, Moscato G. Occupational non-asthmatic eosinophilic bronchitis: current concepts. Med Lav 2012;103(1):17–25.

20. Ferrazzoni S, Scarpa MC, Guarnieri G, et al. Exhaled nitric oxide and breath condensate ph in asthmatic reactions induced by isocyanates. Chest 2009; 136(1):155–62.

21. Dahgam S, Nyberg F, Modig L, et al. Single nucleotide polymorphisms in the NOS2 and NOS3 genes are associated with exhaled nitric oxide. J Med Genet 2012;49(3):200–5.

22. Barbinova L, Baur X. Increase in exhaled nitric oxide (eNO) after work-related isocyanate exposure. Int Arch Occup Environ Health 2006;79(5):387–95.

23. Smit LA, Heederik D, Doekes G, et al. Exhaled nitric oxide in endotoxin-exposed adults: effect modification by smoking and atopy. Occup Environ Med 2009;66(4):251–5.

24. Rouhos A, Kainu A, Piirila P, et al. Repeatability of exhaled nitric oxide measurements in patients with COPD. Clin Physiol Funct Imaging 2011;31(1):26–31.

25. Malinovschi A, Backer V, Harving H, et al. The value of exhaled nitric oxide to identify asthma in smoking patients with asthma-like symptoms. Respir Med 2012;106(6):794–801.

26. de Gouw HW, Hendriks J, Woltman AM, et al. Exhaled nitric oxide (NO) is reduced shortly after bronchoconstriction to direct and indirect stimuli in asthma. Am J Respir Crit Care Med 1998;158(1):315–9.

27. Ho LP, Wood FT, Robson A, et al. Atopy influences exhaled nitric oxide levels in adult asthmatics. Chest 2000;118(5):1327–31.

28. Deykin A, Massaro AF, Coulston E, et al. Exhaled nitric oxide following repeated spirometry or repeated plethysmography in healthy individuals. Am J Respir Crit Care Med 2000;161(4 Pt 1):1237–40.

29. Adisesh LA, Kharitonov SA, Yates DH, et al. Exhaled and nasal nitric oxide is increased in laboratory animal allergy. Clin Exp Allergy 1998;28(7):876–80.

30. Hewitt RS, Smith AD, Cowan JO, et al. Serial exhaled nitric oxide measurements in the assessment of laboratory animal allergy. J Asthma 2008;45(2):101–7.

31. Chan-Yeung M, Obata H, Dittrick M, et al. Airway inflammation, exhaled nitric oxide, and severity of asthma in patients with western red cedar asthma. Am J Respir Crit Care Med 1999;159(5 Pt 1):1434–8.

32. Obata H, Dittrick M, Chan H, et al. Sputum eosinophils and exhaled nitric oxide during late asthmatic reaction in patients with western red cedar asthma. Eur Respir J 1999;13(3):489–95.

33. Tan K, Bruce C, Birkhead A, et al. Nasal and exhaled nitric oxide in response to occupational latex exposure. Allergy 2001;56(7):627–32.

34. Allmers H, Chen Z, Barbinova L, et al. Challenge from methacholine, natural rubber latex, or 4,4- diphenyl-methane diisocyanate in workers with suspected sensitization affects exhaled nitric oxide change in exhaled NO levels after allergen challenges. Int Arch Occup Environ Health 2000;73(3):181–6.

35. Shiryaeva O, Aasmoe L, Straume B, et al. Respiratory impairment in Norwegian salmon industry workers: a cross-sectional study. J Occup Environ Med 2010;52(12):1167–72.

36. Shiryaeva O, Aasmoe L, Straume B, et al. An analysis of the respiratory health status among seafarers in the Russian trawler and merchant fleets. Am J Ind Med 2011;54(12):971–9.

37. van der Walt A, Lopata AL, Nieuwenhuizen NE, et al. Work-related allergy and asthma in spice mill workers–the impact of processing dried spices on IgE reactivity patterns. Int Arch Allergy Immunol 2010;152(3):271–8.

38. Tossa P, Paris C, Zmirou-Navier D, et al. Increase in exhaled nitric oxide is associated with bronchial hyperresponsiveness among apprentices. Am J Respir Crit Care Med 2010;182(6):738–44.

39. Lund MB, Oksne PI, Hamre R, et al. Increased nitric oxide in exhaled air: an early marker of asthma in non-smoking aluminium potroom workers? Occup Environ Med 2000;57(4):274–8.

40. Ulvestad B, Lund MB, Bakke B, et al. Gas and dust exposure in underground construction is associated with signs of airway inflammation. Eur Respir J 2001; 17(3):416–21.

41. Olin AC, Ljungkvist G, Bake B, et al. Exhaled nitric oxide among pulpmill workers reporting gassing incidents involving ozone and chlorine dioxide. Eur Respir J 1999;14(4):828–31.

42. Olin AC, Andersson E, Andersson M, et al. Prevalence of asthma and exhaled nitric oxide are increased in bleachery workers exposed to ozone. Eur Respir J 2004;23(1):87–92.

43. Pronk A, Preller L, Doekes G, et al. Different respiratory phenotypes are associated with isocyanate exposure in spray painters. Eur Respir J 2009; 33(3):494–501.

44. Sue-Chu M, Henriksen AH, Bjermer L. Non-invasive evaluation of lower airway inflammation in hyper-responsive elite cross-country skiers and asthmatics. Respir Med 1999;93(10):719–25.

45. Demange V, Bohadana A, Massin N, et al. Exhaled nitric oxide and airway hyperresponsiveness in workers: a preliminary study in lifeguards. BMC Pulm Med 2009;9:53.

46. Sastre J, Madero MF, Fernandez-Nieto M, et al. Airway response to chlorine inhalation (bleach) among cleaning workers with and without bronchial hyperresponsiveness. Am J Ind Med 2011;54(4):293–9.

47. Fell AK, Noto H, Skogstad M, et al. A cross-shift study of lung function, exhaled nitric oxide and inflammatory markers in blood in Norwegian cement production workers. Occup Environ Med 2011; 68(11):799–805.

48. Carlsten C, de Roos AJ, Kaufman JD, et al. Cell markers, cytokines, and immune parameters in cement mason apprentices. Arthritis Rheum 2007; 57(1):147–53.

49. Mauer MP, Hoen R, Jourd'heuil D. FE NO concentrations in World Trade Center responders and controls, 6 years post-9/11. Lung 2011;189(4):295–303.

50. Piirila P, Wikman H, Luukkonen R, et al. Glutathione S-transferase genotypes and allergic responses to diisocyanate exposure. Pharmacogenetics 2001; 11(5):437–45.

51. Von Essen SG, Scheppers LA, Robbins RA, et al. Respiratory tract inflammation in swine confinement workers studied using induced sputum and exhaled nitric oxide. J Toxicol Clin Toxicol 1998;36(6):557–65.

52. Kolbeck KG, Ehnhage A, Juto JE, et al. Airway reactivity and exhaled NO following swine dust exposure in healthy volunteers. Respir Med 2000;94(11): 1065–72.

53. Sundblad BM, Larsson BM, Palmberg L, et al. Exhaled nitric oxide and bronchial responsiveness in healthy subjects exposed to organic dust. Eur Respir J 2002;20(2):426–31.

54. Hiel D, von Scheele I, Sundblad BM, et al. Evaluation of respiratory effects related to high-pressure cleaning in a piggery with and without robot pre-cleaning. Scand J Work Environ Health 2009; 35(5):376–83.

55. Heldal KK, Madso L, Huser PO, et al. Exposure, symptoms and airway inflammation among sewage workers. Ann Agric Environ Med 2010; 17(2):263–8.

56. Purokivi M, Hirvonen MR, Randell J, et al. Nitric oxide alone is an insufficient biomarker of exposure to microbes in a moisture-damaged building. Inhal Toxicol 2002;14(12):1279–90.

57. Roponen M, Kiviranta J, Seuri M, et al. Inflammatory mediators in nasal lavage, induced sputum and serum of employees with rheumatic and respiratory disorders. Eur Respir J 2001;18(3):542–8.

58. Akpinar-Elci M, Siegel PD, Cox-Ganser JM, et al. Respiratory inflammatory responses among occupants of a water-damaged office building. Indoor Air 2008;18(2):125–30.

59. Franklin P, Dingle P, Stick S. Raised exhaled nitric oxide in healthy children is associated with domestic formaldehyde levels. Am J Respir Crit Care Med 2000;161(5):1757–9.

60. Simpson A, Custovic A, Pipis S, et al. Exhaled nitric oxide, sensitization, and exposure to allergens in patients with asthma who are not taking inhaled steroids. Am J Respir Crit Care Med 1999;160(1):45–9.

61. Langley SJ, Goldthorpe S, Craven M, et al. Exposure and sensitization to indoor allergens: association with lung function, bronchial reactivity, and exhaled nitric oxide measures in asthma. J Allergy Clin Immunol 2003;112(2):362–8.

62. Moore VC, Anees W, Jaakkola MS, et al. Two variants of occupational asthma separable by exhaled breath nitric oxide level. Respir Med 2010;104(6): 873–9.

63. Lehtimaki L, Kankaanranta H, Saarelainen S, et al. Extended exhaled NO measurement differentiates between alveolar and bronchial inflammation. Am J Respir Crit Care Med 2001;163(7):1557–61.

64. Tsoukias NM, George SC. A two-compartment model of pulmonary nitric oxide exchange dynamics. J Appl Physiol 1998;85(2):653–66.

65. Verbanck S, Malinovschi A, George S, et al. Bronchial and alveolar components of exhaled nitric oxide and their relationship. Eur Respir J 2012; 39(5):1258–61.

66. Lehtimaki L, Oksa P, Jarvenpaa R, et al. Pulmonary inflammation in asbestos-exposed subjects with borderline parenchymal changes on HRCT. Respir Med 2010;104(7):1042–9.

67. Sauni R, Oksa P, Lehtimaki L, et al. Increased alveolar nitric oxide and systemic inflammation markers in silica-exposed workers. Occup Environ Med 2012;69(4):256–60.

68. Lemiere C, D'Alpaos V, Chaboillez S, et al. Investigation of occupational asthma: sputum cell counts or exhaled nitric oxide? Chest 2010;137(3):617–22.

69. Swierczynska-Machura D, Krakowiak A, Wiszniewska M, et al. Exhaled nitric oxide levels after specific inahalatory challenge test in subjects with diagnosed occupational asthma. Int J Occup Med Environ Health 2008;21(3): 219–25.

70. Rosias PP, Robroeks CM, Niemarkt HJ, et al. Breath condenser coatings affect measurement of biomarkers in exhaled breath condensate. Eur Respir J 2006;28(5):1036–41.

71. Gessner C, Kuhn H, Seyfarth HJ, et al. Factors influencing breath condensate volume. Pneumologie 2001;55(9):414–9.

72. Effros RM, Biller J, Foss B, et al. A simple method for estimating respiratory solute dilution in exhaled

breath condensates. Am J Respir Crit Care Med 2003;168(12):1500–5.

73. Zetterquist W, Marteus H, Kalm-Stephens P, et al. Oral bacteria- the missing link to ambiguous findings of exhaled nitrogen oxides in cystic fibrosis. Respir Med 2009;103:187–93.

74. Koczulla AR, Noeske S, Herr C, et al. Acute and chronic effects of smoking on inflammation markers in exhaled breath condensate in current smokers. Respiration 2010;79(1):61–7.

75. Koczulla R, Dragonieri S, Schot R, et al. Comparison of exhaled breath condensate pH using two commercially available devices in healthy controls, asthma and COPD patients. Respir Res 2009;10:78.

76. Effros RM. Do low exhaled condensate $NH4+$ concentrations in asthma reflect reduced pulmonary production? Am J Respir Crit Care Med 2003;167(1): 91 [author reply: 91–2].

77. Wells K, Vaughan J, Pajewski TN, et al. Exhaled breath condensate pH assays are not influenced by oral ammonia. Thorax 2005;60(1):27–31.

78. Kullmann T, Barta I, Lazar Z, et al. Exhaled breath condensate pH standardised for $CO2$ partial pressure. Eur Respir J 2007;29(3):496–501.

79. Almstrand AC, Ljungstrom E, Lausmaa J, et al. Airway monitoring by collection and mass spectrometric analysis of exhaled particles. Anal Chem 2009;81(2):662–8.

80. Larsson P, Mirgorodskaya E, Samuelsson L, et al. Surfactant protein A and albumin in particles in exhaled air. Respir Med 2012;106(2):197–204.

81. Bredberg A, Gobom J, Almstrand AC, et al. Exhaled endogenous particles contain lung proteins. Clin Chem 2012;58(2):431–40.

82. Almstrand AC, Josefson M, Bredberg A, et al. TOF-SIMS analysis of exhaled particles from patients with asthma and healthy controls. Eur Respir J 2012; 39(1):59–66.

83. Holmgren H, Ljungström E, Almstrand AC, et al. Size distribution of exhaled particles in the range from 0.01 to 2.0 μm. J Aerosol Sci 2010; 41:439–46.

84. Lemiere C, Chaboilliez S, Trudeau C, et al. Characterization of airway inflammation after repeated exposures to occupational agents. J Allergy Clin Immunol 2000;106(6):1163–70.

85. Fireman E, Lerman Y, Stark M, et al. Detection of occult lung impairment in welders by induced sputum particles and breath oxidation. Am J Ind Med 2008;51(7):503–11.

86. Fireman EM, Lerman Y, Ben Mahor M, et al. Redefining idiopathic interstitial lung disease into occupational lung diseases by analysis of chemical composition of inhaled dust particles in induced sputum and/or lung biopsy specimens. Toxicol Ind Health 2007;23(10):607–15.

Respiratory Protection

Howard J. Cohen, PhD, CIH[a],*, Jeffrey S. Birkner, PhD, CIH[b]

KEYWORDS

- Respirators • Respiratory protection • Occupational exposures • Airborne contaminants

KEY POINTS

- This article focuses on the use and types of personal respiratory protection (respirators) worn by individuals at workplaces where airborne hazardous contaminants may exist.
- Respirators are increasingly also being used in nonindustrial settings such as health care facilities, as concerns regarding infectious epidemics and terrorist threats grow.
- Pulmonologists and other clinicians should understand fundamental issues regarding respiratory protection against airborne contaminants and the use of respirators.

INTRODUCTION

Respiratory protection is used as a method of protecting individuals from inhaling harmful airborne contaminants and in some cases to supply them with breathable air in oxygen-deficient environments. Respiratory protection is not meant to replace other preferred methods of control that can eliminate or reduce airborne hazards, such as substitution, ventilation, enclosures, or process changes. However, there are situations in which respiratory protection must be worn in conjunction with other control methods to adequately protect the wearer. Fundamental issues in protecting workers with respirators are selecting the proper device for the anticipated hazard, ensuring that the wearer is fit and trained to use the respirator properly, and making sure that the device is in working order.

Although respirators are extensively tested in laboratory environments, data regarding the efficacy of respirators in real work environments is limited. For example, despite widespread use of respirators and surgical masks to protect workers from airborne biologic hazards in health care settings, there is little data supporting the clinical efficacy of these practices in preventing infection.[1–4] This has led some to view less costly surgical masks as devices equivalent to more expensive respirators. An examination of laboratory studies clearly demonstrates that respirators are superior to masks in terms of filter efficiency and ability to greatly reduce contaminants from entering the respiratory tract through face seal leakage.

In addition to the respirator device, respirator effectiveness, like all personal protective equipment, depends on certain individual and organizational considerations. Individual issues include knowledge, beliefs, attitudes, and perception of risk. Organizational issues include respirator availability, training and education, management policies, and expectations regarding respirator use. Inattention to these issues can reduce the effectiveness of respirators to protect workers from airborne hazards.[5] Workplace respiratory protection programs aim to address these issues so as to optimize respirator effectiveness.

This review of respiratory protection addresses a brief history of respiratory protection, regulations that govern the manufacturers and users of

Disclosures and conflicts of interest for both authors: none, except that J. Birkner is employed by Moldex-Metric.
[a] Department of Occupational and Environmental Medicine, Yale University School of Medicine, 47 Mustang Drive, Guilford, CT 06437, USA; [b] V.P. Technical Services, Moldex-Metric, 10111 West Jefferson Boulevard, Culver City, CA 90232, USA
* Corresponding author.
E-mail address: howard.cohen@yale.edu

Clin Chest Med 33 (2012) 783–793
http://dx.doi.org/10.1016/j.ccm.2012.09.005

respiratory protection, a description of the types of respirators that exist including their limitations, and the medical evaluation of workers who wear respirators.

HISTORICAL ASPECTS OF RESPIRATORY PROTECTION

Respirators go back to ancient Roman times when a loose-fitting animal bladder was worn by workers in mines to protect against inhaling lead oxide. Leonardo da Vinci recommended the use of a wet cloth as protection against inhaling harmful chemical agents. He also invented a snorkel that connected a breathing tube to a float.[6] In the 1700s, Bernadino Ramazzini, considered the father of occupational medicine, described the inadequacy of respiratory protection in his lifetime against the hazards of arsenic, gypsum, lime, tobacco, and silica (stone cutters).[6]

In the United States, one of the first respirators was the Nealy Smoke Mask, patented in 1877, which filtered out smoke (**Fig. 1**).[7] Advances in respiratory protection that arose from the use of chemical warfare in World War I lead to the forerunners of present-day respirators.

In 1919, the Bureau of Mines initiated the first respirator certification program in the United

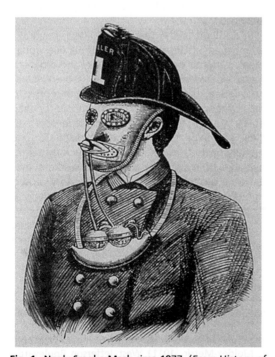

Fig. 1. Nealy Smoke Mask circa 1877. (*From* History of respiratory protective devices in the U.S. Work performed under the auspices of the US Energy, Research & Development Administration under contract No. W-7405-Eng-48.)

States and certified their first respirator in 1920, a self-contained breathing apparatus (SCBA).[8] However, it had no statutory authority to regulate the use of respirators. The use of respirators continued unregulated until the Federal Coal Mine Health and Safety Act was enacted in 1969, resulting in regulations governing the certification and use of respirators in the mining industry.[9]

The Occupational Safety and Health Act, which established the Occupational Safety and Health Administration (OSHA) and the National Institute of Occupational Safety and Health (NIOSH), was promulgated in 1970. OSHA established regulations governing the use of respirators by employers in 29 Code of Federal Regulations Part 1910.134.[10] NIOSH was established as the agency to test respirators and provide certification to manufacturers.[6]

RESPIRATORY PROTECTION REGULATIONS AND STANDARDS

In the United States, the use of respirators in workplaces is governed by OSHA.[10] The OSHA requirements of employers are briefly summarized as follows:

1. Employers must establish a written program that covers the use of respirators at their establishment. The employer must assign a program administrator for the overall responsibility of the respirator program.
2. Respirators must be selected based on the hazard either anticipated or present in the workplace, including routine tasks and foreseeable emergencies. This requires a hazard assessment (quantitative or qualitative) of each task for which respirators may be required. All respirators selected must be NIOSH certified. Only SCBA must be selected for entry into environments that may be immediately hazardous to life and health.
3. Employees must be medically cleared by a physician or other licensed health care professional before being assigned a respirator, discussed later.
4. Employees must be properly fit tested and trained before wearing a respirator in a hazardous environment. Training should include a description of the hazard, signs and symptoms of overexposures, how to properly put on and take off the respirator, how to maintain the device, and an opportunity to acclimate with the respirator before entering a hazardous environment. Fit testing is required for tight-fitting respirators to ensure that the respirator is sized properly for the employee's facial characteristics, discussed later.

5. The employer must provide for the proper storage, inspection, and maintenance of respirators. Emergency use respirators must be inspected at least once a month and a written record maintained. All other respirators must be inspected before and after each time they are worn.

6. The employer must establish change schedules with air-purifying respirators (APRs) so that workers are not overexposed to hazardous contaminants because the filter or sorbent has become exhausted.

7. Supplied-air respirators can be used only with air that meets the Compressed Gas Manufacturer's specification of grade D or higher.

8. An annual evaluation of the employer's respiratory protection is required, including an assessment of how practices compare with the written program's requirements. All deficiencies must be corrected.

Fit testing is performed to determine that an employee can obtain a satisfactory fit with the respirator chosen and also to assign protective factors to respiratory device facepieces. There are 2 basic types of fit testing: qualitative and quantitative. Qualitative fit testing uses a vapor (isoamyl acetate) or aerosol (saccharin or Bitrex) and relies on the wearer to perceive the smell or taste of the challenge agent. When qualitative fit testing is used, the maximum assigned protection factor is 10 regardless of the respirator chosen.

Quantitative fit testing uses a challenge aerosol (usually ambient air) and measures the aerosol leakage inside the respirator to obtain a fit factor. Quantitative fit testing is a more precise method that is usually quicker to perform than qualitative fit testing but requires more expensive instrumentation. Individuals who are quantitatively fit tested can obtain protection factors greater than 10, depending on the respirator selected, discussed later.

NIOSH regulations govern the manufacturers of respirators. Respirator program administrators and others should be aware of how these requirements affect respirator wearers and the common terminology used to describe different types of respirators. NIOSH certification requirements, described in 42 Code of Federal Regulations (CFR) Part 84, include the testing requirements and fees, quality assurance, protection factors, labeling, and instructions to users.[11] NIOSH also provides an online listing of currently certified respirators.[12]

In 1995, NIOSH established a series of criteria and designations for respirators that are certified for protection against particulates, with 3 levels of filter efficiency: 95%, 99%, and 100%. Because many filters in respirators use electrostatically charged media that may be adversely affected by oily substances, they established test conditions to certify filters as "N" for respirators not for use in oily environments, "R" for respirators that can be used for a single shift in oily environments, and "P" for respirators that are oil proof.

NIOSH certifies organic vapor respirators against a single vapor: carbon tetrachloride. Therefore, it is important to understand that some organic vapors, especially those with low molecular weights and low boiling points, such as methylene chloride, are not suitable for use with organic vapor respirators. OSHA established the Advisor Genius, which uses a mathematical model for predicting the service life of various organics with NIOSH-certified organic vapor respirators.[13] NIOSH also investigates reports of respirator failures and malfunctions in the workplace and performs audit testing on a limited number of respirators in the marketplace to determine if they continue to meet certification standards. NIOSH has the authority to revoke any certification of a respirator that fails to continue to meet its requirements.

The US Food and Drug Administration (FDA) has established requirements for manufacturers of surgical masks and respirators that are marketed for health care workers as part of their authority over medical devices. The FDA does not perform testing of these devices but requires that manufacturers meet or prove equivalency to several consensus and military standards, including flammability, fluid resistance, aerosol penetration, breathability, and biocompatibility.[14] Respirators must also be NIOSH certified. The FDA must approve any statement made by respirator manufacturers regarding antiviral coating or similar claims.

OSHA does not require that employers such as hospitals use FDA-cleared respirators, but other organizations, such as the Joint Commission that accredits hospitals, may require employers to use these devices.

The Consumer Product Safety Commission (CPSC) generally has little involvement with respirators. However, they do become involved with fraudulent claims by manufacturers, which has become more prevalent as some offshore manufacturers produce fraudulent NIOSH certification claims. CPSC is also responsible for the general public should they become injured using non-NIOSH-certified respirators.

The American National Standards Institute (ANSI), American Society for Testing and Materials (ASTM) International, and National Fire Protection Association (NFPA) also have standards covering the use of respirators, summarized in **Box 1**.

Box 1
List of consensus standards for respirators

American National Standards Institute (ANSI) Standards

ANSI Z88.2 Practices for respiratory protection

ANSI Z88.6 Respirator physical qualifications for personnel

ANSI Z88.10 Respirator fit testing methods

American Society for Testing and Materials (ASTM) Standards

ASTM F 1862 Resistance of surgical mask to penetration by synthetic blood

ASTM F 1215-89 Initial efficiency of flatsheet filter medium in an airflow using latex spheres

ASTM F2101-01 Evaluating the bacterial filtration efficiency of surgical masks using a biologic aerosol of *Staphylococcus aureus*

National Fire Protection Association (NFPA) Standards

NFPA 1404 Fire service respiratory protection training

NFPA 1984 Wildland fire fighting

NFPA 1981 Open-circuit SCBA for emergency services

ANSI standards are focused primarily on providing accurate information to professionals who make decisions about respirators and respirator programs.[15] ASTM standards are focused on establishing test methods such as the efficacy of surgical masks to prevent penetration by blood or biologic aerosols, which can be cited and adopted by government agencies such as the FDA.[14,16] NFPA standards are focused on fire protection and emergency response workers.[17]

In addition to the US regulations, there are other use and certification standards around the world. Canada has a respirator selection, use, and maintenance standard, CSA Z94.4. The International Standards Organizations, ISO, which has 21 voting member countries, is developing respirator standards that the European Union must adopt and that likely will be adopted by other countries once finalized.

TYPES OF RESPIRATORS

Respirators are generally divided into groups by the means used to prevent contaminants from entering the respiratory system (ie, air purifying and supplied air). They are also divided into the type of facepieces available (eg, half mask and full face). APRs, which use filters or chemical sorbents to remove contaminants from ambient air, are further divided into categories based on the type of contaminant they are designed to remove. Supplied-air respirators (SAR), which use an independent supply of air from a noncontaminated source to provide protection, are generally categorized by the method that the noncontaminated air is delivered to the wearer, as well as the pressure mode that the respirator functions under. Although this summary is meant to be comprehensive, it is not inclusive of every type of device available. Most devices addressed are NIOSH-certified respirators. In this discussion, devices that are NIOSH certified are referred to as respirators, whereas those types of respiratory protection that are used in health care, but not NIOSH certified, are called masks. There are also other devices that provide respiratory protection but are not NIOSH certified, for example, supplied-air suits.

When respirators are used in a workplace, the appropriate type of respirator device must be chosen. Aside from the type of facepiece chosen, as well as its method of removing the contaminant, other factors that should be considered include ease of use, maintenance required, cost, physiologic stress that the device imposes on the individual, as well as environmental conditions such as temperature, humidity, and work load. Psychological effects that the respirator may have on the individual and visibility and communication restrictions that the respirator may present should also be considered.

Industrial Versus Health Care Respirators

Respiratory protection traditionally has been used in industrial settings when adequate control of airborne contaminants cannot be achieved through other preferred controls, such as substitution, ventilation, or engineering controls. Industrial respiratory protective devices, when properly selected and fitted, in accordance with an accepted fit test protocol, are designed to protect workers in settings in which there may be dusts, mists, or chemical vapor/gas contaminants in the work environment. Some higher levels of protection are designed for oxygen-deficient environments. In addition, by virtue of their filter system, they may also block splashes, sprays, and large droplets.

Respiratory protection is increasingly being used in health care and other settings such as prisons, primarily to protect against infectious agents such as tuberculosis, influenza, and other viruses. Both surgical masks and respirators are used, the difference between them from a practical standpoint being what they are designed to accomplish.

Traditionally, surgical masks were used to protect the patient from germs that might be emitted from the mouth or nose of the health care provider. In the United States they are cleared for sale by the FDA. They may be labeled for various uses and medical procedures. They are cleared for different levels of fluid resistance and biologic filter efficiency. Facemasks may be labeled as surgical, laser, isolation, dental, or medical procedure masks. They may come with or without a face shield. They are not designed to filter or block very small particles in the air that may be transmitted by coughs, sneezes, or certain medical procedures. Facemasks also do not provide complete protection from germs and other contaminants because of the loose fit between the surface of the facemask and the face.

Depending on the situation encountered, health care providers may also use NIOSH-certified respirators. Those that are also cleared by the FDA are referred to as Surgical N95 respirators. Making the appropriate selection of the type of facemask or respirator often requires interaction between an occupational safety and health professional,

such as an industrial hygienist, and appropriate health care staff, such as infection control personnel.

Types of Facepieces

The different types of respirator facepieces include half mask, full facepiece, helmet or hood, and loose fitting. Selecting a facepiece type is driven by various factors including the chemical and physical characteristics of the contaminant and the level of the contaminant present. Other considerations are whether the contaminant presents hazards such as eye irritation or an impact hazard. Most facepieces come in varying sizes. Most types of facepieces, except for some filtering facepieces, have exhalation valves. Elastomeric facepieces also may have inhalation valves, talking diaphragms, and other accessories.

Each type of facepiece is associated with the Assigned Protection Factor (APF), the workplace level of respiratory protection that a class of respirator is expected to provide to the wearer when used in accordance with a comprehensive respiratory protection program as outlined by OSHA (see **Table 1**).[10] A protection factor is calculated as the concentration of a contaminant in the ambient environment divided by the concentration inside

Table 1
Assigned protection factors for different respirators

Type of Respirator[a,b]	Type of Facepiece				
	Quarter Mask	Half Mask	Full Facepiece	Helmet/Hood	Loose-fitting Facepiece
Air-purifying respirator	5	10[c]	50		
Powered air-purifying respirator		50	1000	25/1000[d]	25
Supplied-air respirator or airline respirator					
• Demand mode		10	50		.25
• Continuous flow mode		50	1000	25/1000[d]	
• Pressure-demand or other positive pressure mode		50	1000		
Self-contained breathing apparatus					
• Demand mode		10	50	50	
• Pressure-demand or other positive pressure mode (eg, open/closed circuit)			10,000	10,000	

[a] Employers may select respirators assigned for use in higher workplace concentrations of a hazardous substance for use at lower concentrations of that substance or when required respirator use is independent of concentration.
[b] The APFs listed are only effective when the employer implements an effective respirator program, as outlined by OSHA.[10] These APFs do not apply to respirators used solely for escape.
[c] This APF category includes filtering facepieces and half masks with elastomeric facepieces.
[d] The employer must have evidence provided by the respirator manufacturer that testing of these respirators demonstrates performance at a level of protection of 1000 or greater to receive an APF of 1000. Without such testing, PAPRs and SARs with helmets/hoods are to be treated as loose-fitting facepiece respirators and receive an APF of 25.

the respirator or the inverse of the leakage of a respirator. The higher the protection factor, the greater the protection afforded by the respirator.

Quarter Mask Respirators

A Quarter mask respirator covers the nose and mouth with the facepiece extending from the top of the nose to below the mouth, but above the chin. Quarter mask respirators are typically used for protection against particulate hazards. Quarter mask respirators are assigned an APF of 5.

Half-Mask Respirators

A half-mask respirator covers the nose and mouth with the facepiece extending from the top of the nose to below the chin. Half-masks are used for all types of hazards, including particulates, vapors, and gases, and also for supplied air. Half-mask respirators include half-mask filtering facepieces (**Fig. 2**) and elastomeric type facepieces (**Fig. 3**), both of which have an APF of 10. The elastomers used today for half-masks are of varying materials such as thermoplastics and silicones. Choice depends on the chemical characteristics that affect permeability of the hazard through the facepiece, the contaminants' ability to degrade the facepiece, and comfort, although with the multitude of materials available for facepieces most materials are found to be comfortable by the wearer. The advantage is ease of use, but half-masks have limited value in terms of use for supplied-air or airline respirators, as these types of respirators are usually chosen because a higher level of protection is required, yet the half-mask APF always remains at 10.

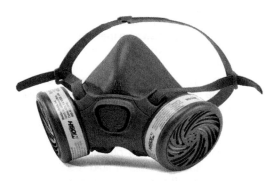

Fig. 3. Elastomeric half-facepiece respirator. (*Courtesy of* Moldex-Metric, Culver City, CA; with permission.)

Full-Facepiece Respirators

A full-facepiece respirator covers from the middle of the forehead to the bottom of the chin (**Fig. 4**). It generally protects the eyes from irritating substances, as well as impact. NIOSH also provides guidance on impact resistance requirements. Full facepieces can be used against all types of contaminants and are commonly used in a supplied-air configuration. Full-facepiece respirators in a negative pressure mode receive an APF of 50 when quantitatively fit tested. They can receive an APF of up to 1000 in some supplied-air configurations and up to 10,000 in some SCBA configurations.

Hoods and Helmets

A hood or helmet respirator completely covers the head and neck and may also cover portions of the shoulders (**Fig. 5**). They come in varying

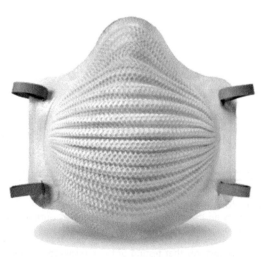

Fig. 2. N95 Filtering facepiece respirator. (*Courtesy of* Moldex-Metric, Culver City, CA; with permission.)

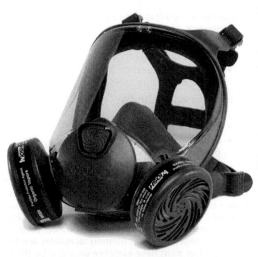

Fig. 4. Full-facepiece respirator. (*Courtesy of* Moldex-Metric, Culver City, CA; with permission.)

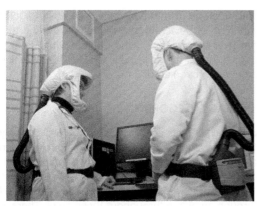

configurations. These types of facepieces may be used in conjunction with air-purifying elements or with some type of supplied-air source that does not filter out the contaminants but rather simply supplies clean and respirable air to the user. The employer must have evidence provided by the respirator manufacturer that demonstrates performance at a level of protection of 1000 or greater to receive an APF of 1000. Without such testing, helmets/hoods are considered a loose-fitting facepiece respirator and receive and APF of 25.

PROTECTIVE SYSTEMS USED BY RESPIRATORS
APRs

An APR is a respirator that uses an air-purifying element to remove a specific type of contaminant from the air. The air is passed through the air-purifying element before entering the respiratory system. The air-purifying element is attached to the respirator body. In filtering facepieces, the filter is an integral part and usually encompasses the facepiece. In elastomeric facepieces the filtering element is usually a separate item that is attached to the facepiece, in the form of a filter pad, cartridge, or canister. There are various types of air-purifying elements. These elements are attached to a negative-pressure APR or powered air-purifying respirator (PAPR), in which air is drawn through the filtering element with the help of a fan and then supplied to the user. PAPRs provide respirable air to the user yet does not require the user to expend energy to draw air through the filtering element.

Particulate Filter

A particulate filter is a filter that mechanically captures solid or liquid particles from the air using a combination of interception, impaction, sedimentation, diffusion, and electrostatic forces. The predominant mechanism of capturing a particle is dictated by a number of factors including particle size, density, velocity of particle, as well as filter characteristics, in particular filter fiber diameter. The filter is an integral part of the respirator, such as a filtering facepiece, in a disc form, or contained in a cartridge, which is attached to the respirator. In some cases, the filter might be contained in or permanently attached to a chemical cartridge.

Chemical Gas and Vapor Filters

Chemical gases and vapors are most commonly filtered using carbon-based materials, which are packed into cartridges or canisters, which are larger capacity cartridges and allow more service time. Chemical cartridges are designed for single gases and vapors or a combination of gases and vapors. NIOSH has certification test requirements that test the service time of cartridges or canisters at certain concentrations, flow rates, and humidities and requires that the cartridge last for a specified period. Service time is determined when the cartridge or canister is challenged with the particular test gas; it must last for a specified period, which is assessed by measuring a breakthrough concentration on the downstream side of the cartridge or canister.

Examples of chemical types that a cartridge or canister might be designed to protect against are organic vapors, various acid gases, ammonia, methylamine, and formaldehyde. The cartridges are certified for a single gas or any combination.

ATMOSPHERE-SUPPLYING RESPIRATORS

Atmosphere-supplying respirators supply a respirable atmosphere independent of the workplace atmosphere. This class includes the SAR and the SCBA (**Fig. 6**). These devices achieve an APF ranging from 10 to 10,000 depending on how the air supply is provided to the facepiece in conjunction with its relationship to the pressure of the outside atmosphere and in conjunction with the type of facepiece. Advantages include high levels of protection and independent air source not requiring the contaminant to be removed from the air. Important limitations include hoses that may have to be carried and dragged through an environment for SARs and the considerable weight, the physical stress associated with carrying such a device, and the limited time that the device can be used (driven by the amount of air available in the tank) for SCBA respirators.

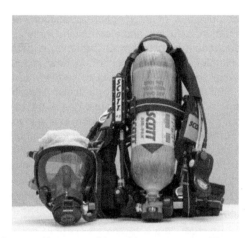

Fig. 6. Self-contained breathing apparatus. (*Courtesy of* Scott Safety, Monroe, NC; with permission.)

NIOSH certifies numerous classes and combinations of these types of respirators.

SARs or airline respirators are those in which the source of breathing air is not designed to be carried by the user; for example, a pump, a compressor, or compressed air tank is not carried by the wearer. A demand mode respirator facepiece receives air when the wearer inhales. The valve is activated when the atmospheric pressure inside the mask drops below the outside atmospheric pressure. A continuous flow mode SAR has air constantly flowing into the mask with the intent of always having a positive atmospheric pressure in relation to the outside atmosphere. A pressure demand mode SAR is intended for the pressure inside the mask to always remain positive relative to the outside atmospheric pressure and deliver more air when the user inhales.

Although continuous mode and pressure demand respirators are designed to provide the requisite volume of air necessary to maintain the atmospheric pressure inside the respirator positive relative to the outside, studies have shown that at high breathing rates under strenuous conditions, even these respirators can become negative relative to the outside air pressure.

The SCBA is an atmosphere-supplying respirator in which the respirable gas source is designed to be carried by the wearer. It is designed to be demand mode, pressure demand mode, or positive pressure mode supplying air with the same relative conditions of inside and outside atmospheric air pressure as previously described. SCBAs are designed to be open circuit in which the exhaled air is expelled to the ambient atmosphere or closed circuit in which the expelled air is processed through catalysts and purifiers to remove exhaled CO_2 and humidity and then mixed

with fresh air from the air tank. The advantage of this type of device is that the length of time that the user can remain in the contaminated area is usually longer than an open-circuit SCBA in which air is not recirculated.

SPECIAL CATEGORIES

Supplied-air suits are devices that protect not only the respiratory system but also the skin from airborne contaminants. They were primarily developed for the nuclear industry. They are made as 1-piece or 2-piece suits, and air is supplied through an airline throughout these suits. There is limited information about their efficacy and the level of protection (APF) that they actually provide.

Escape respirators are designed for one use: to allow a person working under normal working conditions to escape safely from a life-threatening environment that has developed suddenly. There are 2 basic types of escape devices: air purifying and air supplying. They may be mouthpieces, half masks, full facepieces, or hood devices. Choice of these devices requires that the users and employers consider the possible emergency scenarios that could occur in their work environment. In addition to respiratory protection, possible eye irritation must be considered, as a rapid escape would be badly hampered by the inability to see exit routes.

Chemical, biologic, radioactive, nuclear (CBRN) are devices that have been specifically designed to provide resistance against chemical warfare agents. They can be SCBAs, air purifying, powered air purifying, and air-purifying escape devices; can have special features including drinking tubes for extended wear; and must provide protection of the skin and eyes. They are certified by NIOSH.

MEDICAL EVALUATION FOR RESPIRATOR USE

Respirators are used in the workplace in the context of an overall respiratory protection program, which in the United States must meet the requirements detailed by OSHA, as noted earlier. Each employee who wears a respirator must be evaluated by a physician or other licensed health care professional (here also termed provider or clinician) before being assigned a respirator to determine whether use of a respirator poses a risk to the worker. One exception is where workers are allowed to voluntarily wear a filtering facepiece respirator where an airborne hazard does not exist.[10] The health care professional involved in evaluating workers for respirator use should be aware of the potential hazards of concern and should ascertain whether the other components of a respirator protection program have been implemented.

To decide if a worker can safely wear a respirator, the health care provider must be familiar with the physiologic, psychological, and other health and safety issues related to respirators, which depend on several factors, including the type of respirator worn, working conditions, and the health status and other characteristics of the worker.[18,19]

Respirators can have physiologic cost to the wearer, including increased airway resistance, increased dead space volume, and decreased maximal exercise capability, which have been reviewed.[19,20] However, these effects are small for most individuals.[20–22] The physiologic cost of the task that is required to be performed by the wearer is almost always more significant than the wearing of the respirator.

The physiologic cost of wearing a respirator is greater with full-facepiece than half-facepiece respirators.[20] Full-facepiece respirators will add to existing heat burden to wearers who are working in hot environments, one of the reasons that PAPRs were first developed. There is also evidence that wearers of APRs exhibit increased carbon dioxide levels and heart rate; again, those who wear full-facepiece respirators exhibit more of these effects than those who use half-facepiece respirators. The use of PAPRs minimizes the above-mentioned physiologic effects.

Workers who wear SCBA devices must be physically fit to handle the weight of the respirator (around 40 pounds) and perform their task. Because most tanks limit the amount of time that the device can be worn (eg, 20–30 minutes), individuals will normally have time to recover after a short period of wear. This is not true for closed-circuit devices used for prolonged mine rescue activities. Wearers must be trained to respond to such emergencies, and the respirator is less significant than training and psychological capability for most wearers.

Workers' vision and their ability to have their vision corrected affect their wearing of respirators. There was a time when contact lenses were prohibited from use, but they are generally accepted provided that the wearer can safely exit a contaminated workplace should a contact lens problem develop. Special glasses or spectacle kits are required for those who must wear full-facepiece respirators, because temple bars cannot be allowed to interfere with the sealing surface of a respirator.

Psychological and social issues related to wearing a respirator include discomfort, anxiety, claustrophobia, subjective feelings of shortness of breath, and worker acceptability, which have been reviewed.[20,23] Fit testing and a trial with different respirator models can be helpful. For example, claustrophobia will be more likely encountered with a full-facepiece respirator because of its restricted vision. However, individuals with claustrophobia can usually acclimate to wearing a respirator during the training period. On occasion workers are unable to wear a respirator for psychological reasons, despite such efforts.[20]

There are several fit problems encountered by workers with certain facial and dental problems. Workers who use dentures will be required to have their dentures in place while wearing a respirator to obtain an adequate fit. An exception would be an individual who does not wear dentures at work and is capable of achieving an adequate fit. Workers who develop facial scars must have a repeated fit test performed to ensure that they can continue to obtain a proper fit. There are also individuals who cannot shave their skin because of medical conditions (folliculitis), and they may be unsuitable for respirator use. Many of these fit problems can be overcome with the use of a loose-fitting PAPR or loose-fitting SAR. Studies related to respirator effects have been performed primarily on those who wear respirators, generally healthy workers in more industrial work settings. With the potential for more widespread use of respirators in the setting of infectious epidemics, natural disasters, and terrorism, studies have begun to evaluate the psychological and physiologic effects of respirator use by a broader range of users.[18,23]

The medical evaluation for respirator use includes several components, described in greater detail by Szeinuk and colleagues[20] The OSHA respiratory standard requires that a physician or other licensed health professional provide a medical evaluation of each employee who is asked to wear a respirator, before their wearing the device, and that certain information be provided to the health care provider to review.[10] The OSHA questionnaire (Appendix C of the OSHA respirator standard) provides the minimum required information, including the type of respirator, past medical history, symptoms, and prior respirator use (Part A). If the employee is going to wear a full-facepiece respirator or SCBA, several additional questions must be asked. Part B of the OSHA questionnaire is a nonmandatory section and includes questions related to prior jobs and work exposures.

The employer should provide the health care provider who medically clears a respirator wearer the following information about the worker's job before the medical evaluation:

1. The type and weight of the respirator to be used
2. The duration and frequency of respirator use (including use for rescue and escape)
3. The type of work performed and the level of physical effort required while wearing a respirator
4. Additional protective clothing and equipment that must be worn by the worker
5. Special environmental conditions that may be encountered, such as temperature and humidity extremes
6. A written copy of the facility's respiratory protection program

The medical history obtained should focus on the following:

1. Known medical conditions, including seizures, claustrophobia, pulmonary or cardiac diseases, heat intolerance, current smoking, and medications, including nonprescription medications
2. Visual and hearing problems, including use of hearing aid and glasses or contact lens
3. Musculoskeletal problems or past injuries or other physical problems that could interfere with respirator use
4. Current symptoms, including symptoms related to pulmonary and cardiac disease, symptoms with exertion, and symptoms related to work
5. Past problems with the use of a respirator, such as anxiety, rash, and fatigue

A physical examination, although required by OSHA only if the employee answers "yes" on the questionnaire, should be performed as part of the medical examination. The following conditions should be assessed on the examination and history:

1. Musculoskeletal and skin conditions, especially facial deformities, facial hair, or dermatitis that could interfere with or be exacerbated by respirator usage
2. Use of prescription eyeglasses or contact lens and hearing aides
3. Cardiac or pulmonary disease, especially uncontrolled or inadequately treated
4. Endocrine or neurologic conditions such as uncontrolled diabetes or seizures
5. Psychological conditions such as severe anxiety and claustrophobia

The health care professional, based on the results of the overall evaluation, can permit the individual to use all types of respirators or specify restrictions, such as the type of respirator to be worn. For example, the health care provider can specify that a PAPR be used instead of a nonpowered device. The assessment regarding respirator use should take into consideration, in addition to medical or psychological issues, the duration and frequency of respirator usage, the type of work to be performed, the work hazards, and the worker's past experience with respirators.

Workers with substantial cardiopulmonary disease or other major serious health problems need careful assessment, including consideration of special conditions such as extreme temperature or confined space entry. Additional testing, such as spirometry, full pulmonary function tests, chest imaging, or cardiopulmonary exercise testing may be obtained. However, there are no specific medical criteria, such as a certain degree of lung function or maximum oxygen consumption, which indicate that a worker is able (or not able) to wear a respirator. If there are concerns, rather than deny a worker the opportunity to wear a respirator (and potentially a job), a trial of observation at the workplace or in a simulated work setting can be requested. The health care provider can also determine the need for reevaluation of the employee in the future.

The respirator medical evaluation should be considered in the context of the overall workplace protection program and workplace medical surveillance. Periodic spirometry, chest radiography, or other testing may be indicated for surveillance, depending on the work exposures. Although not required by OSHA, spirometry testing frequently is performed as part of respirator medical evaluations. Such testing is encouraged, as it can establish baseline lung function before the job that requires the respirator medical evaluation, in addition to detecting possible early lung disease.

Several additional organizations provide helpful guidelines. The American National Standards Institute maintains ANSI standard Z88.6, which is titled "Respiratory Protection—Respirator Use—Physical Qualifications for Personnel."[15] This standard provides information and rationale for physicians who are responsible for determining the qualifications of respirator wearers. The National Fire Protection Association maintains NFPA standard 1582, which contains medical requirements for firefighters.[17] This standard includes information for those workers who must be prepared to wear SCBAs and perform emergency operations.

REFERENCES

1. Jefferson T, Foxlee R, Mar CD, et al. Physical interventions to interrupt or reduce the spread of respiratory viruses: systematic review. BMJ 2008; 336(7635):77–80.
2. Jaeger JL, Patel M, Dharan N, et al. Transmission of 2009 pandemic influenza A (H1N1) virus among

healthcare personnel—Southern California 2009. Infect Control Hosp Epidemiol 2011;32(12):1149–57.

3. MacIntyre CR, Wang Q, Cauchemez S, et al. A cluster randomized clinical trial comparing fit-tested and non-fit-tested N95 respirators to medical masks to prevent respiratory virus infection in health care workers. Influenza Other Respi Viruses 2011;5(2):170–9.

4. Loeb M, Dafoe N, Mahony J, et al. Surgical mask vs N95 respirator for preventing influenza among health care workers. J Am Med Assoc 2009; 302(17):1865–71.

5. Institute of Medicine. Preventing transmission of pandemic influenza and other viral respiratory diseases: personal protective equipment for healthcare personnel update 2010. Washington, DC: National Academies Press; 2011.

6. Pritchard J. A guide to industrial respiratory protection. HEW Publication #76-189. Cincinnati (OH): NIOSH; 1976.

7. Held BJ. History of respiratory protective devices in the US, University of California. Livermore (CA): Lawrence Livermore Laboratory.

8. Procedure for establishing a test of permissible gas masks, Schedule 13 U.S. Department of the Interior. US: U.S. Gov. Bureau of Mines; 1919. p. 7.

9. Department of Interior, Bureau of Mines. Respiratory protective devices: tests for permissibility; fees. Federal Register 1972;37(59):6244.

10. Respiratory protection, Code of Federal Regulations, Title 29 Part 1910.134. US: U.S. Gov. (CFR document) and Occupational Safety and Health Administration; 2009.

11. Department of Health and Human Services, National Institute of Occupational Safety and Health. Respiratory protective devices: final rules and notice. Federal Register 1995;60(110):30336.

12. NIOSH Certified Equipment List. Available at: http://www2a.cdc.gov/drds/cel/cel_form_code.asp. Accessed March 1, 2012.

13. OSHA Advisor Genius. Calculating the wood equation. Available at: http://www.osha.gov/SLTC/etools/respiratory/mathmodel_advisorgenius.html. Accessed March 1, 2012.

14. Guidance for industry and FDA staff: surgical masks - premarket notification [510(k)] submissions; guidance for industry and FDA. Available at: http://www.fda.gov/MedicalDevices/DeviceRegulationandGuidance/GuidanceDocuments/ucm072549.htm. Accessed March 1, 2012.

15. ANSI Respirator Standards. Available at: http://webstore.ansi.org/RecordDetail.aspx?sku=ANSI/AIHA+Z88.+Respirator+Package. Accessed March 1, 2012.

16. ASTM International Standards. Available at: http://www.astm.org/. Accessed March 1, 2012.

17. NFPA List of Codes and Standards. Available at: http://www.nfpa.org/aboutthecodes/list_of_codes_and_standards.asp?cookie%5Ftest=1. Accessed March 1, 2012.

18. Harber P, Santiago S, Bansal S, et al. Respirator physiologic impact in persons with mild respiratory disease. J Occup Environ Med 2010;52(2):155–62.

19. Harber P, Brown CL, Beck JG. Respirator physiology research: answers in search of the question. J Occup Med 1991;33(1):38–44.

20. Szeinuk J, Beckett WS, Clark N, et al. Medical evaluation for respirator use. Am J Ind Med 2000;37: 142–57.

21. Roberge RJ, Coca A, Williams WJ, et al. Physiological impact of the N95 filtering facepiece respirator on healthcare workers. Respir Care 2010;55(5):569–77.

22. Roberge RJ, Coca A, Williams WJ, et al. Reusable elastomeric air-purifying respirators: physiologic impact on health care workers. Am J Infect Control 2010;38(5):381–6.

23. Harber P, Bansal S, Santiago S, et al. Multidomain subjective response to respirator use during simulated work. J Occup Environ Med 2009;51(1):38–45.

Index

Note: Page numbers of article titles are in **boldface** type.

Clin Chest Med 33 (2012) 795–803
http://dx.doi.org/10.1016/S0272-5231(12)00111-6
0272-5231/12/$ – see front matter © 2012 Elsevier Inc. All rights reserved.

1. Publication Title	2. Publication Number	3. Filing Date
Clinics in Chest Medicine	0 0 0 - 7 0 6	9/14/12

4. Issue Frequency	5. Number of Issues Published Annually	6. Annual Subscription Price
Mar, Jun, Sep, Dec	4	$316.00

7. Complete Mailing Address of Known Office of Publication (Not printer) (Street, city, county, state, and ZIP+4®)

Elsevier Inc.
360 Park Avenue South
New York, NY 10010-1710

Contact Person
Stephen R. Bushing
Telephone (Include area code)
215-239-3688

8. Complete Mailing Address of Headquarters or General Business Office of Publisher (Not printer)

Elsevier Inc., 360 Park Avenue South, New York, NY 10010-1710

9. Full Names and Complete Mailing Addresses of Publisher, Editor, and Managing Editor (Do not leave blank)

Publisher (Name and complete mailing address)

Kim Murphy, Elsevier, Inc., 1600 John F. Kennedy Blvd. Suite 1800, Philadelphia, PA 19103-2899

Editor (Name and complete mailing address)

Katie Hartner, Elsevier, Inc., 1600 John F. Kennedy Blvd. Suite 1800, Philadelphia, PA 19103-2899

Managing Editor (Name and complete mailing address)

Sarah Barth, Elsevier, Inc., 1600 John F. Kennedy Blvd. Suite 1800, Philadelphia, PA 19103-2899

10. Owner (Do not leave blank. If the publication is owned by a corporation, give the name and address of the corporation immediately followed by the names and addresses of all stockholders owning or holding 1 percent or more of the total amount of stock. If not owned by a corporation, give the names and addresses of the individual owners. If owned by a partnership or other unincorporated firm, give its name and address as well as those of each individual owner. If the publication is published by a nonprofit organization, give its name and address.)

Full Name	Complete Mailing Address
Wholly owned subsidiary of	1600 John F. Kennedy Blvd., Ste. 1800
Reed/Elsevier, US holdings	Philadelphia, PA 19103-2899

11. Known Bondholders, Mortgagees, and Other Security Holders Owning or Holding 1 Percent or More of Total Amount of Bonds, Mortgages, or Other Securities. If none, check box. ☐ None

Full Name	Complete Mailing Address
N/A	

12. Tax Status (For completion by nonprofit organizations authorized to mail at nonprofit rates) (Check one)
The purpose, function, and nonprofit status of this organization and the exempt status for federal income tax purposes:
☐ Has Not Changed During Preceding 12 Months
☐ Has Changed During Preceding 12 Months (Publisher must submit explanation of change with this statement)

PS Form 3526, September 2007 (Page 1 of 3 (Instructions Page 3)) PSN 7530-01-000-9931 PRIVACY NOTICE: See our Privacy policy in www.usps.com

13. Publication Title	14. Issue Date for Circulation Data Below
Clinics in Chest Medicine	September 2012

15. Extent and Nature of Circulation		Average No. Copies Each Issue During Preceding 12 Months	No. Copies of Single Issue Published Nearest to Filing Date
a. Total Number of Copies (Net press run)		1495	1359
b. Paid Circulation (By Mail and Outside the Mail)	(1) Mailed Outside-County Paid Subscriptions Stated on PS Form 3541. (Include paid distribution above nominal rate, advertiser's proof copies, and exchange copies)	857	807
	(2) Mailed In-County Paid Subscriptions Stated on PS Form 3541 (Include paid distribution above nominal rate, advertiser's proof copies, and exchange copies)		
	(3) Paid Distribution Outside the Mails Including Sales Through Dealers and Carriers, Street Vendors, Counter Sales, and Other Paid Distribution Outside USPS®	327	330
	(4) Paid Distribution by Other Classes Mailed Through the USPS (e.g. First-Class Mail®)		
c. Total Paid Distribution (Sum of 15b (1), (2), (3), and (4))	▶	1184	1137
d. Free or Nominal Rate Distribution (By Mail and Outside the Mail)	(1) Free or Nominal Rate Outside-County Copies Included on PS Form 3541	71	57
	(2) Free or Nominal Rate In-County Copies Included on PS Form 3541		
	(3) Free or Nominal Rate Copies Mailed at Other Classes Through the USPS (e.g. First-Class Mail)		
	(4) Free or Nominal Rate Distribution Outside the Mail (Carriers or other means)		
e. Total Free or Nominal Rate Distribution (Sum of 15d (1), (2), (3) and (4))	▶	71	57
f. Total Distribution (Sum of 15c and 15e)	▶	1255	1194
g. Copies not Distributed (See instructions to publishers #4 (page #3))	▶	240	165
h. Total (Sum of 15f and g)		1495	1359
i. Percent Paid (15c divided by 15f times 100)	▶	94.34%	95.23%

16. Publication of Statement of Ownership

If the publication is a general publication, publication of this statement is required. Will be printed
in the December 2012 issue of this publication.

Publication not required

17. Signature and Title of Editor, Publisher, Business Manager, or Owner

[signature]

Stephen R. Bushing – Inventory Distribution Coordinator

Date
September 14, 2012

I certify that all information furnished on this form is true and complete. I understand that anyone who furnishes false or misleading information on this form or who omits material or information requested on the form may be subject to criminal sanctions (including fines and imprisonment) and/or civil sanctions (including civil penalties).

PS Form 3526, September 2007 (Page 2 of 3)

Moving?

Make sure your subscription moves with you!

To notify us of your new address, find your **Clinics Account Number** (located on your mailing label above your name), and contact customer service at:

Email: journalscustomerservice-usa@elsevier.com

800-654-2452 (subscribers in the U.S. & Canada)
314-447-8871 (subscribers outside of the U.S. & Canada)

Fax number: 314-447-8029

Elsevier Health Sciences Division
Subscription Customer Service
3251 Riverport Lane
Maryland Heights, MO 63043

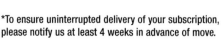

ELSEVIER

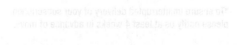

Printed and bound by CPI Group (UK) Ltd, Croydon, CR0 4YY

12/10/2024

01773416-0001